Equine Endocrinology

Equine Endocrinology

Authors

François-René Bertin, DVM, MS, PhD, DACVIM (LAIM)

Senior Lecturer, School of Veterinary Science, The University of Queensland, Gatton, Queensland, Australia

Natalie S. Fraser, DVM, MS, DACT

Senior Lecturer, School of Veterinary Science, The University of Queensland, Gatton, Queensland, Australia

CABI

CABI is a trading name of CAB International

CABI
Nosworthy Way
Wallingford
Oxfordshire OX10 8DE
UK

Tel: +44 (0)1491 832111
Fax: +44 (0)1491 833508
E-mail: info@cabi.org
Website: www.cabi.org

CABI
WeWork
One Lincoln St
24th Floor
Boston, MA 02111
USA

T: +1 (617) 682-9015
E-mail: cabi-nao@cabi.org

A catalogue record for this book is available from the British Library, London, UK.

References to Internet websites (URLs) were accurate at the time of writing.

ISBN-13: 9781789241099 (Paperback)
9781789241105 (ePDF)
9781789241112 (ePub)

Commissioning editor: Alexandra Lainsbury
Editorial assistant: Emma McCann
Production editor: Marta Patiño

Typeset by Exeter Premedia Services Pvt Ltd, Chennai, India
Printed in the USA

Contents

Preface

This first edition of *Equine Endocrinology* is designed for veterinary students and equine practitioners; it aims at providing a comprehensive yet user-friendly tool to approach and manage common endocrine disorders. Equine endocrinology is a very fast moving field and clinical signs of endocrine and metabolic disorders have become dominant presenting complaints in practice.

Equine Endocrinology is divided into an introductory chapter providing the key steps of the clinical approach of equine endocrinology and eight chapters covering the disorders of the main hormonal axes responsible for equine diseases, including female and male reproductive endocrinology. Each chapter is organised in a classic disease-oriented format, briefly presenting the main physiological elements of the key hormonal players and then detailing the epidemiology, clinical signs, diagnostic steps, management and prognosis of each endocrine condition reported in horses. This edition contains more than 50 colour figures and tables to illustrate the physiological mechanisms, clinical findings, diagnostic tests or treatment plans and to allow a better visualisation and understanding of equine metabolic diseases.

The motivation for this first edition of *Equine Endocrinology* stemmed from the inquisitiveness of our students, the dedication of our colleagues in the field and the resilience of horse owners; we hope this book will provide a source of information to improve the management of horses around the world.

We also want to thank Alexandra Lainsbury, Ali Thompson and Jill Northcott at CABI who have guided us along this journey.

François-René Bertin

Acknowledgements

To

Constantin, Annie, Alain, Olivier, Karl and Otto for their love and support.
Thank you to Janice Kritchevsky and Nick Frank for showing me the way and to my students and patients for making it all worthwhile.

Thank you to

Nick Bamford, Chris Elliot, Nick Frank, Jen Gold, Janice Kritchevsky, Sascha Nott, Chiara Palmieri, Allison Stewart and Alex Young for sharing pictures.

Dr François-René Bertin

1 Clinical Approach to Equine Endocrinology

Equine endocrinopathies present with a variety of clinical signs. While some clinical signs, like hypertrichosis, are quite obvious and almost pathognomonic, others, like decreased fertility or weight loss, are subtle and might require a more thorough evaluation (Frank *et al.*, 2010b; McFarlane *et al.*, 2011). In addition, several endocrinopathies can be present in the same animal at the same time, and only early recognition and proper management of both conditions will allow a successful outcome (McGowan *et al.*, 2013b). Therefore, a comprehensive and systematic examination is recommended when evaluating patients.

History

A detailed history is a key step to approach cases in which an endocrinopathy is suspected.

Signalment

Close attention to signalment should be paid as there are age-related endocrinopathies, such as pituitary pars intermedia dysfunction (PPID), and some breeds known to be predisposed to some endocrine disorders, such as insulin dysregulation (ID) in ponies or Morgans (McGowan *et al.*, 2013a; Bamford *et al.*, 2014). Gender can also be an important element to consider as endocrine disorders such as equine metabolic syndrome (EMS) have been shown to decrease conception rates (Sessions-Bresnahan and Carnevale, 2014). Thus, a close examination of a mare's reproductive performance can indicate subclinical endocrinopathies.

Complaint

The primary complaint is often a clear suggestion of an endocrine disorder; however, some owners might overlook minor changes, such as delayed coat shedding or increased water consumption, and only seek veterinary advice when the endocrinopathy impairs the function of the horse and causes more severe signs such as lameness (Horn *et al.*, 2019). Although the awareness of endocrine disorders has increased in the last two decades, early signs of endocrinopathies can be mistaken for normal age-related changes and might not therefore trigger veterinary attention (Miller *et al.*, 2016).

Season

As many hormones have a circannual rhythm, clinical signs can vary with seasons (Frank *et al.*, 2010a; Funk *et al.*, 2011; Borer-Weir *et al.*, 2013). Therefore, collecting history on the previous 12 months and comparing with recent years can be critical when assessing some cases. For example, horses with early signs of PPID can only show delayed coat shedding; comparing the time of shedding over consecutive years might give an indication of early endocrinopathies. Similar considerations are valid for horses with EMS with seasonal episodes of laminitis (Coleman *et al.*, 2018).

Diet

Diet is a paramount element in the assessment of a patient suspected of an endocrine disorder. The clinician should focus on the type of feed offered to the horse (pasture vs hay vs concentrate), the quality of the feed (calcium/phosphorous imbalance can lead to secondary hyperparathyroidism; excessive non-structural carbohydrates, NSC, can lead to ID) and the quantity actually ingested by the horse (Toribio, 2011; Frank and Tadros, 2014). In critical cases such as severely hyperinsulinaemic patients, regular diet analysis is essential to minimize post-prandial hyperinsulinaemic peaks and limit lamellar damage. It is also important to remember that horses and ponies have different eating behaviours and time on pasture might not adequately represent the amount of food ingested: large amounts of grass can be ingested in a short period of time, mainly when the time is restricted. Water intake should also be recorded as increased water intake might suggest a disorder of the hypothalamo–pituitary–adrenal axis (Schott, 2011). Although difficult to properly measure with automatic waterers, a water intake above 3ml/kg/h in an adult horse warrants further investigation.

Concurrent diseases

By nature, endocrine disorders can affect multiple body systems as hormones regulate metabolism, immunity and homeostasis. For example, by modulating immunity, hypothalamo–pituitary–adrenal axis dysregulation can result in recurrent infections or non-healing wounds (Hofberger *et al.*, 2015; McFarlane *et al.*, 2015; Horn *et al.*, 2019). In addition, some endocrinopathies can be the consequence of systemic diseases. For instance, in foals with sepsis, the hypothalamo–pituitary–adrenal axis can be depressed and in adult horses with systemic inflammatory response syndrome, the endocrine pancreas function can be impaired (Hart *et al.*, 2009b; Bertin *et al.*, 2018). Accordingly, a comprehensive evaluation of the horse is required.

Concurrent treatments

Hormones have systemic effects and their action can be modified by drug administration. For example, phenylbutazone has been identified as the cause of endocrine dysregulation in horses: by either altering the protein binding of thyroxine (T4) or by directly decreasing thyroid-stimulating hormone (TSH) secretion, phenylbutazone administration can result in decreased total and free T4 (Ramirez *et al.*, 1997). In addition, phenylbutazone has been shown to extend the preovulatory period of mares by the inhibition of prostaglandin (Lima *et al.*, 2015). As some drugs, such as non-steroidal anti-inflammatory drugs or sedatives, are routinely administered by owners or veterinarians, the clinician should be careful when examining a horse or interpreting a laboratory result (Kritchevsky *et al.*, 2020).

Physical Examination

A thorough physical examination is an essential step of the diagnostic approach for all diseases. For complaints that are likely to have an endocrine cause, particular attention should be paid to level of alertness and activity, body weight and body condition, haircoat, musculoskeletal system and reproductive system.

Alertness and activity

The hypothalamus is the link between the nervous and the endocrine systems. As part of the limbic system, the hypothalamus integrates environmental and intrinsic stimuli and controls alertness, behaviour and emotions through the secretion of releasing hormones (Clarke, 2015). Therefore, changes in activity level can suggest an endocrine disorder at the level of the hypothalamus. For example, in horses with PPID, decreased alertness is reported and can be reversed with proper treatment (Donaldson *et al.*, 2002).

Body weight and body condition

Morphometric measurements and their changes over time are key elements in the evaluation of patients with endocrine disorders. Whether the horse is overweight or underweight, a careful evaluation of fat distribution and muscle mass is warranted. For example, EMS is associated with increased adiposity, whereas PPID is associated with muscle loss (Aleman *et al.*, 2006; Pleasant *et al.*, 2013). Although body weight is a relevant piece of information, it is a poor indicator of muscle/fat ratio and obtaining an accurate body weight can be challenging in equine practice. A 9-point body condition score, initially developed on morphometric measurements from 12 Quarter Horse mares, is now commonly used in practice for all breeds and has been shown to be a useful tool to predict laminitis in horses with EMS (Henneke *et al.*, 1983; Coleman *et al.*, 2018). The score is based on the adiposity in specific areas such as neck, withers, shoulders, ribs, back and tailhead as well as on the density of the fat deposits (Table 1.1 and Figs 1.1–1.9).

In addition to a full body condition score, a cresty neck score has been developed and is mainly relevant in cases of EMS, as the neck is a common site of fat deposition in horses (Table 1.2 and Figs 1.10–1.15) (Carter *et al.*, 2009; Martin-Gimenez *et al.*, 2016).

Haircoat

Aspect, quality, length and shedding pattern of haircoat should be assessed when evaluating patients with endocrine conditions, in which the aspect and

Table 1.1. Description of individual body condition scoring system. From Henneke *et al.*, 1983.

Score	Definition	Description
1	Poor	Animal extremely emaciated. Spinous processes, ribs, tailhead, tuber coxae and ischiae projecting prominently. Bone structure of withers, shoulders and neck easily noticeable. No fatty tissue can be felt.
2	Very thin	Animal emaciated. Slight fat covering over base of spinous processes, transverse processes of lumbar vertebrae feel rounded. Spinous processes, ribs, tailhead, tuber coxae and ischiae prominent. Withers, shoulders and neck structures faintly discernible.
3	Thin	Fat build-up about halfway on spinous processes, transverse processes cannot be felt. Slight fat cover over ribs. Spinous processes and ribs easily discernible. Tailhead prominent, but individual vertebrae cannot be visually identified. Tuber coxae appear rounded, but easily discernible. Tuber ischiae not distinguishable. Withers, shoulders and neck accentuated.
4	Moderately thin	Negative crease along back. Faint outline of ribs discernible. Tailhead prominence depends on conformation; fat can be felt around it. Tuber coxae not discernible. Withers, shoulders and neck not obviously thin.
5	Moderate	Back level. Ribs cannot be visually distinguished but can be easily felt. Fat around tailhead beginning to feel spongy. Withers appear rounded over spinous processes. Shoulders and neck blend smoothly into body.
6	Moderately fleshy	May have slight crease down back. Fat over ribs feels spongy. Fat around tailhead feels soft. Fat beginning to be deposited along side of withers, behind shoulders and along side of neck.
7	Fleshy	May have crease down back. Individual ribs can be felt, but noticeable filling between ribs with fat. Fat around tailhead is soft. Fat deposited along withers, behind shoulders and along neck.
8	Fat	Crease down back. Difficult to feel ribs. Fat around tailhead very soft. Area along withers filled with fat. Area behind shoulders filled with fat. Noticeable thickening of neck. Fat deposited along inner thighs.
9	Extremely fat	Obvious crease down back. Patchy fat appearing over ribs. Bulging fat around tailhead, along withers, behind shoulders and along neck. Fat along inner thighs; may rub together. Flank filled with fat.

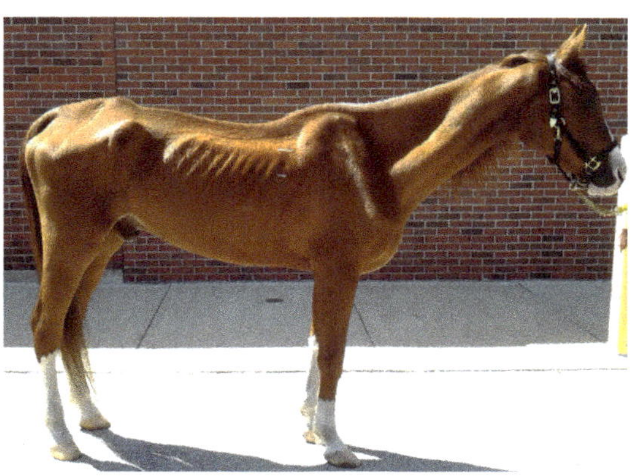

Fig. 1.1. Body condition score of 1/9 in a 12-year-old mixed breed horse (Author's own photograph).

the quality of the hair can be altered. For example, in foals with congenital hypothyroidism, the hair can appear silky; in geriatric patients with PPID, the abnormal ratio of hair in anagen and telogen phases results in hypertrichosis and delayed or absent shedding (Fig. 1.16) (Breuhaus, 2011; Innera *et al.*, 2013). Close examination of the haircoat will also allow the identification of an abnormal sweating pattern with both hyperhidrosis and anhidrosis reported in horses with PPID (Rohrbach *et al.*, 2012; Spelta and Axon, 2012). Finally, close examination of the integument can allow the identification of non-healing wounds or chronic ulcers.

Musculoskeletal system

Examination of the musculoskeletal system is an important part of the assessment of the endocrine

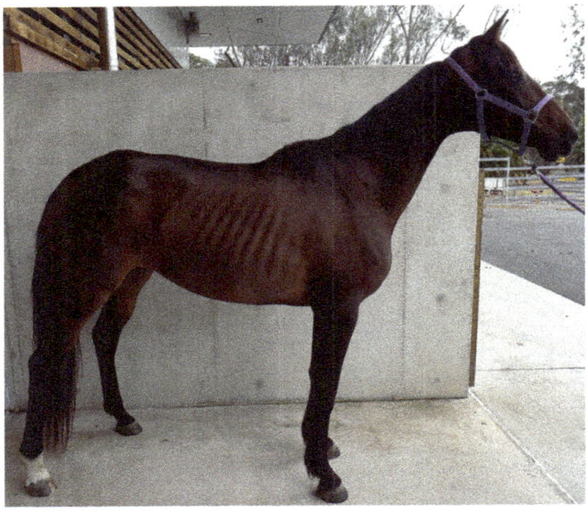

Fig. 1.2. Body condition score of 2/9 in a 9-year-old Thoroughbred mare (Author's own photograph).

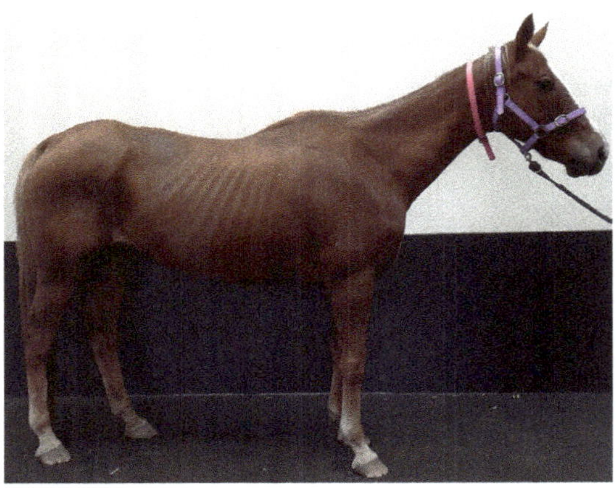

Fig. 1.3. Body condition score of 3/9 in a 15-year-old Australian Stockhorse mare (Author's own photograph).

patient. Lameness is a common presenting complaint for horses with EMS, PPID, hypothyroidism or hyperparathyroidism (Ronen *et al.*, 1992; Frank *et al.*, 2010b; Breuhaus, 2011; Horn *et al.*, 2019). Lameness can have multiple origins such as: laminitis in cases with ID; suspensory ligament degeneration in cases of PPID; poor carpus or tarsus development in premature or dysmature foals with hypothyroidism; or general bone pain in cases of hyperparathyroidism (Ramirez *et al.*, 1997; Asplin *et al.*, 2010; Hofberger *et al.*, 2015; Coleman and Whitfield-Cargile, 2017). In addition, decreased muscle mass and myositis observed in horses with PPID can result in lameness

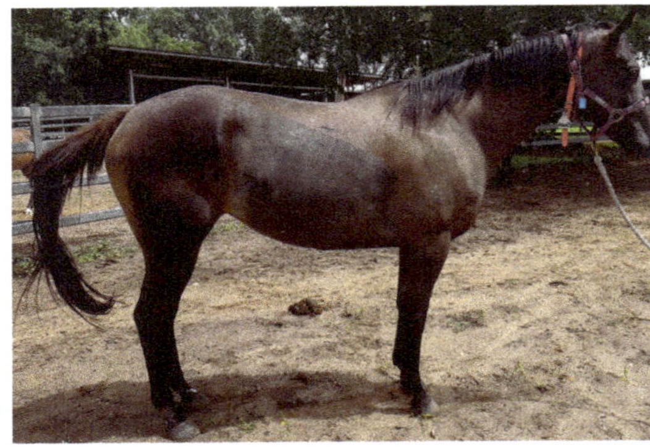

Fig. 1.4. Body condition score of 4/9 in a 4-year-old Thoroughbred mare (Author's own photograph).

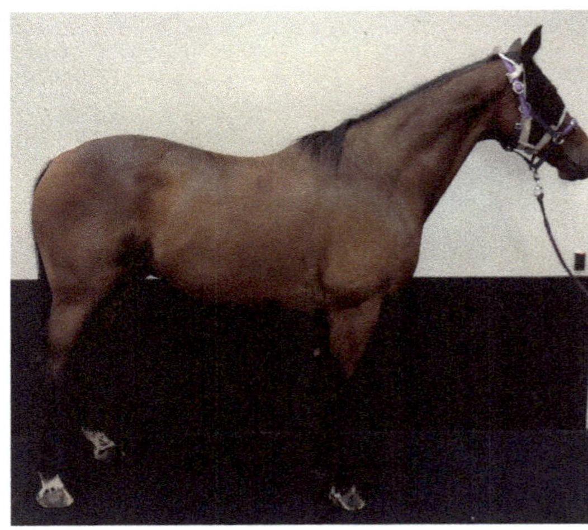

Fig. 1.5. Body condition score of 5/9 in a 13-year-old Thoroughbred gelding (Author's own photograph).

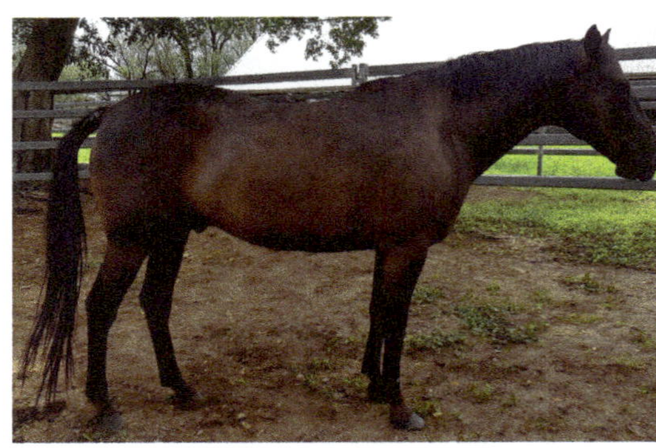

Fig. 1.6. Body condition score of 6/9 in a 16-year-old Australian Stockhorse mare (Author's own photograph).

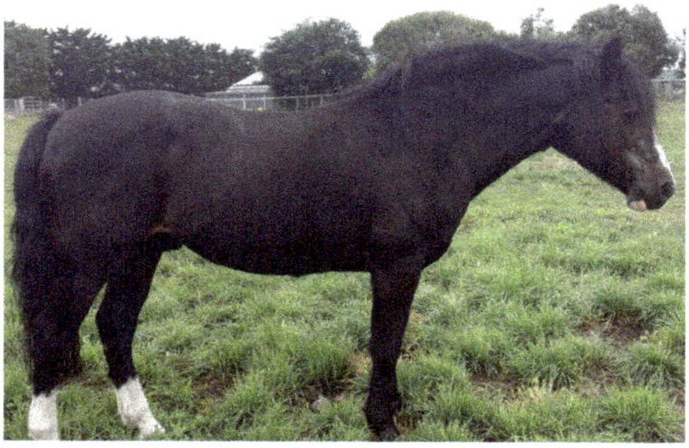

Fig. 1.7. Body condition score of 7/9 in a 12-year-old Welsh pony (courtesy of Dr Allison J. Stewart).

exacerbation (Aleman *et al.*, 2006). In all these cases, a thorough lameness examination and a more detailed evaluation with radiographs, ultrasounds or advanced imaging techniques is indicated.

Reproductive system

The reproductive system and the endocrine system are highly interdependent: an endocrine disorder can present as failure to conceive or subfertility before showing overt signs of endocrinopathy (Frank *et al.*, 2010b). Diseases such as ovarian tumours, cryptorchidism or testicular neoplasia are obvious disorders originating from the reproductive system and are diagnosed by endocrine testing (anti-Müllerian hormone, AMH; human chorionic gonadotropin, hCG; androgens) (Brinsko, 1998; Claes *et al.*, 2013; Murase *et al.*, 2020). However, other endocrine disorders, initially independent of the reproductive system, can alter the equine reproductive function; reproductive disorders, initially independent of the

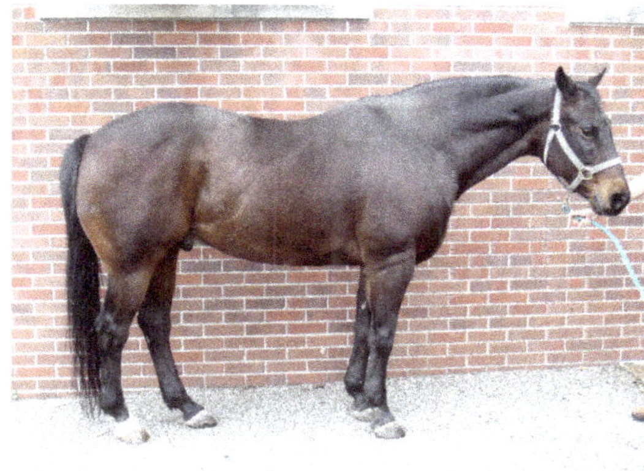

Fig. 1.8. Body condition score of 8/9 in a 14-year-old Quarter Horse gelding (courtesy of Dr Janice E. Kritchevsky).

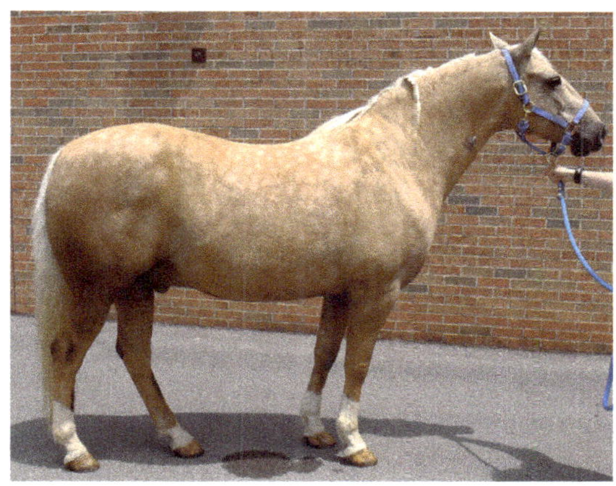

Fig. 1.9. Body condition score of 9/9 in a Quarter Horse gelding (courtesy of Dr Nicholas Frank).

Table 1.2. Cresty neck scoring system. From Carter *et al.*, 2009.

Score	Description
0	No visual appearance of a crest (tissue apparent above the ligamentum nuchae). No palpable crest.
1	No visual appearance of a crest, but slight filling felt with palpation.
2	Noticeable appearance of a crest, but fat deposited fairly evenly from poll to withers. Crest easily cupped in one hand and bent from side to side.
3	Crest enlarged and thickened, so fat deposited more heavily in middle of neck than toward poll and withers, giving mounded appearance. Crest fills cupped hand and begins losing side to side flexibility.
4	Crest grossly enlarged and thickened, and can no longer be cupped in one hand or easily bent from side to side. Crest may have wrinkles/creases perpendicular to top line.
5	Crest is so large it permanently droops to one side.

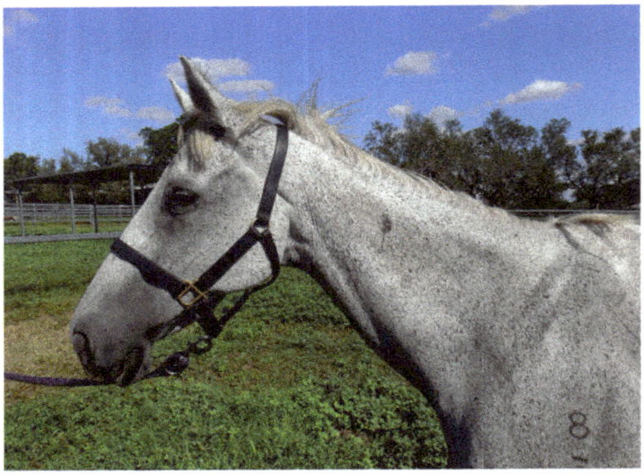

Fig. 1.10. Cresty neck score of 0/5 in a 20-year-old Thoroughbred gelding (Author's own photograph).

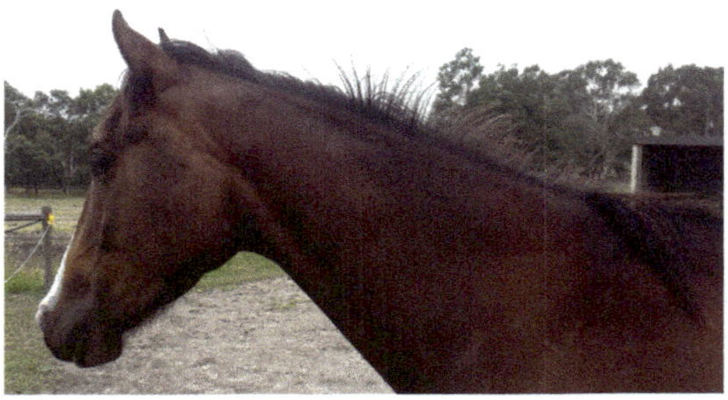

Fig. 1.11. Cresty neck score of 1/5 in an 8-year-old mixed breed pony (courtesy of Dr Allison J. Stewart).

endocrine system, can disturb the hormonal balance (Drew *et al.*, 1975; Boosinger *et al.*, 1995; Buff *et al.*, 2006; Fazio *et al.*, 2016a, b). For example, pregnancy can significantly alter insulin regulation, lipid metabolism and thyroid hormone concentrations and function (Watson *et al.*, 1993; Huszenicza *et al.*, 2000; Gutierrez *et al.*, 2002; Hoffman *et al.*, 2003; Meredith and Dobrinski, 2004; George *et al.*, 2011; Fazio *et al.*, 2016a, b). Thus, careful documentation of a mare's oestrous cycle and a stallion's fertility are recommended when assessing a case suspected of endocrine disorders.

Other relevant body systems

Respiratory system

The respiratory system is not affected by endocrine disorders per se; however, in some cases, the immune system is compromised in endocrine

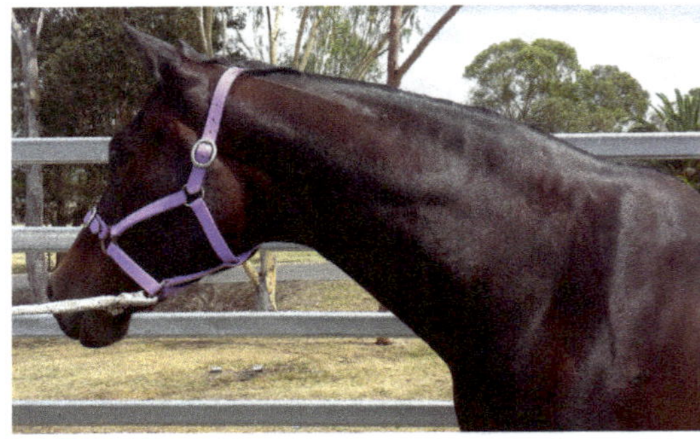

Fig. 1.12. Cresty neck score of 2/5 in a 9-year-old Thoroughbred mare (courtesy of Dr Allison J. Stewart).

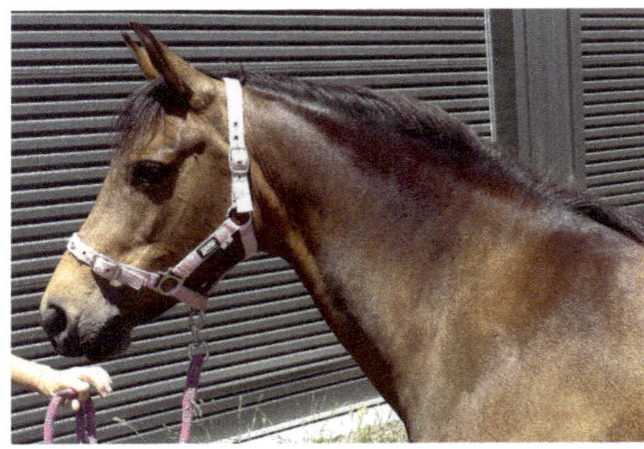

Fig. 1.13. Cresty neck score of 3/5 in a 7-year-old mixed breed pony (courtesy of Dr Allison J. Stewart).

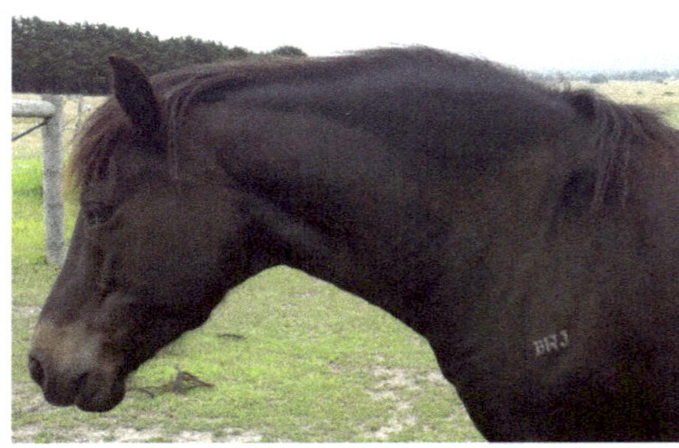

Fig. 1.14. Cresty neck score of 4/5 in an 11-year-old Welsh pony (courtesy of Dr Allison J. Stewart).

conditions such as PPID or relative adrenal insufficiency (RAI), and respiratory infections can develop (Hart and Barton, 2011; McFarlane, 2011). Attention to the respiratory rate should also be paid

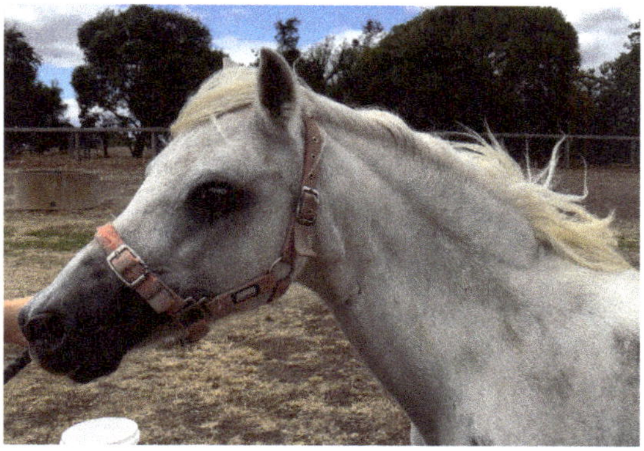

Fig. 1.15. Cresty neck score of 5/5 in an 18-year-old mixed breed pony mare (courtesy of Dr Nicholas J. Bamford).

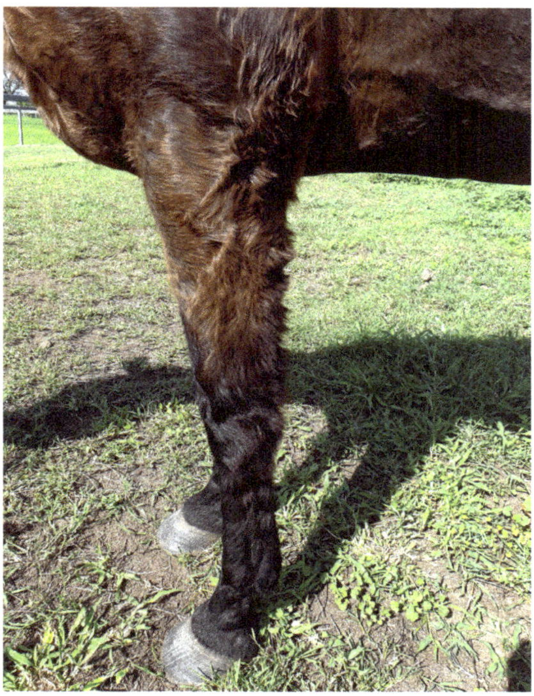

Fig. 1.16. Areas of hypertrichosis associated with pituitary pars intermedia dysfunction (PPID) in a 22-year-old Stockhorse mare (Author's own photograph).

as it has been shown to be a common sign of PPID, mainly in tropical and subtropical climates (Horn *et al.*, 2019).

Alimentary system

Examination of the gastrointestinal system rarely yields abnormal findings in horses with endocrine conditions; however, horses with PPID are more likely to have higher faecal egg counts than age-matched controls and horses with primary hyperparathyroidism can present with clinical signs of colic (Hudson *et al.*, 1999; McFarlane *et al.*, 2010).

Neurological system

Beyond the altered alertness mentioned above, some endocrine disorders can present with neurological signs such as seizures (McFarlane, 2011).

Ocular system

Chronic corneal ulcers are a common alerting sign of PPID as horses suffering from this disorder have a reduced corneal sensitivity and are prone to developing calcific band keratinopathy (Miller *et al.*, 2013; Berryhill *et al.*, 2017).

Haematology and Serum Chemistry

Haematology

A complete blood count can yield subtle changes compatible with an endocrine disorder; however, changes are usually mild and poorly specific (Rohrbach *et al.*, 2012). Nevertheless, the test should be submitted to rule out infectious diseases or malignant haemopathies (Marr *et al.*, 1989; Horn *et al.*, 2019).

Serum chemistry

Specific parameters of a generic chemistry profile can be very valuable when assessing a patient with suspected endocrinopathy. For example, hyperglycaemia can be suggestive of diabetes mellitus, hypercalcaemia can indicate hyperparathyroidism and increased triglyceride concentration is a marker of hyperlipaemia (Peauroi *et al.*, 1998; Durham *et al.*, 2009; McKenzie, 2011). That being said, these changes are usually poorly specific and only considered significant when large or sustained variations are observed. When equivocal results are obtained, additional or more refined testing is warranted. A serum chemistry report should also be submitted to exclude a disease originating from a specific organ, as acute liver or renal diseases can result in similar serum chemistry profiles.

Urinalysis

Endocrine disorders can alter urinary production, urinary specific gravity or urinary composition.

Urine volume and concentration

A urinary production above 30 ml/kg/day in an adult horse is considered abnormal and, if associated with hypo- or isosthenuria, can be suggestive of nephrogenic or neurogenic diabetes insipidus (Schott *et al.*, 1993; Morgan *et al.*, 2012). Other endocrine disorders, such as PPID, have also been shown to alter urinary production and specific gravity (Ireland and McGowan, 2018).

Water deprivation tests have been developed to determine the ability of a horse to concentrate urine and increase urinary specific gravity (Schott, 2011). The standard water deprivation test consists of keeping a horse in a stall overnight with no access to water. A urine specific gravity of less than 1.025 after water deprivation would indicate failure to concentrate urine and suggest a diabetes insipidus (Genetzky *et al.*, 1987). In some cases, when a medullary washout is suspected, longer water deprivation can be required to assess the ability to concentrate urine. The standard test can be extended to up to 2 days or a modified water deprivation test can be used. This modified test is undertaken over 4 days during which the horse has a limited access to water (2 ml/kg/h) (Genetzky *et al.*, 1987; Schott, 2011). Failure to concentrate urine after 4 days of restricted water access would be consistent with a diagnosis of a diabetes insipidus. As there is a risk of significant dehydration, these tests should be stopped if the horse loses more than 5% of body weight. Therefore, water deprivation tests can only be undertaken if a scale is available and after ruling out any primary renal disorder.

Urine composition

Equine urine is rich in calcium; however, in some endocrine conditions, its composition can change. Although diet has a major effect on urinary fractional excretions (FE), calculation of those ratios can be helpful when diseases such as hyperparathyroidism or RAIs are suspected (Table 1.3) (McKeever *et al.*, 2002; Toribio *et al.*, 2005, 2007). In addition, measurement of urine concentrations of specific neurotransmitters or hormones may be useful in some endocrinopathies. For example, measuring urinary catecholamines is diagnostic for pheochromocytoma (Fouché *et al.*, 2016).

Hormone Analysis

Determination of hormone concentration is the most commonly used diagnostic test in equine endocrinology; however, the interpretation of a single value can be complicated as factors such as diet, geographic location, season, time of the day, treatments or assay can confound basal values. The most commonly measured hormones in equine practice are adrenocorticotropic hormone (ACTH), insulin, cortisol, triiodothyronine (T3), T4 and parathormone, but more unusual hormones such as leptin, glucagon-like peptide 1 (GLP-1) or glucose-dependent insulinotropic polypeptide (GIP) can be measured and, to some extent, they can all have results increased or decreased by factors unrelated to the primary endocrine condition. As a result, the clinician should ideally standardize testing protocols to reduce as much as possible variability between results.

Individual variation

In all endocrine studies, there is a significant possibility of factors such as age, gender, breed, oestrous cycle, adiposity or level of activity of the horse having a potential confounding effect (Bamford *et al.*, 2014; Bamford *et al.*, 2016; de Laat *et al.*, 2016a; Beythien *et al.*, 2017; Rapson *et al.*, 2018).

Table 1.3. Urinary fractional excretion (FE) where [X] is the concentration of a given ion in serum or in urine (mmol/l) and [Creatinine] is the concentration of creatinine in serum or urine (μmol/l). From King, 1994.

	Sodium	Potassium	Chloride	Calcium	Phosphorous
FE_X (%)	0.01–1	15–80	0.04–2.1	0–33	0.0–0.5

FE_X (%) = $([X]_{urine} / [X]_{serum}\} \times \{[Creatinine]_{serum} / [Creatinine]_{urine}) \times 100$

Although individual reference intervals cannot be established for all horses, clinicians should keep in mind that interpretation of laboratory results should also be performed in light of the clinical picture and possibly of previous results obtained under similar conditions in the same individual.

Diet

Hormones such as insulin, leptin, GLP-1 or GIP can vary tremendously with changes in type of feed, feeding amounts or feeding schedules. For example, increased carbohydrate intake increases insulin concentrations; acute feed restriction decreases leptin concentrations; and fasting of horses decreases insulin sensitivity (Buff *et al.*, 2006; Bamford *et al.*, 2015; Bertin *et al.*, 2016). Consequently, it is paramount for the clinician to assess the horse with its usual diet to be able to accurately interpret a laboratory result.

Geographic variations

Latitude, altitude and exposure to rainfall, temperatures and daylight amplitude have a specific effect on hormones such as ACTH or alpha-melanocyte-stimulating hormone (α-MSH). For example, the reference intervals for ACTH at lower latitudes (closer to the equator) are wider than the reference intervals at higher latitudes (further from the equator) (Secombe *et al.*, 2017). In addition, elevation, rainfall andtemperatures will interfere with reference intervals in areas with similarlatitude (McFarlane *et al.*, 2011). Therefore, it is recommended that clinicians work with local laboratories that have developed specific reference intervals, as given ACTH results could have very different meanings for a horse living in Michigan (USA) and a horse living in Queensland (Australia). These geographic variations also apply to dynamic testing. For instance, ACTH response to thyrotropin-releasing hormone (TRH) changes with geographical location (Byrne *et al.*, 2018).

Circannual variations

The acknowledgement of seasonal variations in hormone concentrations is critical in the interpretation of laboratory results. ACTH, and its derivates such as α-MSH, are the hormones that have been the most studied with expected increases in autumn, regardless of the geographical location and regardless of the disease status of the horse (Fig. 1.17) (Copas and Durham, 2012; Cordero *et al.*, 2012; Secombe *et al.*, 2017). A similar pattern has also been documented in equine insulin, with higher concentrations in spring and in autumn (Hart *et al.*, 2016; Beythien *et al.*, 2017).

Circadian variations

In addition to circannual variations, some hormones have circadian variations with higher concentrations during specific times of the day. For example,

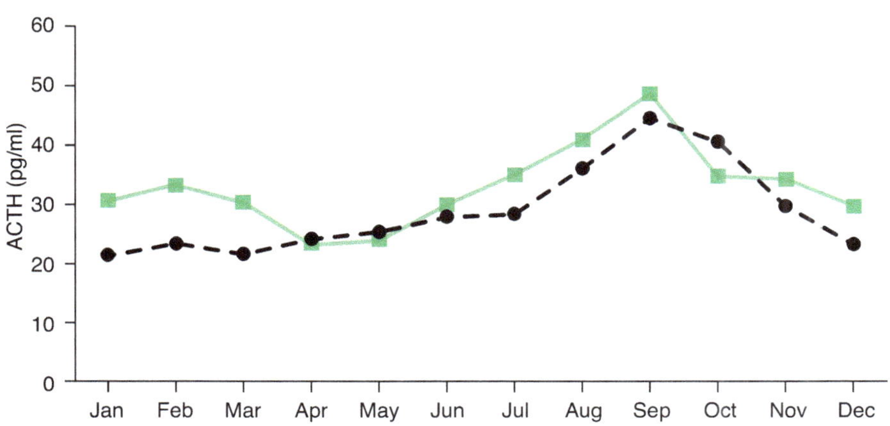

Fig. 1.17. Graphical comparison of the median plasma adrenocorticotropic hormone (ACTH) concentration (pg/ml) by month for healthy horses at two different geographical locations. The line with square markers represents a location closer to the equator than the line with circular markers. Note the geographic and circannual variation in ACTH concentrations. Adapted from Secombe *et al.*, 2017.

the concentration of proopiomelanocortin-derived hormones rises at night-time and the insulin response to a meal varies with time of day (Haritou *et al.*, 2008; Cordero *et al.*, 2012; Bamford *et al.*, 2015). Accordingly, when evaluating a horse with a known endocrine condition, it is advisable to perform testing at similar times to reduce the circadian effect on laboratory results.

Treatment

Many drugs have been shown to interact with hormones. Beyond the ones used to treat specific endocrine conditions, common drugs such as anti-inflammatory drugs or sedatives have been shown to alter hormone effects and secretion. For example, phenylbutazone impairs T4 secretion and alpha-2 agonists directly inhibit insulin secretion by stimulating pancreatic alpha-2-adrenoreceptors (Ramirez *et al.*, 1997; Fagerholm *et al.*, 2011; Yamato Kodera *et al.*, 2013; Lima *et al.*, 2015). Additionally, the duration of the effect can vary depending on the hormone investigated and the drug used. Therefore, it is recommended to discontinue the use of certain drugs when assessing an endocrine patient, or at least to be aware of the use when interpreting a laboratory result.

Hormone stability

Another source of variation to take into account in the interpretation of a laboratory result is the stability of hormones. Some hormones like insulin and T4 have been shown to be stable at room temperature for up to 4 days and up to 8 days when kept at 4°C, and do not require specific precautions (Allen *et al.*, 1997; Carslake *et al.*, 2016; Leschke *et al.*, 2019). On the other hand, ACTH is labile, and concentrations can be altered if the sample is not handled properly. The recommended protocol for the most accurate evaluation of ACTH concentration is to analyse a centrifuged sample within 8 h of collection (Prutton *et al.*, 2015; Stewart *et al.*, 2019). This time frame can be reduced if the sample is kept at temperatures higher than 20°C (Hinrichsen *et al.*, 2019). Freezing samples has been advocated to improve hormone stability; however, freezing does alter hormone concentrations as demonstrated with ACTH concentration changing after prolonged freezing or multiple freeze–thaw cycles (Allen *et al.*, 1997; Haffner *et al.*, 2019; Hu *et al.*, 2020). As changes in hormone concentrations due to poor sample handling result in unpredictable increases or decreases, careful interpretation of results from a sample of unknown origin is warranted to limit the risk of false positive or false negative cases (Allen *et al.*, 1997).

Assay

A large cause of variation in test results is variability between assays. In equine endocrinology, the most commonly used assays are chemiluminescent assays, enzyme-linked immunosorbent assays, radioimmunoassays and, much less frequently, liquid chromatography–mass spectrometry (Reimers *et al.*, 1982; Tinworth *et al.*, 2011; Borer-Weir *et al.*, 2012; Banse *et al.*, 2014; Warnken *et al.*, 2016; Carslake *et al.*, 2017). As most of these assays rely on antigen–antibody affinity, none is specific for equine patients. For example, some enzyme-linked immunosorbent assays used for equine insulin employ porcine, murine or human standards and the frequently used chemiluminescent assays employ human standards (Banse *et al.*, 2014; Karikoski *et al.*, 2015, 2016). Although insulin is relatively well conserved across species, there are some changes in the amino acid sequence that can result in falsely increased or decreased insulin values (Smith, 1966). Therefore, when receiving laboratory results, different reference intervals are to be expected and it is important for clinicians to contact their endocrinology laboratories to ensure that the reference intervals provided are valid for the equine species and for the assay used.

Overall, clinicians should keep in mind that it is paramount to standardize testing, providing as much information as possible to the laboratories to which they are sending samples and to ensure that the laboratories have validated the assay for horses and have developed relevant reference intervals. In order to limit the effect of the factors mentioned above, dynamic testing might be warranted.

Dynamic Testing

Dynamic testing relies on the direct or indirect stimulation or the suppression of an endocrine pathway.

Simple stimulation allows the evaluation of the activity of a specific tissue; for example, in cases of RAI, ACTH is administered intravenously and cortisol is measured to evaluate the function of the zona fasciculata of the adrenal gland (Hart *et al.*, 2009a). On the other hand, more complex stimulation can allow the evaluation of a whole system;

for example, in cases of hyperinsulinaemia, sugar is administered orally and insulin is measured to evaluate the function of the endocrine pancreas but also to assess the activity of incretins (intestinal secretion of insulin) and, to a lesser extent, insulin sensitivity (de Laat *et al.*, 2016b).

Suppression tests rely on the activation of loops of negative feedback. Although no longer recommended for the diagnosis of PPID, dexamethasone suppression is an example of a negative feedback loop. In this test, dexamethasone is administered and cortisol is measured to evaluate how excessive glucocorticosteroids inhibit the production of ACTH by the pituitary gland and decrease cortisol secretion by the adrenal gland (Bertin *et al.*, 2013).

Overall, dynamic testing allows the detection of milder cases of endocrinopathy and is recommended when clinical signs are vague or basal values equivocal. The same limitations regarding assay or hormone stability also exist in dynamic testing; however, the individual variations, circadian variations and, to some extent, geographical variations are often overruled by the use of supraphysiologic doses of hormones.

References

Aleman, M., Watson, J.L., Williams, D.C., LeCouteur, R.A., Nieto, J.E. *et al.* (2006) Myopathy in horses with pituitary pars intermedia dysfunction (Cushing's disease). *Neuromuscular Disorders* 16(11), 737–744. DOI: 10.1016/j.nmd.2006.07.019.

Allen, A.L., Scott, W.M., Cook, S.J., Fretz, P.B. and Doige, C.E. (1997) Effects of delayed serum separation and long-term storage on the measurement of thyroid hormones in equine blood samples. *Veterinary Clinical Pathology* 26(1), 10–12. DOI: 10.1111/j.1939-165X.1997.tb00691.x.

Asplin, K.E., Patterson-Kane, J.C., Sillence, M.N., Pollitt, C.C. and McGowan, C.M. (2010) Histopathology of insulin-induced laminitis in ponies. *Equine Veterinary Journal* 42(8), 700–706. DOI: 10.1111/j.2042-3306.2010.00111.x.

Bamford, N.J., Potter, S.J., Harris, P.A. and Bailey, S.R. (2014) Breed differences in insulin sensitivity and insulinemic responses to oral glucose in horses and ponies of moderate body condition score. *Domestic Animal Endocrinology* 47, 101–107. DOI: 10.1016/j.domaniend.2013.11.001.

Bamford, N.J., Baskerville, C.L., Harris, P.A. and Bailey, S.R. (2015) Postprandial glucose, insulin, and glucagon-like peptide-1 responses of different equine breeds adapted to meals containing micronized maize. *Journal of Animal Science* 93(7), 3377–3383. DOI: 10.2527/jas.2014-8736.

Bamford, N.J., Potter, S.J., Harris, P.A. and Bailey, S.R. (2016) Effect of increased adiposity on insulin sensitivity and adipokine concentrations in horses and ponies fed a high fat diet, with or without a once daily high glycaemic meal. *Equine Veterinary Journal* 48(3), 368–373. DOI: 10.1111/evj.12434.

Banse, H.E., McCann, J., Yang, F., Wagg, C. and McFarlane, D. (2014) Comparison of two methods for measurement of equine insulin. *Journal of Veterinary Diagnostic Investigation* 26(4), 527–530. DOI: 10.1177/1040638714536560.

Berryhill, E.H., Thomasy, S.M., Kass, P.H., Reilly, C.M., Good, K.L. *et al.* (2017) Comparison of corneal degeneration and calcific band keratopathy from 2000 to 2013 in 69 horses. *Veterinary Ophthalmology* 20(1), 16–26. DOI: 10.1111/vop.12338.

Bertin, F.R., Pader, K.S., Lescun, T.B. and Sojka-Kritchevsky, J.E. (2013) Short-term effect of ovariectomy on measures of insulin sensitivity and response to dexamethasone administration in horses. *American Journal of Veterinary Research* 74(12), 1506–1513. DOI: 10.2460/ajvr.74.12.1506.

Bertin, F.R., Taylor, S.D., Bianco, A.W. and Sojka-Kritchevsky, J.E. (2016) The effect of fasting duration on baseline blood glucose concentration, blood insulin concentration, glucose/insulin ratio, oral sugar test, and insulin response test results in horses. *Journal of Veterinary Internal Medicine* 30(5), 1726–1731. DOI: 10.1111/jvim.14529.

Bertin, F.R., Ruffin-Taylor, D. and Stewart, A.J. (2018) Insulin dysregulation in horses with systemic inflammatory response syndrome. *Journal of Veterinary Internal Medicine* 32(4), 1420–1427. DOI: 10.1111/jvim.15138.

Beythien, E., Wulf, M., Ille, N., Aurich, J. and Aurich, C. (2017) Effects of sex, pregnancy and season on insulin secretion and carbohydrate metabolism in horses. *Animal Reproduction Science* 184, 86–93. DOI: 10.1016/j.anireprosci.2017.07.002.

Boosinger, T.R., Brendemuehl, J.P., Bransby, D.L., Wright, J.C., Kemppainen, R.J. *et al.* (1995) Prolonged gestation, decreased triiodothyronine concentration, and thyroid gland histomorphologic features in newborn foals of mares grazing Acremonion coenophialum-infected fescue. *American Journal of Veterinary Research* 56, 66–69.

Borer-Weir, K.E., Bailey, S.R., Menzies-Gow, N.J., Harris, P.A. and Elliott, J. (2012) Evaluation of a commercially available radioimmunoassay and species-specific ELISAs for measurement of high concentrations of insulin in equine serum. *American Journal of Veterinary Research* 73(10), 1596–1602. DOI: 10.2460/ajvr.73.10.1596.

Borer-Weir, K.E., Menzies-Gow, N.J., Bailey, S.R., Harris, P.A. and Elliott, J. (2013) Seasonal and annual influence on insulin and cortisol results from overnight dexamethasone suppression tests in normal ponies and ponies predisposed to laminitis. *Equine Veterinary Journal* 45(6), 688–693. DOI: 10.1111/evj.12053.

Breuhaus, B.A. (2011) Disorders of the equine thyroid gland. *Veterinary Clinics of North America: Equine Practice* 27(1), 115–128. DOI: 10.1016/j.cveq.2010.12.002.

Brinsko, S.P. (1998) Neoplasia of the male reproductive tract. *Veterinary Clinics of North America: Equine Practice* 14(3), 517–533. DOI: 10.1016/S0749-0739(17)30184-0.

Buff, P.R., Johnson, P.J., Wiedmeyer, C.E., Ganjam, V.K., Messer, N.T. *et al*. (2006) Modulation of leptin, insulin, and growth hormone in obese pony mares under chronic nutritional restriction and supplementation with ractopamine hydrochloride. *Vet Ther* 7, 64–72.

Byrne, D.P., Secombe, C.J., Tan, R.H.H., Perera, D.I., Watts, S.P. *et al*. (2018) Circannual variability in adrenocorticotropic hormone responses to administration of thyrotropin-releasing hormone in clinically normal horses in Australia. *The Veterinary Journal* 238, 58–62. DOI: 10.1016/j.tvjl.2018.07.008.

Carslake, H., Karikoski, N., Pinchbeck, G. and McGowan, C. (2016) Serum insulin concentration in horses: effect of storage and handling. *The Veterinary Journal* 211, 94–96. DOI: 10.1016/j.tvjl.2016.02.016.

Carslake, H.B., Pinchbeck, G.L. and McGowan, C.M. (2017) Evaluation of a chemiluminescent immunoassay for measurement of equine insulin. *Journal of Veterinary Internal Medicine* 31(2), 568–574. DOI: 10.1111/jvim.14657.

Carter, R.A., Geor, R.J., Burton Staniar, W., Cubitt, T.A. and Harris, P.A. (2009) Apparent adiposity assessed by standardised scoring systems and morphometric measurements in horses and ponies. *The Veterinary Journal* 179(2), 204–210. DOI: 10.1016/j.tvjl.2008.02.029.

Claes, A., Ball, B.A., Almeida, J., Corbin, C.J. and Conley, A.J. (2013) Serum anti-Müllerian hormone concentrations in stallions: developmental changes, seasonal variation, and differences between intact stallions, cryptorchid stallions, and geldings. *Theriogenology* 79(9), 1229–1235. DOI: 10.1016/j.theriogenology.2013.03.019.

Clarke, I.J. (2015) Hypothalamus as an endocrine organ. *Comprehensive Physiology* 5(1), 217–253. DOI: 10.1002/cphy.c140019.

Coleman, M.C. and Whitfield-Cargile, C. (2017) Orthopedic conditions of the premature and dysmature foal. *Veterinary Clinics of North America: Equine Practice* 33(2), 289–297. DOI: 10.1016/j.cveq.2017.03.001.

Coleman, M.C., Belknap, J.K., Eades, S.C., Galantino-Homer, H.L., Hunt, R.J. *et al*. (2018) Case-control study of risk factors for pasture-and endocrinopathy-associated laminitis in North American horses. *Journal of the American Veterinary Medical Association* 253(4), 470–478. DOI: 10.2460/javma.253.4.470.

Copas, V.E.N. and Durham, A.E. (2012) Circannual variation in plasma adrenocorticotropic hormone concentrations in the UK in normal horses and ponies, and those with pituitary pars intermedia dysfunction. *Equine Veterinary Journal* 44(4), 440–443. DOI: 10.1111/j.2042-3306.2011.00444.x.

Cordero, M., Brorsen, B.W. and McFarlane, D. (2012) Circadian and circannual rhythms of cortisol, ACTH, and α-melanocyte-stimulating hormone in healthy horses. *Domestic Animal Endocrinology* 43(4), 317–324. DOI: 10.1016/j.domaniend.2012.05.005.

de Laat, M.A., Hampson, B.A., Sillence, M.N. and Pollitt, C.C. (2016a) Sustained, low-intensity exercise achieved by a dynamic feeding system decreases body fat in ponies. *Journal of Veterinary Internal Medicine* 30(5), 1732–1738. DOI: 10.1111/jvim.14577.

de Laat, M.A., McGree, J.M. and Sillence, M.N. (2016b) Equine hyperinsulinemia: investigation of the enteroinsular axis during insulin dysregulation. *American Journal of Physiology-Endocrinology and Metabolism* 310(1), E61–E72. DOI: 10.1152/ajpendo.00362.2015.

Donaldson, M.T., LaMonte, B.H., Morresey, P., Smith, G. and Beech, J. (2002) Treatment with pergolide or cyproheptadine of pituitary pars intermedia dysfunction (equine Cushing's disease). *J Vet Intern Med* 16, 742–746.

Drew, B., Barber, W. and Williams, D. (1975) The effect of excess dietary iodine on pregnant mares and foals. *Veterinary Record* 97(5), 93–95. DOI: 10.1136/vr.97.5.93.

Durham, A.E., Hughes, K.J., Cottle, H.J., Rendle, D.I. and Boston, R.C. (2009) Type 2 diabetes mellitus with pancreatic β cell dysfunction in 3 horses confirmed with minimal model analysis. *Equine Veterinary Journal* 41(9), 924–929. DOI: 10.2746/042516409X452152.

Fagerholm, V., Haaparanta, M. and Scheinin, M. (2011) α2-adrenoceptor regulation of blood glucose homeostasis. *Basic & Clinical Pharmacology & Toxicology* 108(6), 365–370. DOI: 10.1111/j.1742-7843.2011.00699.x.

Fazio, E., Medica, P., Cravana, C., Bruschetta, G. and Ferlazzo, A. (2016a) Seasonal thyroid and lipid profiles in Thoroughbred pregnant and nonpregnant mares (Equus caballus). *Theriogenology* 85(9), 1582–1589. DOI: 10.1016/j.theriogenology.2016.01.017.

Fazio, E., Medica, P., Trifiletti, C. and Ferlazzo, A. (2016b) The outcome of the first stages of pregnancy on mares' bloodstream thyroid hormones. *Theriogenology* 86(4), 1036–1041. DOI: 10.1016/j.theriogenology.2016.03.032.

Fouché, N., Gerber, V., Gorgas, D., Marolf, V., Grouzmann, E. *et al*. (2016) Catecholamine metabolism in a Shetland Pony with suspected pheochromocytoma and pituitary pars intermedia dysfunction.

Journal of Veterinary Internal Medicine 30(6), 1872–1878. DOI: 10.1111/jvim.14606.

Frank, N. and Tadros, E.M. (2014) Insulin dysregulation. *Equine Veterinary Journal* 46(1), 103–112. DOI: 10.1111/evj.12169.

Frank, N., Elliott, S.B., Chameroy, K.A., Tóth, F., Chumbler, N.S. *et al.* (2010a) Association of season and pasture grazing with blood hormone and metabolite concentrations in horses with presumed pituitary pars intermedia dysfunction. *Journal of Veterinary Internal Medicine* 24(5), 1167–1175. DOI: 10.1111/j.1939-1676.2010.0547.x.

Frank, N., Geor, R.J., Bailey, S.R., Durham, A.E. and Johnson, P.J. (2010b) Equine metabolic syndrome. *Journal of Veterinary Internal Medicine* 24(3), 467–475. DOI: 10.1111/j.1939-1676.2010.0503.x.

Funk, R.A., Stewart, A.J., Wooldridge, A.A., Kwessi, E., Kemppainen, R.J. *et al.* (2011) Seasonal changes in plasma adrenocorticotropic hormone and α-melanocyte-stimulating hormone in response to thyrotropin-releasing hormone in normal, aged horses. *Journal of Veterinary Internal Medicine* 25(3), 579–585. DOI: 10.1111/j.1939-1676.2011.0712.x.

Genetzky, R.M., Loparco, F. V. and Ledet, A.E. (1987) Clinical pathologic alterations in horses during a water deprivation test. *American Journal of Veterinary Research* 48, 1007–1011.

George, L.A., Staniar, W.B., Cubitt, T.A., Treiber, K.H., Harris, P.A. *et al.* (2011) Evaluation of the effects of pregnancy on insulin sensitivity, insulin secretion, and glucose dynamics in thoroughbred mares. *American Journal of Veterinary Research* 72(5), 666–674. DOI: 10.2460/ajvr.72.5.666.

Gutierrez, C.V., Riddle, W.T. and Bramlage, L.R. (2002) Serum thyroxine concentrations and pregnancy rates 15 to 16 days after ovulation in broodmares. *Journal of the American Veterinary Medical Association* 220(1), 64–66. DOI: 10.2460/javma.2002.220.64.

Haffner, J.C., Neal, D.L., Hoffman, R.M. and Grubbs, S.T. (2019) Plasma adrenocorticotropic hormone concentration in horses decreases after freezing for 60 days. *Journal of Veterinary Diagnostic Investigation* 31(6), 856–858. DOI: 10.1177/1040638719882374.

Haritou, S.J.A., Zylstra, R., Ralli, C., Turner, S. and Tortonese, D.J. (2008) Seasonal changes in circadian peripheral plasma concentrations of melatonin, serotonin, dopamine and cortisol in aged horses with Cushing's disease under natural photoperiod. *Journal of Neuroendocrinology* 20(8), 988–996. DOI: 10.1111/j.1365-2826.2008.01751.x.

Hart, K.A. and Barton, M.H. (2011) Adrenocortical insufficiency in horses and foals. *Veterinary Clinics of North America: Equine Practice* 27(1), 19–34. DOI: 10.1016/j.cveq.2010.12.005.

Hart, K.A., Heusner, G.L., Norton, N.A. and Barton, M.H. (2009a) Hypothalamic-pituitary-adrenal axis assessment in healthy term neonatal foals utilizing a paired low dose/high dose ACTH stimulation test. *Journal of Veterinary Internal Medicine* 23(2), 344–351. DOI: 10.1111/j.1939-1676.2008.00271.x.

Hart, K.A., Slovis, N.M. and Barton, M.H. (2009b) Hypothalamic-pituitary-adrenal axis dysfunction in hospitalized neonatal foals. *Journal of Veterinary Internal Medicine* 23(4), 901–912. DOI: 10.1111/j.1939-1676.2009.0323.x.

Hart, K.A., Wochele, D.M., Norton, N.A., McFarlane, D., Wooldridge, A.A. *et al.* (2016) Effect of age, season, body condition, and endocrine status on serum free cortisol fraction and insulin concentration in horses. *Journal of Veterinary Internal Medicine* 30(2), 653–663. DOI: 10.1111/jvim.13839.

Henneke, D.R., Potter, G.D., Kreider, J.L. and Yeates, B.F. (1983) Relationship between condition score, physical measurements and body fat percentage in mares. *Equine Veterinary Journal* 15(4), 371–372. DOI: 10.1111/j.2042-3306.1983.tb01826.x.

Hinrichsen, S., Stewart, A.J., Yuen, K.Y. and Bertin, F.R. (2019) Effect of various ambient temperatures on the determination of immunoreactive ACTH concentrations in aged horses. *Journal of Veterinary Internal Medicine* 33, 2431–2432.

Hofberger, S., Gauff, F. and Licka, T. (2015) Suspensory ligament degeneration associated with pituitary pars intermedia dysfunction in horses. *The Veterinary Journal* 203(3), 348–350. DOI: 10.1016/j.tvjl.2014.12.037.

Hoffman, R.M., Kronfeld, D.S., Cooper, W.L. and Harris, P.A. (2003) Glucose clearance in grazing mares is affected by diet, pregnancy, and lactation1. *Journal of Animal Science* 81(7), 1764–1771. DOI: 10.2527/2003.8171764x.

Horn, R., Bamford, N.J., Afonso, T., Sutherland, M., Buckerfield, J. *et al.* (2019) Factors associated with survival, laminitis and insulin dysregulation in horses diagnosed with equine pituitary pars intermedia dysfunction. *Equine Veterinary Journal* 51(4), 440–445. DOI: 10.1111/evj.13041.

Hu, K., Stewart, A.J., Yuen, K.Y., Hinrichsen, S., Dryburgh, E.L. *et al.* (2020) The effect of freeze-thaw cycles on determination of immunoreactive plasma adrenocorticotrophic hormone concentrations in horses. *Journal of Veterinary Internal Medicine* 34(3), 1350–1356. DOI: 10.1111/jvim.15771.

Hudson, N.P.H., Church, D.B., Trevena, J., Nielsen, I.L., Major, D. *et al.* (1999) Primary hypoparathyroidism in two horses. *Australian Veterinary Journal* 77(8), 504–508. DOI: 10.1111/j.1751-0813.1999.tb12119.x.

Huszenicza, G., Nagy, P., Juhász, J., Kóródi, P., Kulcsár, M. *et al.* (2000) Relationship between thyroid function and seasonal reproductive activity in mares. *Journal of Reproduction and Fertility. Supplement* (56), 163–172.

Innera, M., Petersen, A.D., Desjardins, D.R., Steficek, B.A., Rosser, E.J. *et al.* (2013) Comparison of hair follicle histology between horses with pituitary pars intermedia dysfunction and excessive hair growth and normal aged horses. *Veterinary Dermatology* 24, 212-7e46-7.

Ireland, J.L. and McGowan, C.M. (2018) Epidemiology of pituitary pars intermedia dysfunction: a systematic literature review of clinical presentation, disease prevalence and risk factors. *The Veterinary Journal* 235, 22–33. DOI: 10.1016/j.tvjl.2018.03.002.

Karikoski, N.P., McGowan, C.M., Singer, E.R., Asplin, K.E., Tulamo, R.-M. *et al.* (2015) Pathology of natural cases of equine Endocrinopathic Laminitis associated with hyperinsulinemia. *Veterinary Pathology* 52(5), 945–956. DOI: 10.1177/0300985814549212.

Karikoski, N.P., Patterson-Kane, J.C., Singer, E.R., McFarlane, D. and McGowan, C.M. (2016) Lamellar pathology in horses with pituitary pars intermedia dysfunction. *Equine Veterinary Journal* 48(4), 472–478. DOI: 10.1111/evj.12450.

King, C. (1994) Practical use of urinary fractional excretion. *Journal of Equine Veterinary Science* 14(9), 464–468. DOI: 10.1016/S0737-0806(06)81968-4.

Kritchevsky, J.E., Muir, G.S., Leschke, D.H.Z., Hodgson, J.K., Hess, E.K. *et al.* (2020) Blood glucose and insulin concentrations after alpha-2-agonists administration in horses with and without insulin dysregulation. *Journal of Veterinary Internal Medicine* 34(2), 902–908. DOI: 10.1111/jvim.15747.

Leschke, D.H., Muir, G.S., Hodgson, J.K., Coyle, M., Horn, R. *et al.* (2019) Immunoreactive insulin stability in horses at risk of insulin dysregulation. *Journal of Veterinary Internal Medicine* 33(6), 2746–2751. DOI: 10.1111/jvim.15629.

Lima, A.G., Costa, L.C.B., Alvarenga, M.A. and Martins, C.B. (2015) Does clinical treatment with phenylbutazone and meloxicam in the pre-ovulatory period influence the ovulation rate in mares? *Reproduction in Domestic Animals* 50(5), 771–775. DOI: 10.1111/rda.12586.

Marr, C.M., Love, S. and Pirie, H.M. (1989) Clinical, ultrasonographic and pathological findings in a horse with splenic lymphosarcoma and pseudohyperparathyroidism. *Equine Veterinary Journal* 21(3), 221–226. DOI: 10.1111/j.2042-3306.1989.tb02152.x.

Martin-Gimenez, T., de Blas, I., Aguilera-Tejero, E., Diez de Castro, E. and Aguirre-Pascasio, C.N. (2016) Endocrine, morphometric, and ultrasonographic characterization of neck adiposity in Andalusian horses. *Domestic Animal Endocrinology* 56, 57–62. DOI: 10.1016/j.domaniend.2016.02.003.

McFarlane, D. (2011) Equine pituitary pars intermedia dysfunction. *Veterinary Clinics of North America: Equine Practice* 27(1), 93–113. DOI: 10.1016/j.cveq.2010.12.007.

McFarlane, D., Hale, G.M., Johnson, E.M. and Maxwell, L.K. (2010) Fecal egg counts after anthelmintic administration to aged horses and horses with pituitary pars intermedia dysfunction. *Journal of the American Veterinary Medical Association* 236(3), 330–334. DOI: 10.2460/javma.236.3.330.

McFarlane, D., Paradis, M.R., Zimmel, D., Sykes, B., Brorsen, B.W. *et al.* (2011) The effect of geographic location, breed, and pituitary dysfunction on seasonal adrenocorticotropin and α-melanocyte-stimulating hormone plasma concentrations in horses. *Journal of Veterinary Internal Medicine* 25(4), 872–881. DOI: 10.1111/j.1939-1676.2011.0745.x.

McFarlane, D., Hill, K. and Anton, J. (2015) Neutrophil function in healthy aged horses and horses with pituitary dysfunction. *Veterinary Immunology and Immunopathology* 165(3–4), 99–106. DOI: 10.1016/j.vetimm.2015.04.006.

McGowan, T.W., Pinchbeck, G.P. and McGowan, C.M. (2013a) Evaluation of basal plasma α-melanocyte-stimulating hormone and adrenocorticotrophic hormone concentrations for the diagnosis of pituitary pars intermedia dysfunction from a population of aged horses. *Equine Veterinary Journal* 45(1), 66–73. DOI: 10.1111/j.2042-3306.2012.00575.x.

McGowan, T.W., Pinchbeck, G.P. and McGowan, C.M. (2013b) Prevalence, risk factors and clinical signs predictive for equine pituitary pars intermedia dysfunction in aged horses. *Equine Veterinary Journal* 45(1), 74–79. DOI: 10.1111/j.2042-3306.2012.00578.x.

McKeever, K.H., Scali, R., Geiser, S. and Kearns, C.F. (2002) Plasma aldosterone concentration and renal sodium excretion are altered during the first days of training. *Equine Veterinary Journal* 34(S34), 524–531. DOI: 10.1111/j.2042-3306.2002.tb05477.x.

McKenzie, H.C. (2011) Equine hyperlipidemias. *Veterinary Clinics of North America: Equine Practice* 27(1), 59–72. DOI: 10.1016/j.cveq.2010.12.008.

Meredith, T.B. and Dobrinski, I. (2004) Thyroid function and pregnancy status in broodmares. *Journal of the American Veterinary Medical Association* 224(6), 892–894. DOI: 10.2460/javma.2004.224.892.

Miller, C., Utter, M.L. and Beech, J. (2013) Evaluation of the effects of age and pituitary pars intermedia dysfunction on corneal sensitivity in horses. *American Journal of Veterinary Research* 74(7), 1030–1035. DOI: 10.2460/ajvr.74.7.1030.

Miller, M.A., Moore, G.E., Bertin, F.R. and Kritchevsky, J.E. (2016) What's new in old horses? Postmortem diagnoses in mature and aged equids. *Veterinary Pathology* 53(2), 390–398. DOI: 10.1177/0300985815608674.

Morgan, R.A., Malalana, F. and McGowan, C.M. (2012) Nephrogenic diabetes insipidus in a 14-year-old gelding. *New Zealand Veterinary Journal* 60(4), 254–257. DOI: 10.1080/00480169.2012.669723.

Murase, H., Ochi, A., Tozaki, T., Kakoi, H., Munkhtuul, T. *et al.* (2020) A case of equine cryptorchidism with undetectable serum anti-Müllerian hormone. *Journal of Veterinary Medical Science* 82(2), 209–211. DOI: 10.1292/jvms.18-0057.

Peauroi, J.R., Fisher, D.J., Mohr, F.C. and Vivrette, S.L. (1998) Primary hyperparathyroidism caused by a functional parathyroid adenoma in a horse. *Journal of the American Veterinary Medical Association* 212(12), 1915–1918.

Pleasant, R.S., Suagee, J.K., Thatcher, C.D., Elvinger, F. and Geor, R.J. (2013) Adiposity, plasma insulin, leptin, lipids, and oxidative stress in mature light breed horses. *Journal of Veterinary Internal Medicine* 27(3), 576–582. DOI: 10.1111/jvim.12056.

Prutton, J.S.W., Kass, P.H., Watson, J.L. and Pusterla, N. (2015) Pre-analytical stability of adrenocorticotrophic hormone from healthy horses in whole blood, plasma and frozen plasma samples. *The Veterinary Journal* 204(1), 123–124. DOI: 10.1016/j.tvjl.2015.02.010.

Ramirez, S., Wolfsheimer, K.J., Moore, R.M., Mora, F., Bueno, A.C. *et al.* (1997) Duration of effects of phenylbutazone on serum total thyroxine and free thyroxine concentrations in horses. *Journal of Veterinary Internal Medicine* 11(6), 371–374. DOI: 10.1111/j.1939-1676.1997.tb00483.x.

Rapson, J.L., Schott, H.C., McCutcheon, L.J., McCutcheon, L.J., Harris, P.A. *et al.* (2018) Effects of age and diet on glucose and insulin dynamics in the horse. *Equine Veterinary Journal* 50(5), 690–696. DOI: 10.1111/evj.12812.

Reimers, T.J., Cowan, R.G., McCann, J.P. and Ross, M.W. (1982) Validation of a rapid solid-phase radioimmunoassay for canine, bovine, and equine insulin. *American Journal of Veterinary Research* 43(7), 1274–1278.

Rohrbach, B.W., Stafford, J.R., Clermont, R.S.W., Reed, S.M., Schott, H.C. *et al.* (2012) Diagnostic frequency, response to therapy, and long-term prognosis among horses and ponies with pituitary pars intermedia dysfunction, 1993–2004. *Journal of Veterinary Internal Medicine* 26(4), 1027–1034. DOI: 10.1111/j.1939-1676.2012.00932.x.

Ronen, N., Van Heerden, J. and Van Amstel, S.R. (1992) Clinical and biochemistry findings, and parathyroid hormone concentrations in three horses with secondary hyperparathyroidism. *Journal of the South African Veterinary Association* 63, 134–136.

Schott, H.C. (2011) Water homeostasis and diabetes insipidus in horses. *Veterinary Clinics of North America: Equine Practice* 27(1), 175–195. DOI: 10.1016/j.cveq.2011.01.002.

Schott, H.C., 2nd., Bayly, W.M., Reed, S.M. and Brobst, D.F. (1993) Nephrogenic diabetes insipidus in sibling colts. *Journal of Veterinary Internal Medicine*7, 68–72.

Secombe, C.J., Tan, R.H.H., Perera, D.I., Byrne, D.P., Watts, S.P. *et al.* (2017) The effect of geographic location on circannual adrenocorticotropic hormone plasma concentrations in horses in Australia. *Journal of Veterinary Internal Medicine* 31(5), 1533–1540. DOI: 10.1111/jvim.14782.

Sessions-Bresnahan, D.R. and Carnevale, E.M. (2014) The effect of equine metabolic syndrome on the ovarian follicular environment. *Journal of Animal Science* 92(4), 1485–1494. DOI: 10.2527/jas.2013-7275.

Smith, L.F. (1966) Species variation in the amino acid sequence of insulin. *The American Journal of Medicine* 40(5), 662–666. DOI: 10.1016/0002-9343(66)90145-8.

Spelta, C.W. and Axon, J.E. (2012) Case series of equine pituitary pars intermedia dysfunction in a tropical climate. *Australian Veterinary Journal* 90(11), 451–456. DOI: 10.1111/j.1751-0813.2012.00997.x.

Stewart, A.J., Yuen, K.A., Hinrichsen, S., Horn, R. and Bertin, F.R. (2019) Effect of sample handling on ACTH concentrations following thyrotropin-releasing hormone stimulation in horses. *Journal of Veterinary Internal Medicine* 33, 2436–2436.

Tinworth, K.D., Wynn, P.C., Boston, R.C., Harris, P.A., Sillence, M.N. *et al.* (2011) Evaluation of commercially available assays for the measurement of equine insulin. *Domestic Animal Endocrinology* 41(2), 81–90. DOI: 10.1016/j.domaniend.2011.05.001.

Toribio, R.E. (2011) Disorders of calcium and phosphate metabolism in horses. *Veterinary Clinics of North America: Equine Practice* 27(1), 129–147. DOI: 10.1016/j.cveq.2010.12.010.

Toribio, R.E., Kohn, C.W., Hardy, J. and Rosol, T.J. (2005) Alterations in serum parathyroid hormone and electrolyte concentrations and urinary excretion of electrolytes in horses with induced endotoxemia. *Journal of Veterinary Internal Medicine* 19(2), 223–231. DOI: 10.1111/j.1939-1676.2005.tb02686.x.

Toribio, R.E., Kohn, C.W., Rourke, K.M., Levine, A.L. and Rosol, T.J. (2007) Effects of hypercalcemia on serum concentrations of magnesium, potassium, and phosphate and urinary excretion of electrolytes in horses. *American Journal of Veterinary Research* 68(5), 543–554. DOI: 10.2460/ajvr.68.5.543

Warnken, T., Huber, K. and Feige, K. (2016) Comparison of three different methods for the quantification of equine insulin. *BMC Veterinary Research* 12(1), 196. DOI: 10.1186/s12917-016-0828-z.

Watson, T.D., Burns, L., Packard, C.J. and Shepherd, J. (1993) Effects of pregnancy and lactation on plasma lipid and lipoprotein concentrations, lipoprotein composition and post-heparin lipase activities in Shetland pony mares. *Reproduction* 97(2), 563–568. DOI: 10.1530/jrf.0.0970563.

Yamato Kodera, S., Yoshida, M., Dezaki, K., Yada, T., Murayama, T. *et al.* (2013) Inhibition of insulin secretion from rat pancreatic islets by dexmedetomidine and medetomidine, two sedatives frequently used in clinical settings. *Endocrine Journal* 60(3), 337–346. DOI: 10.1507/endocrj.EJ12-0308.

2 Diseases of the Thyroid Gland and the Hypothalamo–Pituitary–Thyroid Axis

Thyroid hormones (thyroxine, T4 and triiodothyronine, T3) are involved in key metabolic steps such as cellular oxygen consumption, protein and lipid metabolism and body heat regulation (Breuhaus, 2011). Although they are not considered indispensable for adult life, they play a tremendous role in growing animals as they stimulate organ development and maturation. True thyroid gland dysfunction is rare in horses but both hyper- and hypothyroidism have been described.

Hypothalamo–Pituitary–Thyroid Axis Physiology

The thyroid gland is under the regulation of the hypothalamo–pituitary–thyroid axis. Neurons of the paraventricular nucleus of the hypothalamus synthesize the thyrotropin-releasing hormone (TRH), a polypeptide that is released in the hypophyseal portal system where it binds to the thyrotropes of the anterior pituitary gland to induce the release of the thyroid-stimulating hormone (TSH or thyrotropin) (Taylor *et al.*, 1990). TSH is a glycopeptide composed of two subunits and stimulates the thyroid follicular cells to induce the synthesis and release of thyroid hormones (Parmentier *et al.*, 1989). Both TRH and TSH are released in a pulsatile manner, have short half-lives, are down regulated by thyroid hormones, dopamine and somatostatin and up regulated by alpha-adrenergic agonists (Greenspan *et al.*, 1986).

Under the stimulation of TSH, thyroid follicular cells increase their iodine uptake and thyroglobulin synthesis to form monoiodotyrosine (MIT) and diiodotyrosine (DIT). These iodized thyroglobulins are then combined to form T4 or T3 (Breuhaus, 2011). Thyroid hormones are finally released in the bloodstream (80% as T4 and 20% as T3), mainly bound to proteins such as thyroid hormone-binding globulins or albumin. Only the free fractions of T4 and T3 are metabolically active and the protein-bound fractions are considered as a pool of readily available hormone protected from renal filtration (Breuhaus, 2011). T4 is released in larger amounts than T3 and binds more tightly to proteins, resulting in an increased half-life (Frank *et al.*, 2002). In addition, T4 has less affinity for thyroid hormone receptors resulting in T4 being less metabolically active than T3; however, T4 can be deiodized in target tissues by deiodinases (type-1 and/or type-2) to form T3. As very little T3 is directly released by the follicular cells of the thyroid gland, deiodination of T4 is the main source of T3 (Frank *et al.*, 2002; Breuhaus, 2011). Another deiodinase (type-3) cleaves T4 into reverse triiodothyronine (rT3) which has very little metabolic activity. This third deiodinase is an important regulator of thyroid hormone function (Breuhaus, 2011).

Thyroid hormones enhance aerobic metabolism and virtually all tissues can respond to thyroid hormone stimulation. The thyroid hormone actions can be initiated within the cell nucleus (genomic action by regulation of transcription factors) or at the plasma membrane, the cytoplasm and the mitochondrion (non-genomic action by stimulation of transmembrane receptors and downstream effectors) (Cheng *et al.*, 2010). Regardless of the pathway, thyroid hormones promote protein synthesis, energy metabolism, cell division and heat production resulting in organ growth and maturation. In horses, thyroid hormones have been shown to play a key role in adaptation to age, season, feed availability and activity (Malinowski *et al.*, 1996; Christensen *et al.*, 1997; Graves *et al.*, 2006; Brinkmann *et al.*, 2016; Fazio *et al.*, 2016a).

Assessment of the Equine Thyroid Function

The thyroid gland is composed of two lobes located caudally to the larynx, on each side of the trachea. In normal horses, the thyroid gland

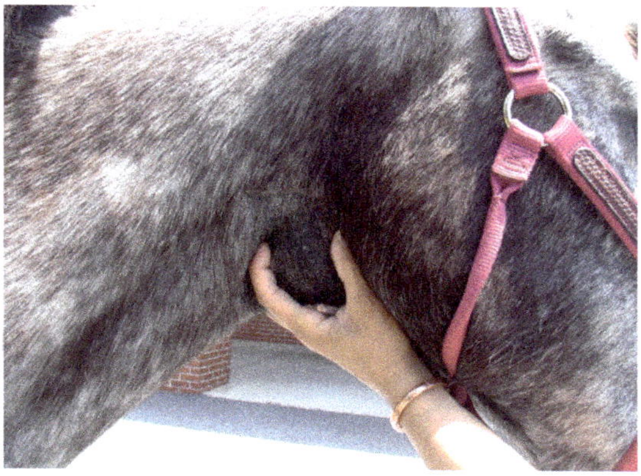

Fig. 2.1. Enlarged thyroid gland in a 17-year-old mixed breed gelding (courtesy of Dr Allison J. Stewart).

is non-visible, barely palpable and measures approximately 2.5 cm × 2.5 cm × 5 cm; however, in older horses, the gland can be enlarged and easily identified (Fig. 2.1) (Frank *et al.*, 2002). A pathological enlargement of the thyroid gland is named *goitre* but changes in thyroid gland size are poorly correlated to a diagnosis of hyper- or hypothyroidism, justifying the need to investigate the hypothalamo–pituitary–thyroid axis function (Dalefield and Palmer, 1994; Frank *et al.*, 2002).

Thyroid hormone measurement

T4 and T3 can be easily measured by diagnostic laboratories from serum or heparinized plasma; however, the challenge for the clinician is to be able to recognize false positive cases, mainly in the diagnosis of hypothyroidism (Beech, 1987; Sojka *et al.*, 1993; Thompson *et al.*, 1997). Several assays have been developed and validated to measure equine thyroid hormones including a radioimmunoassay and a chemiluminescent assays and reference ranges have been developed for total and free fractions of thyroid hormones (Table 2.1) (Ramirez *et al.*, 1997; Singh *et al.*, 1997; Breuhaus, 2011; Tangyuenyong *et al.*, 2017). These ranges are, however, quite large, as thyroid hormones are secreted in a pulsatile manner with higher concentrations of T3 in the morning and higher concentrations of T4 in the afternoon, making thyroid hormone measurements poorly repeatable (Duckett *et al.*, 1989; Thompson *et al.*, 1997). In addition, T4 measurement by direct methods reportedly underestimates T4 concentrations, compared with concentrations obtained by dialysis methods (Breuhaus *et al.*, 2006). The use of a thyroid panel including total and free fractions of both T4 and T3 is therefore recommended to limit false positive diagnoses (Frank *et al.*, 2002). If only limited evaluation is available, free fractions are to be preferred as thyroid hormone protein binding can be altered in some disease states or after drug administration; however, it is reported that, in healthy subjects, total and free fractions are correlated (Breuhaus, 2011; Li *et al.*, 2014). Unlike other hormones, thyroid hormones are quite stable and samples can be left for 24 h in whole blood at room temperature; however, freezing could result in false increases in T4 (Allen *et al.*, 1997).

In interpreting a thyroid panel at a single timepoint, it can be difficult to ascertain a diagnosis of hyper- or hypothyroidism as many factors have been shown to durably alter thyroid hormone concentrations. Decreases in food availability, changes in diet composition (energy, protein, zinc or copper), administration of phenylbutazone, administration of dexamethasone (systemic or topical), administration of trimethoprim sulfadiazine, exercise, transport and gestation have all been shown to change thyroid hormone concentrations (Morris and Garcia, 1983, 1985; Sojka *et al.*, 1993; Messer *et al.*, 1995a, b; Ramirez *et al.*, 1997; Gonzalez *et al.*, 1998; Rothschild *et al.*, 2004; Abraham *et al.*, 2011; Fazio *et al.*, 2016b, 2017). Therefore, caution should be used when interpreting a thyroid hormone panel from a horse that has received any kind of medication or supplement in the 2 weeks prior to testing (Breuhaus, 2011).

Table 2.1. Baseline concentrations of thyroid hormones (thyroxine, T4 and triiodothyronine, T3) in adult horses based on 71 subjects. Adapted from Breuhaus, 2011.

	Total T4 nmol/l	Free T4 pmol/l	Free T4 (dialysis) pmol/l	Total T3 nmol/l	Free T3 pmol/	TSH ng/ml
Median	19	11	22	0.9	1.7	0.23
95% CI	18–22	10–12	21–25	0.9–1.1	1.8–2.4	0.21–0.37

Dynamic testing

As interpretation of a single thyroid hormone concentration is often challenging, stimulation and suppression tests provide a better assessment of the hypothalamo–pituitary–thyroid axis. These tests are poorly compatible with ambulatory practice and often require referral.

Thyrotropin-releasing hormone stimulation test

Intravenous injection of TRH (1 mg for adult horses or 0.5 mg for ponies) is used to stimulate the thyrotropes of the anterior pituitary gland to trigger the release of TSH, resulting in the release of T4 and T3 (Beech and Garcia, 1985; Lothrop and Nolan, 1986; Harris *et al.*, 1992). In euthyroid horses, the injection should result in a twofold increase in TSH within 45 min, a twofold increase in T3 within 2 h and a twofold increase in T4 within 4 h (Lothrop and Nolan, 1986; Breuhaus, 2002, 2011).

Thyroid-stimulating hormone stimulation test

Intravenous injection of TSH (5 IU for an adult horse) is used to stimulate the release of T4 and T3 from the thyroid gland (Held and Oliver, 1984; Harris *et al.*, 1992; Sojka *et al.*, 1993; Graves *et al.*, 2006). In euthyroid horses, the injection should result in a sixfold increase in total T3 within 2 h, a two- to threefold increase in total T4 within 4 h and a fourfold increase in free T4 within 4 h (Morris and Garcia, 1983; Held and Oliver, 1984; Sojka *et al.*, 1993).

Triiodothyronine suppression test

Administration of T3 is used to suppress the hypothalamo–pituitary–thyroid axis and decrease the release of T4 by activating a loop of negative feedback (Alberts *et al.*, 2000). The protocol requires hospitalization of the horse and consists in the intramuscular administration of 2.5 mg of T3 twice daily for 4 days with blood sampling 5 min before each injection, twice daily on days 5 and 7 and in the morning on day 10. In euthyroid horses, administration of T3 should result in a rapid and marked (10- to 20-fold) increase in T3 and in a gradual but sustained decrease in T4 observed until day 10 (Alberts *et al.*, 2000; Breuhaus, 2011).

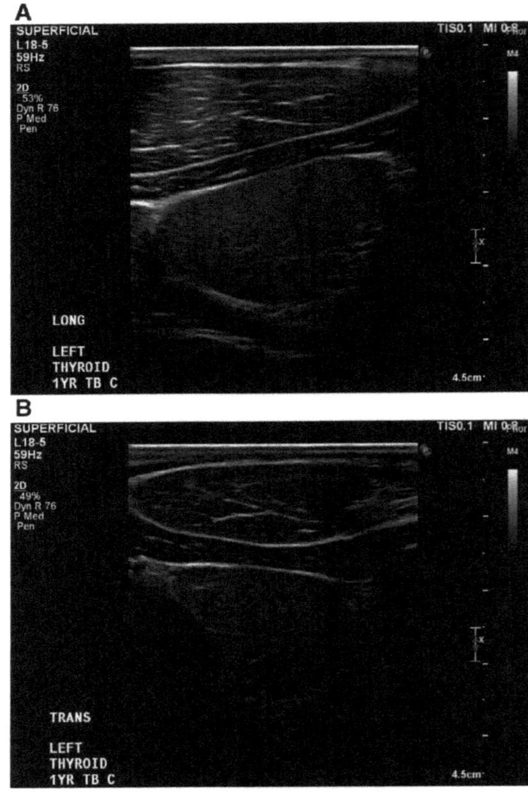

Fig. 2.2. Longitudinal (A) and transverse (B) ultrasound images of the left thyroid lobe of an 18-month-old Thoroughbred colt (courtesy of Dr Alex Young).

Diagnostic imaging

In addition to providing information regarding the structure of the thyroid gland, diagnostic imaging can assess its activity. Ultrasonographic examination can be used to document the nature of the enlargement of the thyroid gland, detect the presence of cysts or nodules, identify a biopsy site and compare the sizes and echogenicity of the right and left lobe of the gland. Thyroid lobes are reported to have a volume ranging from 13.5 to 18.9 cm^3, depending on the age of the horse, and are said to be hyper- to isoechoic to the sternocephalicus muscle (Fig. 2.2) (Davies *et al.*, 2010). Nuclear scintigraphy allows an evaluation of the function of the thyroid gland by determining a differential radiopharmaceutical uptake between lobes (Hillidge *et al.*, 1982; Held *et al.*, 1985; Tan *et al.*, 2008; Davies *et al.*, 2010; Daniel and Neelis, 2014).

Hypothyroidism in Adult Horses

Hypothyroidism refers to a hypothalamo–pituitary–thyroid axis dysfunction. Depending on the origin of the disorder, hypothyroidism has been classified into four types:

- *primary hypothyroidism*, referring to an impaired secretion of T4 and T3 caused by disorder of the thyroid gland itself;
- *secondary hypothyroidism*, referring to an impaired secretion of TSH caused by a disorder of the anterior pituitary gland;
- *tertiary hypothyroidism*, referring to an impaired secretion of TRH caused by a disorder of the hypothalamus; and
- *quaternary hypothyroidism*, referring to an impaired binding of thyroid hormones to thyroid hormone receptors located in peripheral tissues.

Although these endocrinopathies are well described in people and in other companion animals, the existence of true hypothyroidism in adult horses is rather controversial, as clinical signs are vague and a diagnosis is often made without enough evidence (Frank *et al.*, 2002).

Primary hypothyroidism

Spontaneous cases of primary hypothyroidism are rare, and the clinical description is often limited to experimentally induced primary hypothyroidism. Iodine deficiency, or ingestion of goitrogens such as sulfurated organic compounds, thiocyanates and isothiocyanates, are reported to be possible causes of primary hypothyroidism; however, horses on low iodine or goitrogenic diets fail to show evidence of hypothyroidism after a TRH stimulation test (Frank *et al.*, 2002; Breuhaus, 2003). Immune-mediated diseases are also reported as common causes of primary hypothyroidism in other species (Kaptein *et al.*, 1994). In horses, however, there is limited evidence indicating that a Hashimoto thyroiditis-like disease, characterized by lymphocytic infiltration and fibrosis of the thyroid gland associated with increased anti-thyroglobulin and anti-thyroid peroxidase antibody titres, would exist in horses showing a macroscopically enlarged thyroid gland (Perillo *et al.*, 2005). Most cases of primary hypothyroidism are therefore considered idiopathic (Frank *et al.*, 2002).

In the absence of clear evidence of spontaneous primary hypothyroidism, the description of the clinical presentation of this disorder is based on anecdotal reports and on horses that have undergone surgical thyroidectomy or propylthiouracil (PTU) administration. In these reports, clinical signs associated with decreased thyroid gland activity are mild and include decreased heart rate, decreased respiratory rate, decreased body temperature (possibly associated with cold intolerance), alopecia or coarse haircoat, myopathy, agalactia and keratoconjunctivitis sicca (Lowe *et al.*, 1974, 1987; Stanley and Hillidge, 1982; Thompson *et al.*, 1986; Harris *et al.*, 1992; Vischer *et al.*, 1999; Johnson *et al.*, 2003; Schwarz *et al.*, 2008). Changes in clinical pathology panels are also mild and include decreases in packed cell volume, hypophosphataemia and increases in both triglycerides and cholesterol (Lowe *et al.*, 1974; Frank *et al.*, 2003, Frank *et al.*, 2004). It is important to note that none of the clinical signs traditionally associated with primary hypothyroidism, such as obesity, regional adiposity, decreased fertility, laminitis and anhidrosis, have been observed in thyroidectomized horses and that these signs have been shown to be caused by other endocrinopathies, including equine metabolic syndrome (EMS) (Gutierrez *et al.*, 2002; Meredith and Dobrinski, 2004; Breuhaus, 2009, 2011).

A definitive diagnosis of primary hypothyroidism relies on the demonstration of an inability of the thyroid gland to respond to stimulus. Low concentrations of thyroid hormones can raise a suspicion of hypothyroidism; however, a diagnosis of primary hypothyroidism is based on a negative TSH stimulation test (Morris and Garcia, 1983; Held and Oliver, 1984; Sojka *et al.*, 1993; Schwarz *et al.*, 2008).

Management of primary hypothyroidism is possible using thyroid hormone replacement therapy with synthetic T4 (Vischer *et al.*, 1999). Oral administration of levothyroxine sodium (20 µg/kg) once daily can restore T4 and T3 concentrations within reference intervals and resolve clinical signs (Vischer *et al.*, 1999; Schwarz *et al.*, 2008). Long-term administration of levothyroxine to euthyroid horses, even at high doses (100 µg/kg), does not appear to adversely affect health and would be limited to hyperexcitability and weight loss; however, only limited data are available (Sommardahl *et al.*, 2005; Frank *et al.*, 2008a; Bertin *et al.*, 2019). In humans, oversupplementation is associated with cardiovascular disorders such as atrial fibrillation, myocardial infarction and congestive heart failure (Gomberg-Maitland and Frishman, 1998;

Vale *et al.*, 2019). For prolonged treatments, gradual weaning is recommended if therapy is to be discontinued.

Secondary hypothyroidism

This disorder is characterized by an impaired TSH secretion and multiple factors have been shown to alter the hypothalamo–pituitary–thyroid axis and present as secondary hypothyroidism. Therefore, most cases of secondary hypothyroidism are caused by non-thyroidal factors such as drug administration (phenylbutazone, trimethoprim sulfadiazine), diet changes or food deprivation, exercise or gestation (Morris and Garcia, 1985; Flisińska-Bojanowska *et al.*, 1991; Messer *et al.*, 1995b; Rothschild *et al.*, 2004; Graves *et al.*, 2006). There is no report of spontaneous secondary hypothyroidism.

The clinical presentation is similar to primary hypothyroidism and thyroid hormone concentrations are low. A diagnosis is reached by obtaining a good history and by performing stimulation tests. Since secondary hypothyroidism is caused by an anterior pituitary gland disorder resulting in an impaired TSH secretion, the combination of a TRH stimulation test and a TSH stimulation test is required. The TRH stimulation test will be consistent with hypothyroidism, with no increase in T4 or T3 concentrations, whereas the TSH stimulation test will be normal, indicating a normal thyroid gland function (Sojka *et al.*, 1993; Messer *et al.*, 1995a). As TSH is not routinely measured and might be difficult to obtain, diagnosis is often limited to history and the TRH stimulation test (Frank *et al.*, 2002).

Thyroid hormone supplementation should only be initiated if non-thyroidal factors have been eliminated and the results of the TRH stimulation test are consistent with hypothyroidism. In these cases, careful supplementation is warranted.

Tertiary and quaternary hypothyroidism

Neither tertiary nor quaternary hypothyroidism have been clearly described in horses. Decreases in T4 and T3 concentrations observed in mares in seasonal anoestrus could be the result of a decreased hypothalamic stimulation consistent with tertiary hypothyroidism; however, more research in this area is required (Huszenicza *et al.*, 2000).

Non-thyroidal illness syndrome or euthyroid sick syndrome in adult horses

This syndrome is well recognized in other species but documentation in horses is limited (De Groot, 1999; Hilderbran *et al.*, 2014). Four mechanisms reducing thyroid function have been described in dogs and humans and it is assumed that they also occur in horses. These mechanisms include an increased free fraction to bound fraction, a decreased conversion of T4 into T3, a decreased clearance in rT3 and a decreased thyrotrope activity (similar to tertiary hypothyroidism) (Berger *et al.*, 2001; Frank *et al.*, 2002; Warner and Beckett, 2010; Breuhaus, 2011). Sepsis, stress, trauma, fasting or systemic inflammation are associated with non-thyroidal illness syndrome in other species. One study documented a decrease in T3 followed by a decrease in T4 in hospitalized horses and, in human medicine, these decreases are associated with disease severity and non-survival (Slag *et al.*, 1981; Kaptein *et al.*, 1982; De Groot, 1999; Hilderbran *et al.*, 2014). In an equine study, those changes were not associated with an increase in TSH indicating a hypothalamo–pituitary–thyroid axis dysfunction (Hilderbran *et al.*, 2014). This syndrome could be mistaken for true hypothyroidism; however, treatment should focus on the underlying condition rather than on thyroid hormone supplementation.

Hypothyroidism in Foals

Thyroid hormones are involved in organ development and maturation, and concentrations of T4 and T3 in neonates are much higher than in adult horses (Table 2.2) (Irvine and Evans, 1975; Murray and Luba, 1993; Breuhaus, 2014). Therefore, low concentrations of T4 and T3 have much more severe effects on growing foals than on adults and hypothyroidism in foals is much more common than in adults.

Congenital goitre

During gestation, the fetal thyroid gland is unable to regulate iodine uptake. Therefore, excessive or deficient iodine ingestion by the mare inhibits the synthesis of T4 and T3 in the fetal thyroid gland (Drew *et al.*, 1975; Osame and Ichijo, 1994). This low production of thyroid hormone activates a feedback loop, stimulating TRH and TSH secretion and resulting in an enlarged thyroid gland and a

Table 2.2. Baseline concentrations of thyroid hormones (thyroxine, T4 and triiodothyronine, T3) in 24–36-h-old foals based on 20 healthy subjects. Adapted from Breuhaus, 2014.

	Total T4 nmol/l	Free T4 (dialysis) pmol/l	Total T3 nmol/l	Free T3 pmol/l	TSH ng/ml
Median	260.5	97.5	8.2	10.0	0.24
95% CI	191–318	49–144	6.0–11.8	5.6–24.2	0.10–0.68

congenital goitre (Doige and McLaughlin, 1981; Eroksuz *et al.*, 2004). Possible dietary goitrogens include mustard, seaweed and selenium-deficient diets. As the mare's thyroid gland can regulate iodine uptake and excretion, the mare does not exhibit clinical signs of hypothyroidism (Doige and McLaughlin, 1981; Eroksuz *et al.*, 2004). Clinical signs in the foal depend on the gestational stage and range from mild to severe, with a goitre, weakness, hypothermia, sparse haircoat and delayed bone development (Drew *et al.*, 1975; Irvine, 1984; Murray, 1990).

Prognosis for this condition in foals depends on the severity of the clinical signs, which can improve or resolve once dietary iodine is addressed. Supportive care is paramount and thyroid hormone supplementation can be used. Daily oral administration of 20–50 µg/kg of levothyroxine and 1 µg/kg of T3 would be recommended; however, the doses for foals have not been specifically established (Irvine, 1984).

Thyroid gland hyperplasia and musculoskeletal deformity syndrome

This congenital syndrome consists in hypothyroidism and severe musculoskeletal deformities in foals delivered after prolonged gestation (340–400 days) (Allen *et al.*, 1996). The syndrome was initially documented in northern Pacific regions but has now been described in central regions of the American continent (Vivrette *et al.*, 1984; McLaughlin *et al.*, 1986; Allen *et al.*, 1996; Gawrylash, 2004).

Foals with thyroid gland hyperplasia and musculoskeletal deformities appear weak and are unable to stand, with severe flexural deformities, prognathism and a short and silky haircoat (Fig. 2.3) (Vivrette *et al.*, 1984; Gawrylash, 2004). In these foals, T3 and T4 concentrations are normal to low and the thyroid gland does not respond to stimulation (McLaughlin *et al.*, 1986). The syndrome has no sex or breed predisposition and has been experimentally induced by *in utero* thyroidectomy (Allen *et al.*, 1998). The syndrome would be endemic and associated with low iodine intake and high nitrate intake during gestation (Allen *et al.*, 1996). Prognosis is poor and signs do not respond to thyroid hormone supplementation.

Non-thyroidal illness syndrome or euthyroid sick syndrome in foals

Systemically ill foals exhibit non-thyroidal illness syndrome (Pirrone *et al.*, 2013). Premature and systemically ill foals have lower T3 concentrations than healthy foals and premature foals have lower T4 concentrations than healthy and systemically ill foals (Breuhaus, 2014). TSH response to a TRH stimulation test in premature foals is higher than in healthy foals, suggesting an impaired thyroid gland responsiveness (Breuhaus, 2014). However, results of thyroid hormone testing in foals appears variable and might need to be interpreted thoughtfully before establishing a prognosis or implementing thyroid hormone supplementation (Furr *et al.*, 1992; Pirrone *et al.*, 2013).

Other diseases associated with hypothyroidism in foals

Ingestion of fescue infected with *Epichloë coenophiala* (previously known as *Acremonium coenophialum*) by pregnant mares has been associated with the delivery of small, weak, dysmature foals after prolonged gestation (Boosinger *et al.*, 1995). The endophytic fungus has some dopamine-agonist properties that inhibit TSH and lead to secondary hypothyroidism (Evans, 2002; Breuhaus, 2003). Clinical signs are similar to thyroid gland hyperplasia and musculoskeletal deformity syndrome (Fig. 2.4). Such foals have low T3 concentrations but normal T4 concentrations. Supportive care is indicated but thyroid hormone supplementation is not required. In non-pregnant animals, ingestion of endophyte-infected fescue did not impair thyroid function (Breuhaus, 2003).

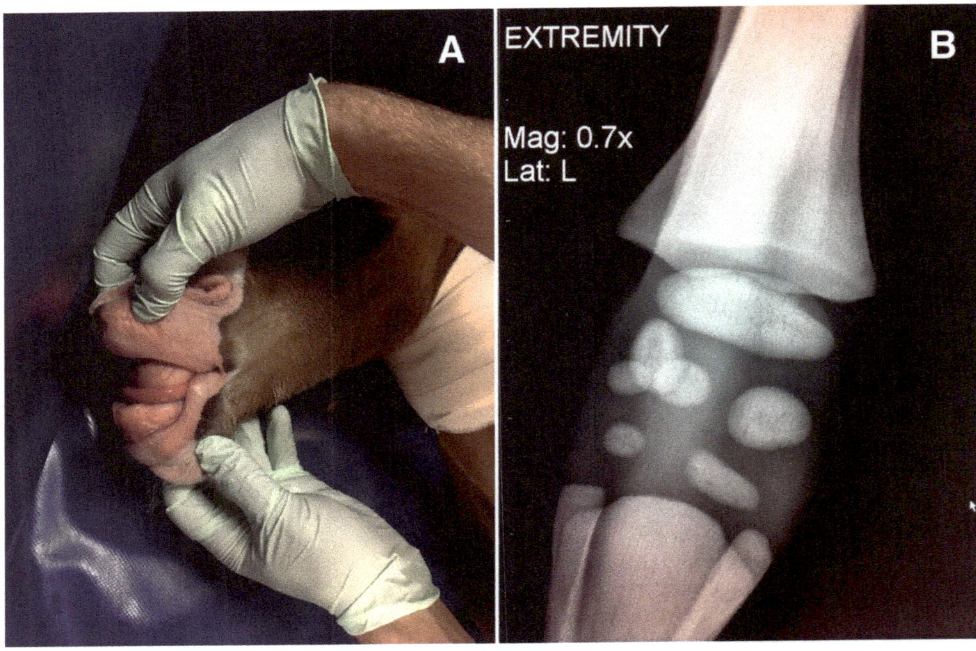

Fig. 2.3. Neonatal foal with congenital hypothyroidism (thyroidgland hyperplasia and musculoskeletal deformity syndrome). Note the prognathism(A) and the incomplete ossification of the left carpus (B) (courtesy Dr JenGold).

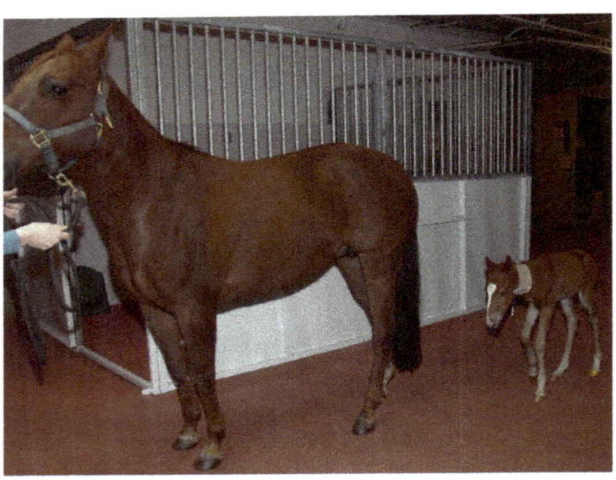

Fig. 2.4. Three-day-old foal born from a mare fed with fescue infected with Epichloë coenophiala (previously known as Acremonium coenophialum) after 13 months of gestation (Author's own photograph).

Hyperthyroidism

Thyroid tumours are common in older horses and their incidence increases after 17 years of age (Turk *et al.*, 1983; van der Velden and Meulenaar, 1986; Hovda *et al.*, 1990; Dalefield and Palmer, 1994; Ramirez *et al.*, 1998; Alberts *et al.*, 2000; Tan *et al.*, 2008). Most tumours are non-functional adenomas that do not progress into adenocarcinomas and do not impair the thyroid gland function (Dalefield and Palmer, 1994). In some rare cases, however, hyperthyroidism is reported (Alberts *et al.*, 2000; Tan *et al.*, 2008).

Clinical signs of hyperthyroidism include weight loss, tachycardia, tachypnoea, hyperactivity and polyphagia (Ramirez *et al.*, 1998; Alberts *et al.*, 2000). In one case, failure to completely shed haircoat and heat intolerance were reported (Tan *et al.*, 2008). Total T4 and T3 concentrations are normal to increased but concentrations of free fraction of T4 are markedly increased (Ramirez *et al.*, 1998; Tan *et al.*, 2008). Additional diagnostics such as a T3 suppression test, ultrasonography, scintigraphy and biopsy are recommended to confirm the diagnosis of hyperthyroidism.

Confirmed cases of hyperthyroidism can be managed by surgical thyroidectomy, PTU administration or a combination of both. Surgical unilateral thyroidectomy can be performed on standing horses with no major complication. Ultrasonographic examination before resection is recommended to limit risks of haemorrhage and damage to the recurrent laryngeal nerve (Elce *et al.*, 2003; Troillet *et al.*, 2016; Marcatili *et al.*, 2018). If bilateral thyroidectomy is required, thyroid hormone supplementation is recommended and should be adjusted to maintain thyroid hormone concentrations within reference intervals. If the tumour is large, prior treatment with PTU is also indicated. PTU can be administered orally, daily at 4–8 mg/kg for 2–4 weeks with biweekly reassessment (Tan *et al.*, 2008). If the tumour cannot be resected, PTU treatment can be continued until thyroid hormones are within the reference intervals. The PTU dose can then be reduced to maintain thyroid hormone concentrations within the reference intervals. As a precaution, a mask and gloves should be worn when administering PTU.

If the tumour is non-functional, resection might not be required as metastases are rare and the tumours progress slowly (Dalefield and Palmer, 1994). However, if the tumour is large and compressing the oesophagus or trachea, surgical hemithyroidectomy followed by thyroid hormone supplementation is indicated.

Other Disorders Associated, or Reportedly Associated, with Diseases of the Thyroid Gland

Tumours of the parafollicular cells (C-cells) are also common in older horses (Ueki *et al.*, 2004). These cells are responsible for calcitonin secretion; however, there is no report of a functional C-cell adenoma leading to increased calcitonin secretion (van der Velden and Meulenaar, 1986; Kuwamura *et al.*, 1998; Ueki *et al.*, 2004; Fortin *et al.*, 2018). Clinical signs are limited to the presence of a paralaryngeal mass (Lucke and Lane, 1984). Resection is only indicated if the mass is associated with dysphagia or dyspnoea.

Anhidrosis is a disease of unknown origin resulting in the inability to sweat (Stanley and Hillidge, 1982; Mayhew and Ferguson, 1987). The disease has been associated with thyroid dysfunction, but the evidence is weak as, in these horses, thyroid hormone concentrations are within normal limits and responses to TRH stimulation are also within normal limits (Breuhaus, 2009). Thyroid hormone supplementation has also shown disappointing results and does not seem to help horses with anhidrosis (Hillyer and Taylor, 1992; Breuhaus, 2009).

Obesity and laminitis were associated with thyroid dysfunction before EMS and insulin dysregulation (ID) were recognized as pathological entities (Frank *et al.*, 2010). The thyroid function of horses with these conditions is normal and thyroid supplementation is only used in cases of weight loss resistance (Frank *et al.*, 2008a, b).

Equine rhabdomyolysis was also considered to possibly be associated with thyroid dysfunction before polysaccharide storage myopathy was characterized (Harris *et al.*, 1992; Valberg *et al.*, 1999). Again, the evidence is weak and the pathophysiology unclear.

References

Abraham, G., Allersmeier, M., Schusser, G.F. and Ungemach, F.R. (2011) Serum thyroid hormone, insulin, glucose, triglycerides and protein concentrations in normal horses: association with topical dexamethasone usage. *The Veterinary Journal* 188(3), 307–312. DOI: 10.1016/j.tvjl.2010.05.033.

Alberts, M.K., McCann, J.P. and Woods, P.R. (2000) Hemithyroidectomy in a horse with confirmed hyperthyroidism. *Journal of the American Veterinary Medical Association* 217(7), 1009–1054. DOI: 10.2460/javma.2000.217.1051.

Allen, A.L., Townsend, H.G., Doige, C.E. and Fretz, P.B. (1996) A case-control study of the congenital hypothyroidism and dysmaturity syndrome of foals. *The Canadian Veterinary Journal* 37(349–51), 354–358.

Allen, A.L., Scott, W.M., Cook, S.J., Fretz, P.B. and Doige, C.E. (1997) Effects of delayed serum separation and long-term storage on the measurement of thyroid hormones in equine blood samples. *Veterinary Clinical Pathology* 26(1), 10–12. DOI: 10.1111/j.1939-165X.1997.tb00691.x.

Allen, A.L., Fretz, P.B., Card, C.E. and Doige, C.E. (1998) The effects of partial thyroidectomy on the development of the equine fetus. *Equine Veterinary Journal* 30(1), 53–59. DOI: 10.1111/j.2042-3306.1998.tb04088.x.

Beech, J. (1987) Evaluation of thyroid, adrenal, and pituitary function. *Veterinary Clinics of North America: Equine Practice* 3(3), 649–660. DOI: 10.1016/S0749-0739(17)30669-7.

Beech, J. and Garcia, M. (1985) Hormonal response to thyrotropin-releasing hormone in healthy horses and in horses with pituitary adenoma. *American Journal of Veterinary Research* 46(9), 1941–1943.

Berger, M., Reymond, M., Shenkin, A., Rey, F., Wardle, C. *et al.* (2001) Influence of selenium supplements on the post-traumatic alterations of the thyroid axis: a placebo-controlled trial. *Intensive Care Medicine* 27(1), 91–100. DOI: 10.1007/s001340000757.

Bertin, F.R., Eichstadt Forsythe, L. and Kritchevsky, J.E. (2019) Effects of high doses of levothyroxine sodium on serum concentrations of triiodothyronine and thyroxine in horses. *American Journal of Veterinary Research* 80(6), 565–571. DOI: 10.2460/ajvr.80.6.565.

Boosinger, T.R., Brendemuehl, J.P., Bransby, D.L., Wright, J.C., Kemppainen, R.J. *et al.* (1995) Prolonged gestation, decreased triiodothyronine concentration, and thyroid gland histomorphologic features in newborn foals of mares grazing Acremonion coenophialum-infected fescue. *American Journal of Veterinary Research* 56(1), 66–69.

Breuhaus, B.A. (2002) Thyroid-stimulating hormone in adult euthyroid and hypothyroid horses. *Journal of Veterinary Internal Medicine* 16(1), 109–115. DOI: 10.1111/j.1939-1676.2002.tb01615.x.

Breuhaus, B.A. (2003) Thyroid function in mature horses ingesting endophyte-infected fescue seed. *Journal of the American Veterinary Medical Association* 223(3), 340–345. DOI: 10.2460/javma.2003.223.340.

Breuhaus, B.A. (2009) Thyroid function in anhidrotic horses. *Journal of Veterinary Internal Medicine* 23(1), 168–173. DOI: 10.1111/j.1939-1676.2008.0217.x.

Breuhaus, B.A. (2011) Disorders of the equine thyroid gland. *Veterinary Clinics of North America: Equine Practice* 27(1), 115–128. DOI: 10.1016/j.cveq.2010.12.002.

Breuhaus, B.A. (2014) Thyroid function and dysfunction in term and premature equine neonates. *Journal of Veterinary Internal Medicine* 28(4), 1301–1309. DOI: 10.1111/jvim.12382.

Breuhaus, B.A., Refsal, K.R. and Beyerlein, S.L. (2006) Measurement of free thyroxine concentration in horses by equilibrium dialysis. *Journal of Veterinary Internal Medicine* 20(2), 371–376. DOI: 10.1111/j.1939-1676.2006.tb02870.x.

Brinkmann, L., Gerken, M., Hambly, C., Speakman, J.R. and Riek, A. (2016) Thyroid hormones correlate with field metabolic rate in ponies, *Equus ferus caballus*. *The Journal of Experimental Biology* 219(16), 2559–2566. DOI: 10.1242/jeb.138784.

Cheng, S.-Y., Leonard, J.L. and Davis, P.J. (2010) Molecular aspects of thyroid hormone actions. *Endocrine Reviews* 31(2), 139–170. DOI: 10.1210/er.2009-0007.

Christensen, R.A., Malinowski, K., Massenzio, A.M., Hafs, H.D. and Scanes, C.G. (1997) Acute effects of short-term feed deprivation and refeeding on circulating concentrations of metabolites, insulin-like growth factor I, insulin-like growth factor binding proteins, somatotropin, and thyroid hormones in adult geldings. *Journal of Animal Science* 75(5), 1351–1358. DOI: 10.2527/1997.7551351x.

Dalefield, R.R. and Palmer, D.N. (1994) The frequent occurrence of thyroid tumours in aged horses. *Journal of Comparative Pathology* 110(1), 57–64. DOI: 10.1016/S0021-9975(08)80270-8.

Daniel, G.B. and Neelis, D.A. (2014) Thyroid scintigraphy in veterinary medicine. *Seminars in Nuclear Medicine* 44(1), 24–34. DOI: 10.1053/j.semnuclmed.2013.08.007.

Davies, S., Barber, D.O.N., Crisman, M., Tan, R., Larson, M. *et al.* (2010) Quantitative pertechnetate thyroid scintigraphy and the ultrasonographic appearance of the thyroid gland in clinically normal horses. *Veterinary Radiology & Ultrasound* 51(6), 674–680. DOI: 10.1111/j.1740-8261.2010.01721.x.

De Groot, L.J. (1999) Dangerous dogmas in medicine: the nonthyroidal illness syndrome. *The Journal of Clinical Endocrinology & Metabolism* 84(1), 151–164. DOI: 10.1210/jcem.84.1.5364.

Doige, C.E. and McLaughlin, B.G. (1981) Hyperplastic goitre in newborn foals in Western Canada. *The Canadian Veterinary Journal* 22(2), 42–45.

Drew, B., Barber, W. and Williams, D. (1975) The effect of excess dietary iodine on pregnant mares and foals. *Veterinary Record* 97(5), 93–95. DOI: 10.1136/vr.97.5.93.

Duckett, W.M., Manning, J.P. and Weston, P.G. (1989) Thyroid hormone periodicity in healthy adult geldings. *Equine Veterinary Journal* 21(2), 123–125. DOI: 10.1111/j.2042-3306.1989.tb02115.x.

Elce, Y.A., Ross, M.W., Davidson, E.J. and Tulleners, E.P. (2003) Unilateral thyroidectomy in 6 horses. *Veterinary Surgery* 32(2), 187–190. DOI: 10.1053/jvet.2003.50017.

Eroksuz, H., Eroksuz, Y., Ozer, H., Ceribasi, A.O., Yaman, I. *et al.* (2004) Equine goiter associated with excess dietary iodine. *Veterinary and Human Toxicology* 46(3), 147–149.

Evans, T.J. (2002) Endocrine alterations associated with ergopeptine alkaloid exposure during equine pregnancy. *Veterinary Clinics of North America: Equine Practice* 18(2), 371–378 DOI: 10.1016/S0749-0739(02)00019-6.

Fazio, E., Medica, P., Cravana, C., Bruschetta, G. and Ferlazzo, A. (2016a) Seasonal thyroid and lipid profiles in Thoroughbred pregnant and nonpregnant mares (*Equus caballus*). *Theriogenology* 85(9), 1582–1589. DOI: 10.1016/j.theriogenology.2016.01.017.

Fazio, E., Medica, P., Trifiletti, C. and Ferlazzo, A. (2016b) The outcome of the first stages of pregnancy on mares' bloodstream thyroid hormones. *Theriogenology* 86(4), 1036–1041. DOI: 10.1016/j.theriogenology.2016.03.032.

Fazio, E., Medica, P., Cravana, C. and Ferlazzo, A. (2017) Total and free iodothyronine changes in response to transport of Equidae (Equus asinus and Equus caballus). *Veterinaria Italiana* 53(1), 55–60. DOI: 10.12834/VetIt.55.155.2.

Flisińska-Bojanowska, A., Komosa, M. and Gill, J. (1991) Influence of pregnancy on diurnal and seasonal changes in cortisol, T3 and T4 levels in the mare blood serum. *Comparative Biochemistry and Physiology Part A: Physiology* 98(1), 23–30. DOI: 10.1016/0300-9629(91)90571-S.

Fortin, J.S., Royal, A.B. and Kuroki, K. (2018) Concurrent thoracic mesothelioma and thyroid C-cell adenoma with amyloid deposition in an aged horse. *Veterinary Medicine and Science* 4(1), 63–70. DOI: 10.1002/vms3.87.

Frank, N., Sojka, J. and Messer, N.T. (2002) Equine thyroid dysfunction. *Veterinary Clinics of North America: Equine Practice* 18(2), 305–319. DOI: 10.1016/S0749-0739(02)00007-X.

Frank, N., Sojka, J.E., Patterson, B.W., Wood, K.V., Bonham, C.C. *et al.* (2003) Effect of hypothyroidism on kinetics of metabolism of very-low-density lipoprotein in mares. *American Journal of Veterinary Research* 64(8), 1052–1058. DOI: 10.2460/ajvr.2003.64.1052.

Frank, N., Sojka, J.E. and Latour, M.A. (2004) Effect of hypothyroidism on the blood lipid response to higher dietary fat intake in mares. *Journal of Animal Science* 82(9), 2640–2646. DOI: 10.2527/2004.8292640x.

Frank, N., Buchanan, B.R. and Elliott, S.B. (2008a) Effects of long-term oral administration of levothyroxine sodium on serum thyroid hormone concentrations, clinicopathologic variables, and echocardiographic measurements in healthy adult horses. *American Journal of Veterinary Research* 69(1), 68–75. DOI: 10.2460/ajvr.69.1.68.

Frank, N., Elliott, S.B. and Boston, R.C. (2008b) Effects of long-term oral administration of levothyroxine sodium on glucose dynamics in healthy adult horses. *American Journal of Veterinary Research* 69(1), 76–81. DOI: 10.2460/ajvr.69.1.76.

Frank, N., Geor, R.J., Bailey, S.R., Durham, A.E. and Johnson, P. (2010) Equine metabolic syndrome. *Journal of Veterinary Internal Medicine* 24(3), 467–475. DOI: 10.1111/j.1939-1676.2010.0503.x.

Furr, M.O., Murray, M.J. and Ferguson, D.C. (1992) The effects of stress on gastric ulceration, T3, T4, reverse T3 and cortisol in neonatal foals. *Equine Veterinary Journal* 24(1), 37–40. DOI: 10.1111/j.2042-3306.1992.tb02776.x.

Gawrylash, S.K. (2004) Thyroid hyperplasia and musculoskeletal deformity in a standardbred filly in Ontario. *The Canadian Veterinary Journal* 45(5), 424–426.

Gomberg-Maitland, M. and Frishman, W.H. (1998) Thyroid hormone and cardiovascular disease. *American Heart Journal* 135(2), 187–196. DOI: 10.1016/S0002-8703(98)70081-X.

Gonzalez, O., Gonzalez, E.M.A., Sanchez, C., Pinto, J., Gonzalez, I. *et al.* (1998) Effect of exercise on erythrocyte β-adrenergic receptors and plasma concentrations of catecholamines and thyroid hormones in thoroughbred horses. *Equine Veterinary Journal* 30(1), 72–78. DOI: 10.1111/j.2042-3306.1998.tb04091.x.

Graves, E.A., Schott, H.C., Marteniuk, J.V., Refsal, K.R. and Nachreiner, R.F. (2006) Thyroid hormone responses to endurance exercise. *Equine Veterinary Journal* 38(36), 32–36. DOI: 10.1111/j.2042-3306.2006.tb05509.x.

Greenspan, S.L., Klibanski, A., Schoenfeld, D. and Ridgway, E.C. (1986) Pulsatile secretion of thyrotropin in man. *The Journal of Clinical Endocrinology & Metabolism* 63(3), 661–668. DOI: 10.1210/jcem-63-3-661.

Gutierrez, C.V., Riddle, W.T. and Bramlage, L.R. (2002) Serum thyroxine concentrations and pregnancy rates 15 to 16 days after ovulation in broodmares. *Journal of the American Veterinary Medical Association* 220(1), 64–66. DOI: 10.2460/javma.2002.220.64.

Harris, P., Marlin, D. and Gray, J. (1992) Equine thyroid function tests: a preliminary investigation. *British Veterinary Journal* 148(1), 71–80. DOI: 10.1016/0007-1935(92)90069-D.

Held, J.P. and Oliver, J.W. (1984) A sampling protocol for the thyrotropin-stimulation test in the horse. *Journal of the American Veterinary Medical Association* 184(3), 326–327.

Held, J.P., Patton, C.S., Toal, R.L. and Geiser, D.R. (1985) Work intolerance in a horse with thyroid carcinoma. *Journal of the American Veterinary Medical Association* 187(10), 1044–1045

Hilderbran, A.C., Breuhaus, B.A. and Refsal, K.R. (2014) Nonthyroidal illness syndrome in adult horses. *Journal of Veterinary Internal Medicine* 28(2), 609–617. DOI: 10.1111/jvim.12274.

Hillidge, C.J., Sanecki, R.K. and Theodorakis, M.C. (1982) Thyroid carcinoma in a horse. *Journal of the American Veterinary Medical Association* 181(7), 711–714.

Hillyer, M.H. and Taylor, F.G.R. (1992) Cutaneous manifestations of suspected hypothyroidism in a horse. *Equine Veterinary Education* 4(3), 116–118. DOI: 10.1111/j.2042-3292.1992.tb01590.x.

Hovda, L.R., Shaftoe, S., Rose, M.L. and Clemmons, L.H. (1990) Mediastinal squamous cell carcinoma and thyroid carcinoma in an aged horse. *Journal of the American Veterinary Medical Association* 197(9), 1187–1189.

Huszenicza, G., Nagy, P., Juhász, J., Kóródi, P., Kulcsár, M. *et al.* (2000) Relationship between thyroid function and seasonal reproductive activity in mares. *Journal of Reproduction and Fertility. Supplement* (56), 163–172.

Irvine, C.H.G. (1984) Hypothyroidism in the foal. *Equine Veterinary Journal* 16(4), 302–306. DOI: 10.1111/j.2042-3306.1984.tb01932.x.

Irvine, C.H. and Evans, M.J. (1975) Postnatal changes in total and free thyroxine and triiodothyronine in foal serum. *Journal of Reproduction and Fertility. Supplement* (23), 709–715.

Johnson, P.J., Messer, N.T., Ganjam, V.K., Thompson, D.L., Refsal, K.R. *et al.* (2003) Effects of propylthiouracil and bromocryptine on serum concentrations of thyrotrophin and thyroid hormones in normal female horses. *Equine Veterinary Journal* 35(3), 296–301. DOI: 10.2746/042516403776148309.

Kaptein, E.M., Weiner, J.M., Robinson, W.J., Wheeler, W.S. and Nicoloff, J.T. (1982) Relationship of altered thyroid hormone indices to survival in nonthyroidal illnesses. *Clinical Endocrinology* 16(6), 565–574. DOI: 10.1111/j.1365-2265.1982.tb03173.x.

Kaptein, E.M., Hays, M.T. and Ferguson, D.C. (1994) Thyroid hormone metabolism. A comparative evaluation. *The Veterinary Clinics of North America. Small Animal Practice* 24(3), 431–466. DOI: 10.1016/s0195-5616(94)50051-2.

Kuwamura, M., Shirota, A., Yamate, J., Kotani, T., Ohashi, F. *et al.* (1998) C-cell adenoma containing variously sized thyroid follicles in a horse. *Journal of Veterinary Medical Science* 60(3), 387–389. DOI: 10.1292/jvms.60.387.

Li, H., Yuan, X., Liu, L., Zhou, J., Li, C. *et al.* (2014) Clinical evaluation of various thyroid hormones on thyroid function. *International Journal of Endocrinology* 2014(2), 618572–5. DOI: 10.1155/2014/618572.

Lothrop, C.D. and Nolan, H.L. (1986) Equine thyroid function assessment with the thyrotropin-releasing hormone response test. *American Journal of Veterinary Research* 47(4), 942–944.

Lowe, J.E., Baldwin, B.H., Foote, R.H., Hillman, R.B. and Kallfelz, F.A. (1974) Equine hypothyroidism: the long term effects of thyroidectomy on metabolism and growth in mares and stallions. *The Cornell Veterinarian* 64(2), 276–295.

Lowe, J.E., Foote, R.H., Baldwin, B.H., Hillman, R.B. and Kallfelz, F.A. (1987) Reproductive patterns in cyclic and pregnant thyroidectomized mares. *Journal of Reproduction and Fertility. Supplement* 35, 281–288.

Lucke, V.M. and Lane, J.G. (1984) C-cell tumours of the thyroid in the horse. *Equine Veterinary Journal* 16(1), 28–30. DOI: 10.1111/j.2042-3306.1984.tb01843.x.

Malinowski, K., Christensen, R.A., Hafs, H.D. and Scanes, C.G. (1996) Age and breed differences in thyroid hormones, insulin-like growth factor (IGF)-I and IGF binding proteins in female horses. *Journal of Animal Science* 74(8), 1936–1942. DOI: 10.2527/1996.7481936x.

Marcatili, M., Voss, S.J. and Pollock, P.J. (2018) Standing thyroidectomy in 10 horses. *Veterinary Surgery* 47(1), 86–92. DOI: 10.1111/vsu.12744.

Mayhew, I.G. and Ferguson, H.O. (1987) Clinical, clinicopathologic, and epidemiologic features of anhidrosis in central Florida thoroughbred horses. *Journal of Veterinary Internal Medicine* 1(3), 136–141. DOI: 10.1111/j.1939-1676.1987.tb02001.x.

McLaughlin, B.G., Doige, C.E. and McLaughlin, P.S. (1986) Thyroid hormone levels in foals with congenital musculoskeletal lesions. *The Canadian Veterinary Journal* 27(7), 264–267.

Meredith, T.B. and Dobrinski, I. (2004) Thyroid function and pregnancy status in broodmares. *Journal of the American Veterinary Medical Association* 224(6), 892–894. DOI: 10.2460/javma.2004.224.892.

Messer, N.T., Ganjam, V.K., Nachreiner, R.F. and Krause, G.F. (1995a) Effect of dexamethasone administration on serum thyroid hormone concentrations in clinically normal horses. *Journal of the American Veterinary Medical Association* 206(1), 63–66.

Messer, N.T., Johnson, P.J., Refsal, K.R., Nachreiner, R.F., Ganjam, V.K. *et al.* (1995b) Effect of food deprivation on baseline iodothyronine and cortisol concentrations in healthy, adult horses. *American Journal of Veterinary Research* 56(1), 116–121.

Morris, D.D. and Garcia, M. (1983) Thyroid-stimulating hormone: response test in healthy horses, and effect of phenylbutazone on equine thyroid hormones. *American Journal of Veterinary Research* 44(3), 503–507.

Morris, D.D. and Garcia, M.C. (1985) Effects of phenylbutazone and anabolic steroids on adrenal and thyroid gland function tests in healthy horses. *American Journal of Veterinary Research* 46(2), 359–364.

Murray, M.J. (1990) Hypothyroidism and respiratory insufficiency in a neonatal foal. *Journal of the American Veterinary Medical Association* 197(12), 1635–1638.

Murray, M.J. and Luba, N.K. (1993) Plasma gastrin and somatostatin, and serum thyroxine (T4), triiodothyronine (T3), reverse triiodothyronine (rT3) and cortisol concentrations in foals from birth to 28 days of age. *Equine Veterinary Journal* 25(3), 237–239. DOI: 10.1111/j.2042-3306.1993.tb02951.x.

Osame, S. and Ichijo, S. (1994) Clinicopathological observations on thoroughbred foals with enlarged thyroid gland. *The Journal of Veterinary Medical Science* 56(4), 771–772. DOI: 10.1292/jvms.56.771.

Parmentier, M., Libert, F., Maenhaut, C., Lefort, A., Gerard, C. *et al.* (1989) Molecular cloning of the thyrotropin receptor. *Science* 246(4937), 1620–1622. DOI: 10.1126/science.2556796.

Perillo, A., Passantino, G., Passantino, L., Cianciotta, A., Mastrosimini, A.M. *et al.* (2005) First observation of an Hashimoto thyroiditis-like disease in horses from eastern Europe: histopathological and immunological findings. *Immunopharmacology and Immunotoxicology* 27(2), 241–253. DOI: 10.1081/IPH-200067743.

Pirrone, A., Panzani, S., Govoni, N., Castagnetti, C. and Veronesi, M.C. (2013) Thyroid hormone concentrations in foals affected by perinatal asphyxia syndrome. *Theriogenology* 80(6), 624–629. DOI: 10.1016/j.theriogenology.2013.06.003.

Ramirez, S., Wolfsheimer, K.J., Moore, R.M., Mora, F., Bueno, A.C. *et al.* (1997) Duration of effects of phenylbutazone on serum total thyroxine and free thyroxine concentrations in horses. *Journal of Veterinary Internal Medicine* 11(6), 371–374. DOI: 10.1111/j.1939-1676.1997.tb00483.x.

Ramirez, S., McClure, J.J., Moore, R.M., Wolfsheimer, K.J., Gaunt, S.D. *et al.* (1998) Hyperthyroidism associated with a thyroid adenocarcinoma in a 21-year-old gelding. *Journal of Veterinary Internal Medicine* 12(6), 475–477. DOI: 10.1111/j.1939-1676.1998.tb02153.x.

Rothschild, C.M., Hines, M.T., Breuhaus, B., Gay, J. and Sellon, D.C. (2004) Effects of trimethoprim-sulfadiazine on thyroid function of horses. *Journal of Veterinary Internal Medicine* 18(3), 370–373. DOI: 10.1111/j.1939-1676.2004.tb02563.x.

Schwarz, B.C., Sallmutter, T. and Nell, B. (2008) Keratoconjunctivitis sicca attributable to parasympathetic facial nerve dysfunction associated with hypothyroidism in a horse. *Journal of the American Veterinary Medical Association* 233(11), 1761–1766. DOI: 10.2460/javma.233.11.1761.

Singh, A.K., Jiang, Y., White, T. and Spassova, D. (1997) Validation of nonradioactive chemiluminescent immunoassay methods for the analysis of thyroxine and cortisol in blood samples obtained from dogs, cats, and horses. *Journal of Veterinary Diagnostic Investigation* 9(3), 261–268. DOI: 10.1177/104063879700900307.

Slag, M.F., Morley, J.E., Elson, M.K., Crowson, T.W., Nuttall, F.Q. (1981) Hypothyroxinemia in critically ill patients as a predictor of high mortality. *JAMA: The Journal of the American Medical Association* 245(1), 43–45. DOI: 10.1001/jama.1981.03310260021020.

Sojka, J.E., Johnson, M.A. and Bottoms, G.D. (1993) Serum triiodothyronine, total thyroxine, and free thyroxine concentrations in horses. *American Journal of Veterinary Research* 54(1), 52–55.

Sommardahl, C.S., Frank, N., Elliott, S.B., Webb, L.L., Refsal, K.R. *et al.* (2005) Effects of oral administration of levothyroxine sodium on serum concentrations of thyroid gland hormones and responses to injections of thyrotropin-releasing hormone in healthy adult mares. *American Journal of Veterinary Research* 66(6), 1025–1031. DOI: 10.2460/ajvr.2005.66.1025.

Stanley, O. and Hillidge, C.J. (1982) Alopecia associated with hypothyroidism in a horse. *Equine Veterinary Journal* 14(2), 165–167. DOI: 10.1111/j.2042-3306.1982.tb02378.x.

Tan, R.H.H., Davies, S.E., Crisman, M.V., Coyle, L. and Daniel, G.B. (2008) Propylthiouracil for treatment of hyperthyroidism in a horse. *Journal of Veterinary Internal Medicine* 22(5), 1253–1258. DOI: 10.1111/j.1939-1676.2008.0169.x.

Tangyuenyong, S., Nambo, Y., Nagaoka, K., Tanaka, T. and Watanabe, G. (2017) Sensitive radioimmunoassay of total thyroxine (T4) in horses using a simple extraction method. *Journal of Veterinary Medical Science* 79(7), 1294–1300. DOI: 10.1292/jvms.17-0133.

Taylor, T., Wondisford, F.E., Blaine, T. and Weintraub, B.D. (1990) The paraventricular nucleus of the hypothalamus has a major role in thyroid hormone feedback regulation of thyrotropin synthesis and secretion. *Endocrinology* 126(1), 317–324. DOI: 10.1210/endo-126-1-317.

Thompson, F.N., Caudle, A.B., Kemppainen, R.J., Nett, T.M., Brown, J. *et al.* (1986) Thyroidal and prolactin secretion in agalactic mares. *Theriogenology* 25(4), 575–580. DOI: 10.1016/0093-691X(86)90141-X.

Thompson, J.C., Ellison, R.S. and Kirk, J. (1997) Serum thyroid hormone concentrations in New Zealand horses. *New Zealand Veterinary Journal* 45(1), 11–14. DOI: 10.1080/00480169.1997.35981.

Troillet, A., Böttcher, D., Brehm, W. and Scharner, D. (2016) Retrospective evaluation of hemithyroidectomy in 14 horses. *Veterinary Surgery* 45(7), 949–954. DOI: 10.1111/vsu.12540.

Turk, J.R., Nakata, Y.J., Leathers, C.W. and Gallina, A.M. (1983) Ultimobranchial adenoma of the thyroid gland in a horse. *Veterinary Pathology* 20(1), 114–117. DOI: 10.1177/030098588302000113.

Ueki, H., Kowatari, Y., Oyamada, T., Oikawa, M. and Yoshikawa, H. (2004) Non-functional C-cell adenoma in aged horses. *Journal of Comparative Pathology* 131(2–3), 157–165. DOI: 10.1016/j.jcpa.2004.03.001.

Valberg, S.J., Mickelson, J.R., Gallant, E.M., Macleay, J.M., Lentz, L. *et al.* (1999) Exertional rhabdomyolysis in quarter horses and thoroughbreds: one syndrome, multiple aetiologies. *Equine Veterinary Journal* 31(S30), 533–538. DOI: 10.1111/j.2042-3306.1999.tb05279.x.

Vale, C., Neves, J.S., von Hafe, M., Borges-Canha, M. and Leite-Moreira, A. (2019) The role of thyroid hormones in heart failure. *Cardiovascular Drugs and Therapy* 33(2), 179–188. DOI: 10.1007/s10557-019-06870-4.

van der Velden, M.A. and Meulenaar, H. (1986) Medullary thyroid carcinoma in a horse. *Veterinary Pathology* 23(5), 622–624. DOI: 10.1177/030098588602300512.

Vischer, C.M., Foreman, J.H., Constable, P.D., Benson, G.J., Kline, K.H. *et al.* (1999) Hemodynamic effects of thyroidectomy in sedentary horses. *American Journal of Veterinary Research* 60(1), 14–21.

Vivrette, S.L., Reimers, T.J. and Krock, L. (1984) Skeletal disease in a hypothyroid foal. *The Cornell Veterinarian* 74(4), 373–386.

Warner, M.H. and Beckett, G.J. (2010) Mechanisms behind the non-thyroidal illness syndrome: an update. *Journal of Endocrinology* 205(1), 1–13. DOI: 10.1677/JOE-09-0412.

3 Calcium Regulation and Diseases of the Parathyroid Gland

Calcium is required for many physiological functions such as muscle contraction, enzyme activation, cell division and migration, blood coagulation and hormone secretion (Toribio, 2011). In addition to a functional role, calcium also has a structural role as about 99% of total calcium is found in the skeleton. The remaining calcium is distributed between cell membranes (90%, including cellular plasma membrane, endoplasmic reticulum, mitochondria) and extracellular fluid (10%, including plasma). Circulating calcium is either found as ionized (or free calcium) representing about 55% of circulating calcium, bound to proteins (mainly albumin) representing about 40% of circulating plasma or complexed with anions (calcium citrate, calcium bicarbonate, calcium lactate, calcium phosphate) representing about 5% of circulating calcium (Lopez *et al.*, 2006). The balance between ionized, bound and complexed calcium varies with plasma protein concentration and blood pH: a lower pH decreases calcium binding to protein and increases the ionized fraction of circulating calcium.

Calcium metabolism is tied to phosphorous metabolism and is tightly regulated by parathyroid hormone, vitamin D and calcitonin. As a divalent cation, calcium is poorly absorbed through the gastrointestinal tract, whereas phosphorous, as an anion, passes easily through the enterocyte (Schryver *et al.*, 1970, 1974). Therefore, facilitation of gastrointestinal calcium absorption is required to ensure constant blood calcium concentrations (Wilkens *et al.*, 2017).

Parathyroid Physiology and Calcium Regulation

Parathyroid hormone

The parathyroid hormone is the main hormone involved in calcium and phosphorus homeostasis. The hormone is secreted by the chief cells of the parathyroid gland in response to a decrease in circulating calcium as detected by calcium-sensing receptors (Aguilera-Tejero *et al.*, 1998, 2001; Toribio *et al.*, 2003a). The complete parathyroid hormone once released in the circulation contains 84 amino acids and is rapidly removed within minutes by the liver (about 75%) and the kidneys (about 25%); however, smaller compounds of 34 amino acids that exhibit full parathyroid hormone activity stay in the circulation for hours (Martin *et al.*, 1979). Therefore, some of the observed parathyroid hormone activity is caused by these smaller compounds which can complicate parathyroid hormone measurements. Parathyroid hormone secretion is mainly triggered by hypocalcaemia. Horses have quite a high calcium set-point for parathyroid hormone secretion (around 1.37 mmol/l) indicating that they maintain circulating calcium at high concentrations and that even slight hypocalcaemia increases parathyroid hormone secretion (Toribio *et al.*, 2003a, c). It is clinically relevant to note, however, that release of parathyroid hormone and activation of the parathyroid hormone receptor are magnesium dependent; therefore, hypomagnesaemia inhibits both parathyroid hormone release and activity, even in the presence of hypocalcaemia (Toribio, 2011). In many species, including humans, the parathyroid gland is well defined and is located immediately behind the thyroid gland. In horses, however, the parathyroid tissue is quite diffuse and often difficult to localize. Several studies have reported failure of localizing the parathyroid gland or variability in anatomic location from the thyroid gland area to the thoracic inlet (Wong *et al.*, 2004; Gorenberg *et al.*, 2020). In cases of chronic hypocalcaemia, such as pregnancy, lactation or poor diet, the parathyroid gland can become hyperplastic to maintain parathyroid hormone production.

The main effects of the parathyroid hormone are to increase circulating calcium (hypercalcaemic effect) and decrease circulating phosphorus (hypophosphataemic effect). The increases in circulating calcium associated with parathyroid hormone

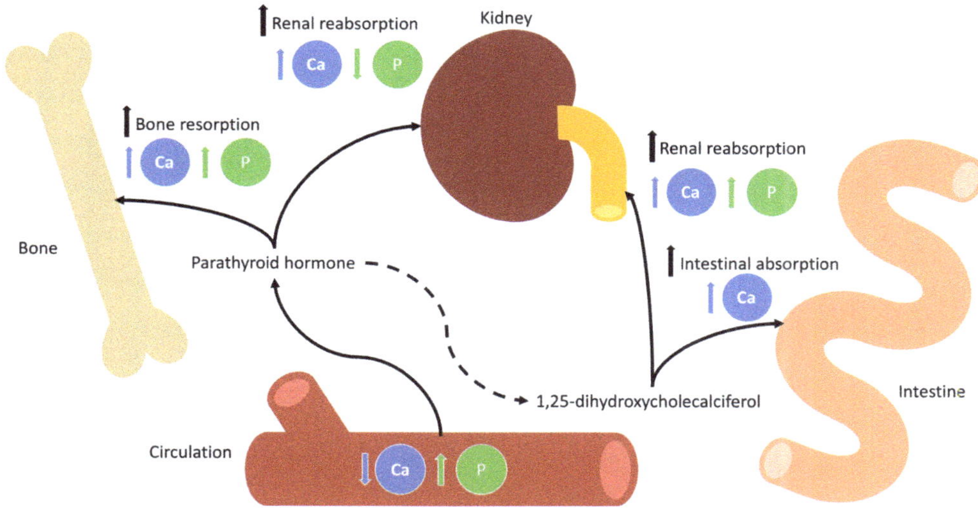

Fig. 3.1. Calcium regulation: mechanisms involved in the resolution of hypocalcaemia (where Ca is calcium and P is phosphorous) (Author's own diagram).

are caused by two direct mechanisms: bone resorption mobilizing both calcium and phosphorous from the bone to the circulation and renal reabsorption reducing the amount of calcium excreted by the kidneys in the urine (Fig. 3.1). Along with the second mechanism, parathyroid hormone also increases phosphorous excretion by the kidneys that overrides the mobilization of phosphorus from bone resorption. A third, indirect, mechanism by which parathyroid hormone increases circulating blood calcium is by promoting the conversion of vitamin D_3 into 1,25-dihydroxycholecalciferol in the kidney. This mechanism is regulated by both phosphorous and 1,25-dihydroxycholecalciferol, as hyperphosphataemia directly inhibits the conversion of vitamin D_3 into 1,25-dihydroxycholecalciferol and 1,25-dihydroxycholecalciferol inhibits the secretion of parathyroid hormone.

1,25-dihydroxycholecalciferol

Vitamin D is a lipophilic vitamin that, after a succession of enzymatic transformations, is converted into 1,25-dihydroxycholecalciferol, a pseudo hormone that increases transcellular transport of calcium in the intestinal tract and in the kidneys (Fig. 3.1). This transport is facilitated by calcium-binding proteins expressed at the border of epithelial cells that increase the rate of calcium absorption (Friedman and Gesek, 1995; Wasserman and Fullmer, 1995). The hypercalcaemic effect of 1,25-dihydroxycholecalciferol is prolonged as the calcium-binding proteins have a half-life of a few weeks. To a much lesser extent, 1,25-dihydroxycholecalciferol also increases phosphorus and magnesium absorption from the intestinal tract and from the kidney (hyperphosphataemic effect and hypermagnesaemic effect) (Ritchie *et al.*, 2001; Toribio, 2011). Finally, 1,25-dihydroxycholecalciferol, similar to parathyroid hormone, is also involved in bone resorption mobilizing calcium and phosphorus from the bone to the circulation.

Calcitonin

Hypercalcaemia triggers the secretion of calcitonin, a peptide released by the parafollicular C-cells of the thyroid gland. Like hypocalcaemia, hypercalcaemia is detected by calcium-sensing receptors (Garrett *et al.*, 1995). Calcitonin decreases circulating calcium concentration by suppressing bone resorption and by increasing urinary calcium excretion (Fig. 3.2). Although equine C-cells are highly responsive to hypercalcaemia, the role of calcitonin in horses is poorly understood except in the prevention of bone resorption during lactation (Woodrow *et al.*, 2006; Rourke *et al.*, 2010). Of interest, gastrin is another trigger for calcitonin secretion and

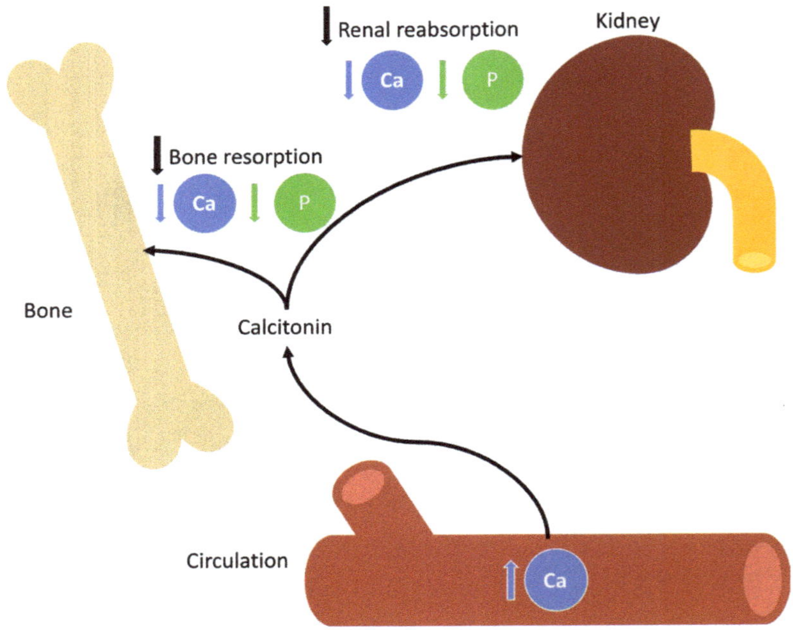

Fig. 3.2. Calcium regulation: mechanisms involved in the resolution of hypercalcaemia (where Ca is calcium and P is phosphorous) (Author's own diagram).

post-prandial increases in calcitonin have been documented.

Other regulators of calcium metabolism

In addition to circadian and circannual rhythms of parathyroid hormone and 1,25-dihydroxycholecalciferol, that can have a significant effect on calcium regulation in horses at high latitudes (further from the equator), other factors have been shown to impact calcium metabolism (Azarpeykan *et al.*, 2016a, b).

The parathyroid hormone-related peptide (PTHrP) shares the first 13 amino acids of its sequence with the parathyroid hormone and can act through the same receptors. This peptide can be produced by a range of tissue and has a series of functions (Wysolmerski and Stewart, 1998; Mundy and Guise, 1999). In healthy adult horses, the PTHrP has a limited effect on calcium regulation with restricted promotion of bone resorption and inhibition of renal calcium excretion; however, excessive PTHrP secretion is reported in cases of tumours (humoral hypercalcaemia of malignancy) (McCoy and Beasley, 1986; Suva *et al.*, 1987; Karcher *et al.*, 1990; Rosol *et al.*, 1994; Semevolos *et al.*, 2002; Barton *et al.*, 2004).

The fibroblast growth factor 23 (FGF-23) klotho axis plays a central function in regulation of calcium, phosphorous, parathyroid hormone and 1,25-dihydroxycholecalciferol, and is considered as the main phosphorous-regulating hormone (Berndt and Kumar, 2007; Kuro-o, 2010, 2013). FGF-23 is secreted by osteocytes and osteoblasts and enhances renal excretion of phosphorous (Schiavi and Kumar, 2004; Berndt and Kumar, 2007; Lanske and Razzaque, 2014). Klotho acts as a coreceptor for FGF-23 and enhances renal excretion of phosphorous but also decreases parathyroid hormone and 1,25-dihydroxycholecalciferol secretion (Hu *et al.*, 2012; Kuro-o, 2013). Not much is known about the clinical relevance of this axis in horses; however, it is suspected that FGF-23–klotho axis dysregulation could contribute to mineral metabolism disorders in critically ill foals (Kamr *et al.*, 2018).

Hyperparathyroidism

The diagnosis of hyperparathyroidism is usually based on high parathyroid hormone concentrations associated with sustained hypercalcaemia (Toribio, 2011). In addition to primary, secondary and pseudo hyperparathyroidism, hypercalcaemia can result from chronic renal failure, plant intoxication (hypervitaminoses D), calcinosis and neonatal hypercalcaemia. Primary hyperparathyroidism is relatively rare in horses and should be suspected in cases of persistent hypercalcaemia (Roussel and Thatcher, 1987; Cottle *et al.*, 2016). Secondary hyperparathyroidism of nutritional origin is a well-described disease of horses in specific geographical locations and has a characteristic clinical presentation (Ronen *et al.*, 1992). Pseudohyperparathyroidism refers to a paraneoplastic condition associated with different types of tumour (Suva *et al.*, 1987).

Primary hyperparathyroidism

Parathyroid adenomas are the main cause of parathyroid hyperplasia resulting in increased parathyroid hormone secretion not responsive to calcium negative feedback (Peauroi *et al.*, 1998; Wong *et al.*, 2004). Excessive parathyroid hormone secretion results in increased bone resorption, increased renal reabsorption of calcium and decreased renal reabsorption of phosphorous leading to persistent hypercalcaemia and hypophosphataemia (Frank *et al.*, 1998; Peauroi *et al.*, 1998; Tomlinson *et al.*, 2014).

Clinical signs of primary hyperparathyroidism are initially subtle, and hypercalcaemia is often considered as an incidental finding for a few months before lethargy, inappetence, weight loss, shifting-leg lameness or shivering become obvious (Roussel and Thatcher, 1987; Peauroi *et al.*, 1998; Wong *et al.*, 2004; Tomlinson *et al.*, 2014; Cottle *et al.*, 2016). In more advanced cases, poor dentition, malocclusion, tooth resorption and progressive enlargement of facial bone are described (Frank *et al.*, 1998; Wong *et al.*, 2004; Earley *et al.*, 2017).

The diagnosis of primary hyperparathyroidism is based on persistent hypercalcaemia (total and ionized calcium), hypophosphataemia, low urinary fractional excretion (FE) of calcium, high FE of phosphorous, high parathyroid hormone concentrations with exclusion of chronic renal disease (absence of azotaemia) and paraneoplastic syndrome (absence of tumour and low PTHrP) (Frank *et al.*, 1998; Wong *et al.*, 2004; Gorenberg *et al.*, 2020). Diagnostic imaging has produced inconsistent results. Radiographs can reveal loss of periodontal lamina dura denta, stenosis of the nasal passages and osteopenia (Fig. 3.3) (Frank *et al.*, 1998; Cottle *et al.*, 2016). Ultrasonographic examination of the parathyroid gland is complicated by the poor definition of the parathyroid tissue in horses by individual variations. The parathyroid gland can be found around the thyroid gland, in the mid-neck region or at the thoracic inlet (Gorenberg *et al.*, 2020). In many cases, the gland cannot be found but when identified, small areas of heterogeneous echogenicity within the gland are described (Frank *et al.*, 1998; Cottle *et al.*, 2016; Gorenberg *et al.*, 2020). Technetium 99 m sestamibi scintigraphy of the neck from the ramus of the jaw to the thoracic inlet has been used to identify the parathyroid gland with variable success; however, more recent studies have had a higher success rate using 70–200 mCi (2.5–7.5 GBq) of technetium 99 m sestamibi per horse and scanning at 10–15 min, 2.5 h, 4–5.5 h and 24 h (Wong *et al.*, 2004; Tomlinson *et al.*, 2014; Cottle *et al.*, 2016).

Medical therapy of primary hyperparathyroidism is based on dietary changes to reduce calcium intake and calciuresis by combining intravenous fluid therapy and diuretics; however, prognosis for medical management alone is usually poor and euthanasia might be necessary (Frank *et al.*, 1998). Surgical exploration of the neck and excision of the parathyroid adenoma is the recommended treatment; however, in the absence of clear localization of the parathyroid tissue, surgical exploration can be unrewarding (Wong *et al.*, 2004; Cottle *et al.*, 2016). Post-operative complications of successful excision of the parathyroid tissue include muscle tremors, stiffness and cardiac arrhythmias resulting from hypocalcaemia, acute kidney injury, hypomagnesaemia and hypophosphataemia, resolved over time with proper supplementation (Tomlinson *et al.*, 2014). Prognosis for horses with post-operative improvement of circulating calcium and parathyroid hormone concentration is good (Gorenberg *et al.*, 2020).

Secondary hyperparathyroidism

Renal secondary hyperparathyroidism is described in small animals where phosphorous retention reduces circulating calcium leading to increased parathyroid hormone secretion. In horses, chronic kidney disease is associated with hypercalcaemia. Parathyroid concentrations in these horses is usually within reference range indicating that hypercalcaemia is more likely due to impaired renal

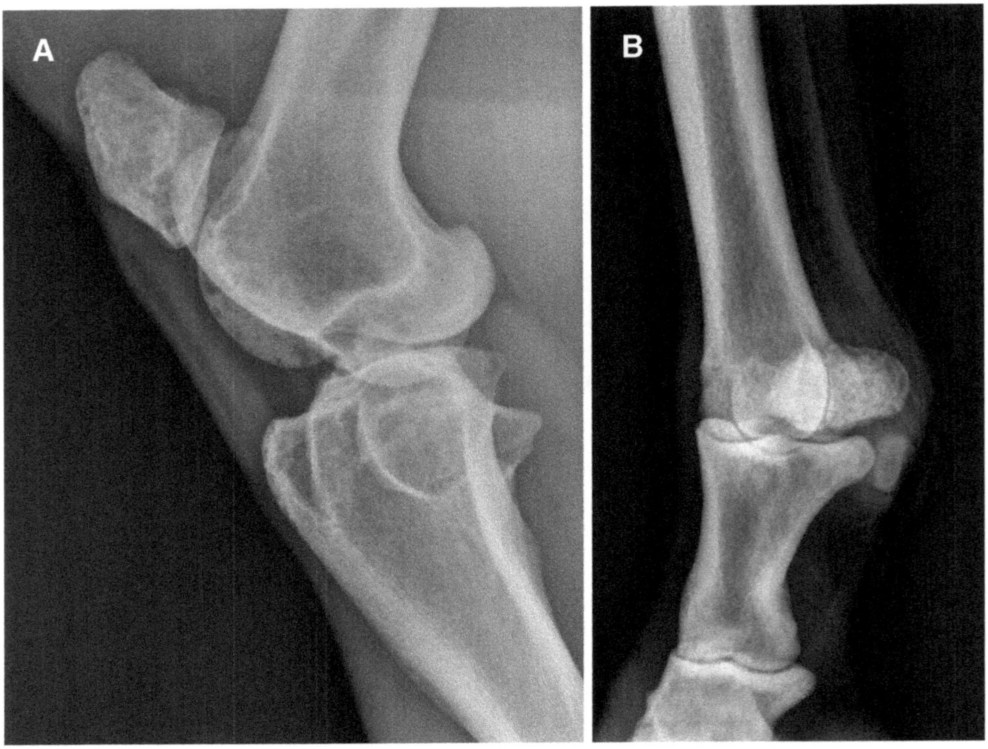

Fig. 3.3. Lateromedial projection of the right stifle (A) and dorsolateral–palmaromedial oblique projection of the left front fetlock (B), in a 17-year-old pony mare with a history of acute onset left front and right hind lameness, diagnosed with primary hyperparathyroidism. Note the polyostotic pathology with coarse trabecular pattern and multiple, variably-sized punctate lucencies scattered throughout the epiphyseal/metaphyseal regions of multiple bones. Irregular sclerosis surrounds the regions of lysis, contributing to the markedly heterogeneous opacity in these locations (courtesy of Dr Chris Elliot and Dr Alex Young).

excretion of calcium rather than calcium mobilization by parathyroid hormone (Bayly *et al.*, 1986). That being said, although there is no evidence of increased parathyroid secretion in horses with renal disease, prolongation of parathyroid hormone half-life due to renal tubular damage might contribute to the observed hypercalcaemia (Elfers *et al.*, 1986a).

Nutritional secondary hyperparathyroidism is described in horses fed diets low in calcium and rich in phosphorous (with a phosphorous/calcium ratio above 3/1) or in horses fed on pastures with plants rich in oxalate (Joyce *et al.*, 1971). The disease was common in the past and named ‘big head’, Miller’s disease, bran disease, equine osteoporosis, osteitis fibrosa or osteodistrophia fibrosa; however, with improvement of animal nutrition, the disease is now less common in developed countries and more commonly associated with ingestion of oxalate-rich plants (McKenzie, 1988; Benders *et al.*, 2001). When ingested, oxalate binds dietary calcium to form an insoluble calcium oxalate, with decreasing calcium available for absorption and an increase in calcium faecal output (Blaney *et al.*, 1981a, b; McKenzie *et al.*, 1981a). A diet containing 1% oxalate can reduce intestinal absorption of calcium by about 70%, potentially leading to negative calcium balance when horses are fed on such pastures (Swartzman *et al.*, 1978). Therefore, it is considered that horses fed on pastures in which calcium/oxalate ratio is below 1/2 or fed grasses in which total oxalate is above 0.5%, are at risk of developing nutritional secondary hyperparathyroidism (Blaney *et al.*, 1981a). To a lesser extent, oxalate can also bind to dietary magnesium; however, magnesium oxalate is more soluble than calcium oxalate and can be absorbed. Hyperphosphataemia and

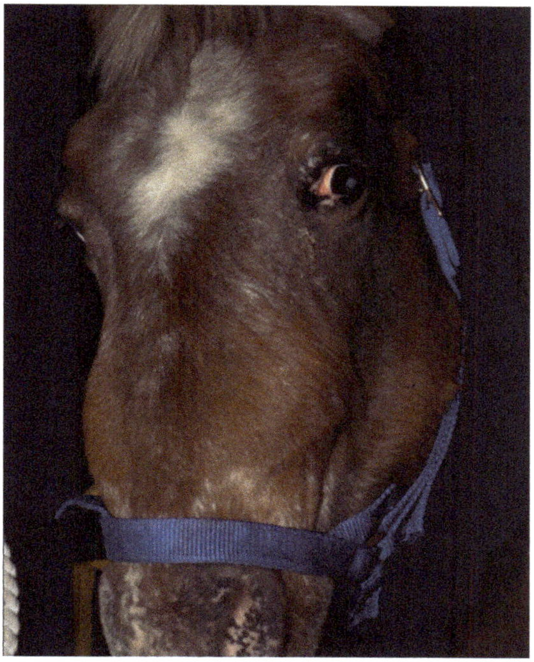

Fig. 3.4. Severe enlargement of facial bones in a 13-year-old gelding with nutritional secondary hyperparathyroidism ('big head') (courtesy of Dr Janice E. Kritchevsky).

hypocalcaemia stimulate parathyroid hormone secretion resulting in bone resorption and leading to osteodystrophy. As mentioned above, hyperphosphataemia inhibits the conversion of vitamin D_3 into 1,25-dihydroxycholecalciferol, leading to sustained parathyroid hormone secretion (hyperparathyroidism) and sustained bone resorption (Krook and Barrett, 1962). The disease develops over periods of inadequate diet; therefore, the regulators of calcium metabolism maintain calcium concentrations in these animals within reference intervals. This normocalcaemia, however, is maintained at the expense of skeletal reserves.

Clinically, the typical features of nutritional secondary hyperparathyroidism include thickening of the maxillary and mandibular bones, lameness, stiffness, weight loss, anorexia and tachypnoea with or without an inspiratory stridor (Fig. 3.4) (Joyce *et al.*, 1971; Ronen *et al.*, 1992; Benders *et al.*, 2001; Lacitignola *et al.*, 2018). Clinical signs of hypocalcaemia are relatively uncommon in secondary hyperparathyroidism; however, the combination of low calcium and high oxalate can lead to intestinal absorption of oxalate that chelates circulating calcium, leading to hypocalcaemia (Herbert and Dittmer, 2017).

A diagnosis of nutritional secondary hyperparathyroidism is based on history, diet analysis and laboratory findings including hyperphosphataemia, hypo- or normocalcaemia, hypocalciuria, hyperphosphaturia and increased parathyroid hormone concentrations (Ronen *et al.*, 1992; Benders *et al.*, 2001). As described with primary hyperparathyroidism, bone resorption can be apparent in more severe and chronic cases; it is usually more evident on the facial bones but can also result in long-bone fractures (Benders *et al.*, 2001; Lacitignola *et al.*, 2018).

Management of nutritional secondary hyperparathyroidism relies on calcium supplementation and diet analysis. Calcium carbonate or dicalcium phosphate at 100 to 300 g/day and diets with a calcium/phosphate ratio above 3/1 have resulted in clinical improvement (Ronen *et al.*, 1992). Addition of lucerne hay, reduction in grain intake and removal of oxalate-containing plants might also be beneficial. In horses fed grasses potentially high in oxalate, supplementation should provide at least 20 mg/kg/day of calcium and 10 mg/kg/day of phosphorous to limit the risk of nutritional secondary hyperparathyroidism (Gartner *et al.*, 1981). If, despite supplementation, new cases are detected on the property, the supplementation can be doubled and mixed with molasses to improve palatability (McKenzie *et al.*, 1981b). Severe cases of osteodystrophy should be confined, and non-structural anti-inflammatory drugs can be administered to relieve pain (Benders *et al.*, 2001; Lacitignola *et al.*, 2018). The prognosis for severely affected cases with marked osteodystrophy and dental loss is poor; however, in younger animals with milder clinical signs, prognosis is fair to good (Benders *et al.*, 2001; Herbert and Dittmer, 2017; Lacitignola *et al.*, 2018).

Pseudohyperparathyroidism

Hypercalcaemia is reported in neoplastic diseases in horses (humoral hypercalcaemia of malignancy) (McCoy and Beasley, 1986; Rosol *et al.*, 1994). The condition has been documented with multiple myeloma, lymphosarcoma, ovarian tumours, genital squamous cell carcinomas and ameloblastomas (Marr *et al.*, 1989; Karcher *et al.*, 1990; Mair *et al.*, 1990; Rosol *et al.*, 1994; Barton *et al.*, 2004).

Rather than an increase in parathyroid hormone, hypercalcaemia is induced by excessive production of PTHrP (Barton *et al.*, 2004). Clinical signs are mostly the result of the initiating tumour and are usually vague, including weight loss and changes in demeanour; however, more advanced cases can show reduced bone density and soft tissue calcification (Mair *et al.*, 1990). A diagnosis of pseudohyperparathyroidism is made by demonstration of hypercalcaemia, hypophosphataemia, reduced FE of calcium, increased FE of phosphorous, normal parathyroid hormone concentration and increased PTHrP (Karcher *et al.*, 1990; Barton *et al.*, 2004). Prognosis is usually guarded as the disease is caused by a neoplasm.

Hypoparathyroidism

The diagnosis of hypoparathyroidism is usually based on the presence of hypocalcaemia and hyperphosphataemia in the absence of renal disease (Hudson *et al.*, 1999). Primary hypoparathyroidism is a rare disorder that can result in life-threatening hypocalcaemia; however, other disorders classified as secondary hypoparathyroidism associated with systemic inflammation can be more common and result in milder hypocalcaemia. Additional causes of hypocalcaemia, not developed here but leading to similar clinical signs, include lactation, tetany, malignant hyperthermia, myopathy and toxicoses such as cantharidin, cadmium and oxalate (Toribio, 2011).

Primary hypoparathyroidism

There are only a few reports of equine primary hypoparathyroidism, but the disease should be suspected in cases of recurrent and severe hypocalcaemia (Couëtil *et al.*, 1998; Hudson *et al.*, 1999; Durie *et al.*, 2010). Primary hypoparathyroidism is caused by an absence of functional parathyroid activity; however, unlike what is described in humans where genetic mutations and iatrogenic causes have been documented, no clear aetiology has been identified in horses (Hudson *et al.*, 1999; Toribio, 2011; Mannstadt *et al.*, 2017).

Clinical manifestations of primary hypoparathyroidism include synchronous diaphragmatic flutter with tachycardia and tachypnoea; restlessness, muscle twitching and ataxia possibly progressing to recumbency and seizure-like activity; as well as gastrointestinal ileus with or without signs of colic (Couëtil *et al.*, 1998; Hudson *et al.*, 1999; Durie *et al.*, 2010). All these signs are consistent with severe hypocalcaemia.

Table 3.1. Parathyroid stimulation test used to diagnose primary hypoparathyroidism. Disodium ethylenediaminetetraacetic acid is administered intravenously at increasing doses to achieve a linear decrease in blood calcium and a blood sample is drawn before each dose increment. A diagnosis of primary hypoparathyroidism is achieved when ethylenediaminetetraacetic acid-induced hypocalcaemia fails to elicit a parathyroid hormone response. Adapted from Durie *et al.*, 2010.

Time	Disodium ethylenediaminetetraacetic acid
0–5 min	30 mg/kg/h
5–10 min	40 mg/kg/h
10–15 min	60 mg/kg/h
15–20 min	90 mg/kg/h
20–25 min	120 mg/kg/h
25–30 min	180 mg/kg/h

Serum chemistry for primary hypoparathyroidism reveals severe hypocalcaemia, hyperphosphataemia and hypomagnesaemia with albumin, creatinine and blood urea nitrogen within normal limits excluding acute kidney injury (Couëtil *et al.*, 1998; Hudson *et al.*, 1999). Parathyroid hormone concentrations, as measured with a radioimmunoassay, are usually low (Couëtil *et al.*, 1998; Hudson *et al.*, 1999; Durie *et al.*, 2010). In one case, a parathyroid hormone stimulation test has been used to induce hypocalcaemia by intravenous infusion of ethylenediaminetetraacetic acid and confirm the absence of parathyroid activity (Table 3.1).

In the absence of a parathyroid stimulation test, the combination of refractory hypocalcaemia, hyperphosphataemia and low parathyroid hormone concentrations is diagnostic for primary hypoparathyroidism.

Management of primary hypoparathyroidism involves intravenous and oral calcium supplementation. Depending on the severity of hypocalcaemia, the initial parenteral calcium supplementation ranges from 400 to 1500 mEq of calcium gluconate administered over 20 min to 4 h (Couëtil *et al.*, 1998; Hudson *et al.*, 1999; Durie *et al.*, 2010). In cases of mild hypocalcaemia, a maintenance rate of 10 mEq of calcium gluconate per litre of balanced electrolytic solution can then be used; however, a maintenance rate of up to 30 mEq of calcium gluconate per litre of balanced electrolytic solution might be necessary in more severe cases (Toribio, 2011). Frequent monitoring of ionized calcium concentration is important to correctly adjust the dose, as excessive supplementation can result in cardiovascular disorders, mainly in systematically sick animals. Long-term management relies on oral calcium supplementation with calcium carbonate (limestone powder, 100–300 g daily) or dicalcium phosphate (100–200 g daily) (Couëtil *et al.*, 1998; Hudson *et al.*, 1999; Toribio, 2011). In addition, as magnesium is essential for calcium homeostasis and common in primary hypoparathyroidism, hypocalcaemia might not correct until magnesium supplementation is provided orally or parenterally. There would be low value in vitamin D supplementation as, in cases of primary hypoparathyroidism, the concentrations of parathyroid hormone required for conversion of vitamin D_3 into 1,25-dihydroxycholecalciferol in the kidney are low (Couëtil *et al.*, 1998).

Secondary hypoparathyroidism

The definition of secondary hypoparathyroidism is controversial in equine endocrinology and includes three distinct mechanisms: (i) low to normal parathyroid hormone concentration with hypocalcaemia; (ii) normal to high parathyroid hormone concentration with hypocalcaemia; and (iii) low parathyroid hormone concentration with hypercalcaemia. In the absence of a clear definition, there are currently no clear reports of secondary hypoparathyroidism in horses; however, several studies have documented impaired parathyroid hormone activity in systemically ill horses that could be consistent with secondary hypoparathyroidism (Toribio *et al.*, 2001, 2005; Hurcombe *et al.*, 2009).

In the first definition, of low to normal parathyroid hormone concentration and hypocalcaemia, inflammatory mediators (tumour necrosis factor α, interleukin 1 and interleukin 6) inhibit parathyroid gland secretions resulting in low parathyroid hormone concentrations (Toribio *et al.*, 2003b, 2005). This mechanism has been documented in horses with systemic inflammatory response syndrome, in which hypocalcaemia and hypomagnesaemia are common and associated with poor survival, as well as in horses with experimentally induced endotoxaemia (Dart *et al.*, 1992; Garcia-Lopez *et al.*, 2001; Toribio *et al.*, 2005).

In the second definition, of normal to high parathyroid hormone concentration and hypocalcaemia, peripheral tissues would have a decreased sensitivity to parathyroid hormone (parathyroid hormone resistance) resulting in persistent hypocalcaemia despite high parathyroid hormone concentrations (Lind *et al.*, 2000; Zaloga, 2000; Toribio *et al.*, 2001, 2005). This mechanism, similar to idiopathic hypocalcaemia in foals, has been documented in septic foals as well as in adult horses with enterocolitis and is associated with poor survival (Toribio *et al.*, 2001, 2005; Hurcombe *et al.*, 2009; Kamr *et al.*, 2018).

These two mechanisms have been described in horses with identical conditions (enterocolitis and experimentally induced endotoxaemia), suggesting more complex calcium–parathyroid hormone dynamics (Dart *et al.*, 1992; Garcia-Lopez *et al.*, 2001; Toribio *et al.*, 2005).

In the third definition, of low parathyroid hormone concentration and hypercalcaemia, the low parathyroid hormone concentration results from an inhibitory effect of parathyroid hormone-independent hypercalcaemia (Elfers *et al.*, 1986b). This form of secondary hypoparathyroidism, more described in human medicine, is similar to pseudohyperparathyroidism described above, where tumours with secretion of PTH-P, renal diseases and toxicants such as vitamin A or D induce hypercalcaemia that suppresses parathyroid hormone secretion (Aguilera-Tejero *et al.*, 2000; Barton *et al.*, 2004).

Management of secondary hypoparathyroidism relies on the management of the primary cause, sepsis, enterocolitis or renal disease, and on regulation of calcium concentrations (hyper- or hypocalcaemia) as detailed above. In all these cases, magnesium monitoring is recommended as persistent hypomagnesaemia prevents proper calcium regulation (Toribio, 2011).

Pseudohypoparathyroidism and idiopathic hypocalcaemia in foals

The condition is poorly described in horses and has only been reported in foals (Beyer *et al.*, 1997; Kamr *et al.*, 2018). In such foals, the clinical presentation is similar to primary hypoparathyroidism with tachycardia, ataxia, recumbency, ileus, hypocalcaemia and hyperphosphataemia; however, parathyroid hormone concentrations are variable and can be below or above reference intervals suggesting a possible peripheral tissue parathyroid hormone insensitivity (Beyer *et al.*, 1997; Kamr *et al.*, 2018). Although no aetiology has been identified, prognosis for survival is poor despite calcium supplementation (Beyer *et al.*, 1997).

References

Aguilera-Tejero, E., Garfia, B., Estepa, J.C., López, I., Mayer-Valor, R. *et al.* (1998) Effects of exercise and EDTA administration on blood ionized calcium and parathyroid hormone in horses. *American Journal of Veterinary Research* 59(12), 1605–1607.

Aguilera-Tejero, E., Estepa, J.C., López, I., Bas, S. and Rodríguez, M. (2000) Polycystic kidneys as a cause of chronic renal failure and secondary hypoparathyroidism in a horse. *Equine Veterinary Journal* 32(2), 167–169. DOI: 10.2746/042516400777591552.

Aguilera-Tejero, E., Estepa, J.C., López, I., Bas, S., Garfia, B. *et al.* (2001) Plasma ionized calcium and parathyroid hormone concentrations in horses after endurance rides. *Journal of the American Veterinary Medical Association* 219(4), 488–490. DOI: 10.2460/javma.2001.219.488.

Azarpeykan, S., Dittmer, K.E., Gee, E.K., Marshall, J.C., Elder, P. *et al.* (2016a) Circadian rhythm of calciotropic hormones, serum calcium, phosphorus and magnesium during the shortest and longest days of the year in horses in New Zealand. *Journal of Animal Physiology and Animal Nutrition* 100(6), 1058–1066. DOI: 10.1111/jpn.12477.

Azarpeykan, S., Dittmer, K.E., Gee, E.K., Marshall, J.C., Wallace, J. *et al.* (2016b) Influence of blanketing and season on vitamin D and parathyroid hormone, calcium, phosphorus, and magnesium concentrations in horses in New Zealand. *Domestic Animal Endocrinology* 56, 75–84. DOI: 10.1016/j.domaniend.2016.03.003.

Barton, M.H., Sharma, P., LeRoy, B.E. and Howerth, E.W. (2004) Hypercalcemia and high serum parathyroid hormone-related protein concentration in a horse with multiple myeloma. *Journal of the American Veterinary Medical Association* 225(3), 409–413. DOI: 10.2460/javma.2004.225.409.

Bayly, W.M., Brobst, D.F., Elfers, R.S. and Reed, S.M. (1986) Serum and urinary biochemistry and enzyme changes in ponies with acute renal failure. *The Cornell Veterinarian* 76(3), 306–316.

Benders, N.A., Junker, K., Wensing, T., van den Ingh, T.S. and van der Kolk, J.H. (2001) Diagnosis of secondary hyperparathyroidism in a pony using intact parathyroid hormone radioimmunoassay. *Veterinary Record* 149(6), 185–187. DOI: 10.1136/vr.149.6.185.

Berndt, T. and Kumar, R. (2007) Phosphatonins and the regulation of phosphate homeostasis. *Annual Review of Physiology* 69, 341–359. DOI: 10.1146/annurev.physiol.69.040705.141729.

Beyer, M.J., Freestone, J.F., Reimer, J.M., Bernard, W.V. and Rueve, E.R. (1997) Idiopathic hypocalcemia in foals. *Journal of Veterinary Internal Medicine* 11(6), 356–360. DOI: 10.1111/j.1939-1676.1997.tb00480.x.

Blaney, B.J., Gartner, R.J.W. and McKenzie, R.A. (1981a) The effects of oxalate in some tropical grasses on the availability to horses of calcium, phosphorus and magnesium. *The Journal of Agricultural Science* 97(3), 507–514. DOI: 10.1017/S0021859600036820.

Blaney, B.J., Gartner, R.J.W. and McKenzie, R.A. (1981b) The inability of horses to absorb calcium from calcium oxalate. *The Journal of Agricultural Science* 97(3), 639–641. DOI: 10.1017/S0021859600036984.

Cottle, H.J., Hughes, K.J., Thompson, H., Johnston, P.E.J. and Philbey, A.W. (2016) Primary hyperparathyroidism in a 17-year-old Arab × Welsh cob pony mare with a functional parathyroid adenoma. *Equine Veterinary Education* 28(9), 477–485. DOI: 10.1111/eve.12183.

Couëtil, L.L., Sojka, J.E. and Nachreiner, R.F. (1998) Primary hypoparathyroidism in a horse. *Journal of Veterinary Internal Medicine* 12(1), 45–49. DOI: 10.1111/j.1939-1676.1998.tb00496.x.

Dart, A.J., Snyder, J.R., Spier, S.J. and Sullivan, K.E. (1992) Ionized calcium concentration in horses with surgically managed gastrointestinal disease: 147 cases (1988–1990). *Journal of the American Veterinary Medical Association* 201(8), 1244–1248.

Durie, I., van Loon, G., Hesta, M., Bauwens, C. and Deprez, P. (2010) Hypocalcemia caused by primary hypoparathyroidism in a 3-month-old filly. *Journal of Veterinary Internal Medicine* 24(2), 439–442. DOI: 10.1111/j.1939-1676.2009.0463.x.

Earley, E.T., Rawlinson, J.R., Baratt, R.M., Galloway, S.S., Smedley, R.C. *et al.* (2017) Hematologic, biochemical, and endocrine parameters in horses with tooth resorption and Hypercementosis. *Journal of Veterinary Dentistry* 34(3), 155–160. DOI: 10.1177/0898756417717039.

Elfers, R.S., Bayly, W.M., Brobst, D.F., Reed, S.M., Liggitt, H.D. *et al.* (1986a) Alterations in calcium, phosphorus and C-terminal parathyroid hormone levels in equine acute renal disease. *The Cornell Veterinarian* 76, 317–329.

Elfers, R.S., Bayly, W.M., Brobst, D.F., Reed, S.M., Liggitt, H.D. *et al.* (1986b) Alterations in calcium, phosphorus and C-terminal parathyroid hormone levels in equine acute renal disease. *The Cornell Veterinarian* 76(3), 317–329.

Frank, N., Hawkins, J.F., Couëtil, L.L. and Raymond, J.T. (1998) Primary hyperparathyroidism with osteodystrophia fibrosa of the facial bones in a pony. *Journal of the American Veterinary Medical Association* 212(1), 84–86.

Friedman, P.A. and Gesek, F.A. (1995) Cellular calcium transport in renal epithelia: measurement, mechanisms, and regulation. *Physiological Reviews* 75(3), 429–471. DOI: 10.1152/physrev.1995.75.3.429.

Garcia-Lopez, J.M., Provost, P.J., Rush, J.E., Zicker, S.C., Burmaster, H. *et al.* (2001) Prevalence and prognostic importance of hypomagnesemia and hypocalcemia in horses that have colic surgery. *American Journal of Veterinary Research* 62(1), 7–12. DOI: 10.2460/ajvr.2001.62.7.

Garrett, J.E., Tamir, H., Kifor, O., Simin, R.T., Rogers, K.V. *et al.* (1995) Calcitonin-secreting cells of the thyroid express an extracellular calcium receptor gene. *Endocrinology* 136(11), 5202–5211. DOI: 10.1210/endo.136.11.7588259.

Gartner, R.J.W., Blaney, B.J. and McKenzie, R.A. (1981) Supplements to correct oxalate-induced negative calcium and phosphorus balances in horses fed tropical grass hays. *The Journal of Agricultural Science* 97(3), 581–589. DOI: 10.1017/S002185960003690X.

Gorenberg, E.B., Johnson, A.L., Magdesian, K.G., Bertin, F.-R., Costa, L.R.R. *et al.* (2020) Diagnosis and treatment of confirmed and suspected primary hyperparathyroidism in equids: 17 cases (1999–2016). *Equine Veterinary Journal* 52(1), 83–90. DOI: 10.1111/evj.13120.

Herbert, E.W. and Dittmer, K.E. (2017) Acute and chronic oxalate toxicity in Miniature Horses associated with soursob (*Oxalis pes-caprae*) ingestion. *Equine Veterinary Education* 29(10), 549–557. DOI: 10.1111/eve.12605.

Hu, M.C., Kuro-o, M. and Moe, O.W. (2012) The emerging role of klotho in clinical nephrology. *Nephrology Dialysis Transplantation* 27(7), 2650–2657. DOI: 10.1093/ndt/gfs160.

Hudson, N.P., Church, D.B., Trevena, J., Nielsen, I.L., Major, D. *et al.* (1999) Primary hypoparathyroidism in two horses. *Australian Veterinary Journal* 77(8), 504–508. DOI: 10.1111/j.1751-0813.1999.tb12119.x.

Hurcombe, S.D.A., Toribio, R.E., Slovis, N.M., Saville, W.J., Mudge, M.C. *et al.* (2009) Calcium regulating hormones and serum calcium and magnesium concentrations in septic and critically ill foals and their association with survival. *Journal of Veterinary Internal Medicine* 23(2), 335–343. DOI: 10.1111/j.1939-1676.2009.0275.x.

Joyce, J.R., Pierce, K.R., Romane, W.M. and Baker, J.M. (1971) Clinical study of nutritional secondary hyperparathyroidism in horses. *Journal of the American Veterinary Medical Association* 158(12), 2033

Kamr, A.M., Dembek, K.A., Hildreth, B.E., Morresey, P.R., Rathgeber, R.A. *et al.* (2018) The FGF-23/klotho axis and its relationship with phosphorus, calcium, vitamin D, PTH, aldosterone, severity of disease, and outcome in hospitalised foals. *Equine Veterinary Journal* 50(6), 739–746. DOI: 10.1111/evj.12946.

Karcher, L.F., Le Net, J.L., Turner, B.F., Reimers, T.J. and Tennant, B.C. (1990) Pseudohyperparathyroidism in a mare associated with squamous cell carcinoma of the vulva. *The Cornell Veterinarian* 80(2), 153–162.

Krook, L. and Barrett, R.B. (1962) Simian bone disease – a secondary hyperparathyroidism. *The Cornell Veterinarian* 52, 459.

Kuro-o, M. (2010) Overview of the FGF23-klotho axis. *Pediatric Nephrology* 25(4), 583–590. DOI: 10.1007/s00467-009-1260-4.

Kuro-o, M. (2013) Klotho, phosphate and FGF-23 in ageing and disturbed mineral metabolism. *Nature Reviews Nephrology* 9(11), 650–660. DOI: 10.1038/nrneph.2013.111.

Lacitignola, L., Luca, P.D., Santovito, R., Comite, M.S.D. and Crovace, A. (2018) Nutritional secondary hyperparathyroidism in two ponies. *Open Veterinary Journal* 8(2), 149–153. DOI: 10.4314/ovj.v8i2.6.

Lanske, B. and Razzaque, M.S. (2014) Molecular interactions of FGF23 and PTH in phosphate regulation. *Kidney International* 86(6), 1072–1074. DOI: 10.1038/ki.2014.316.

Lind, L., Carlstedt, F., Rastad, J., Stiernström, H., Stridsberg, M. *et al.* (2000) Hypocalcemia and parathyroid hormone secretion in critically ill patients. *Critical Care Medicine* 28(1), 93–99. DOI: 10.1097/00003246-200001000-00015.

Lopez, I., Estepa, J.C., Mendoza, F.J., Mayer-Valor, R. and Aguilera-Tejero, E. (2006) Fractionation of calcium and magnesium in equine serum. *American Journal of Veterinary Research* 67(3), 463–466. DOI: 10.2460/ajvr.67.3.463.

Mair, T.S., Yeo, S.P. and Lucke, V.M. (1990) Hypercalcaemia and soft tissue mineralisation associated with lymphosarcoma in two horses. *The Veterinary Record* 126(5), 99–101.

Mannstadt, M., Bilezikian, J.P., Thakker, R.V., Hannan, F.M., Clarke, B.L. *et al.* (2017) Hypoparathyroidism. *Nature Reviews Disease Primers* 3(1). DOI: 10.1038/nrdp.2017.55.

Marr, C.M., Love, S. and Pirie, H.M. (1989) Clinical, ultrasonographic and pathological findings in a horse with splenic lymphosarcoma and pseudohyperparathyroidism. *Equine Veterinary Journal* 21(3), 221–226. DOI: 10.1111/j.2042-3306.1989.tb02152.x.

Martin, K.J., Hruska, K.A., Freitag, J.J., Klahr, S. and Slatopolsky, E. (1979) The peripheral metabolism of parathyroid hormone. *New England Journal of Medicine* 301(20), 1092–1098. DOI: 10.1056/NEJM197911153012005.

McCoy, D.J. and Beasley, R. (1986) Hypercalcemia associated with malignancy in a horse. *Journal of the American Veterinary Medical Association* 189(1), 87–89.

McKenzie, R.A. (1988) Purple pigeon grass (Setaria incrassata): a potential cause of nutritional secondary hyperpharathyroidism of grazing horses. *Australian Veterinary Journal* 65(10), 329–330. DOI: 10.1111/j.1751-0813.1988.tb14520.x.

McKenzie, R.A., Blaney, B.J. and Gartner, R.J.W. (1981a) The effect of dietary oxalate on calcium, phosphorus and magnesium balances in horses. *The Journal of Agricultural Science* 97(1), 69–74. DOI: 10.1017/S0021859600035851.

McKenzie, R.A., Gartner, R.J., Blaney, B.J. and Glanville, R.J. (1981b) Control of nutritional secondary hyperparathyroidism in grazing horses with calcium plus phosphorus supplementation. *Australian Veterinary Journal* 57(12), 554–557. DOI: 10.1111/j.1751-0813.1981.tb00433.x.

Mundy, G.R. and Guise, T.A. (1999) Hormonal control of calcium homeostasis. *Clinical Chemistry* 45(8, Pt 2), 1347–1352. DOI: 10.1093/clinchem/45.8.1347.

Peauroi, J.R., Fisher, D.J., Mohr, F.C. and Vivrette, S.L. (1998) Primary hyperparathyroidism caused by a functional parathyroid adenoma in a horse. *Journal of the American Veterinary Medical Association* 212(12), 1915–1918.

Ritchie, G., Kerstan, D., Dai, L.J., Kang, H.S., Canaff, L. *et al.* (2001) 1,25(OH)(2)D(3) stimulates Mg2+ uptake into MDCT cells: modulation by extracellular Ca2+ and Mg2+. *American Journal of Physiology. Renal Physiology* 280(5), F868–878. DOI: 10.1152/ajprenal.2001.280.5.F868.

Ronen, N., van Heerden, J. and van Amstel, S.R. (1992) Clinical and biochemistry findings, and parathyroid hormone concentrations in three horses with secondary hyperparathyroidism. *Journal of the South African Veterinary Association* 63(3), 134–136.

Rosol, T.J., Nagode, L.A., Robertson, J.T., Leeth, B.D., Steinmeyer, C.L. *et al.* (1994) Humoral hypercalcemia of malignancy associated with ameloblastoma in a horse. *Journal of the American Veterinary Medical Association* 204(12), 1930–1933.

Rourke, K.M., Coe, S., Kohn, C.W., Rosol, T.J., Mendoza, F.J. *et al.* (2010) Cloning, comparative sequence analysis and mRNA expression of calcium-transporting genes in horses. *General and Comparative Endocrinology* 167(1), 6–10. DOI: 10.1016/j.ygcen.2010.02.022.

Roussel, A.J. and Thatcher, C.D. (1987) Primary hyperparathyroidism in a Pony mare. *Compendium on Continuing Education for the Practicing Veterinarian* 9, 781–783.

Schiavi, S.C. and Kumar, R. (2004) The phosphatonin pathway: new insights in phosphate homeostasis. *Kidney International* 65(1), 1–14. DOI: 10.1111/j.1523-1755.2004.00355.x.

Schryver, H.F., Craig, P.H., Hintz, H.F., Hogue, D.E. and Lowe, J.E. (1970) The site of calcium absorption in the horse. *The Journal of Nutrition* 100(10), 1127–1131. DOI: 10.1093/jn/100.10.1127.

Schryver, H.F., Hintz, H.F. and Lowe, J.E. (1974) Calcium and phosphorus in the nutrition of the horse. *The Cornell Veterinarian* 64(4), 493–515.

Semevolos, S.A., Brower-Toland, B.D., Bent, S.J. and Nixon, A.J. (2002) Parathyroid hormone-related peptide and Indian hedgehog expression patterns in naturally acquired equine osteochondrosis. *Journal of Orthopaedic Research* 20(6), 1290–1297. DOI: 10.1016/S0736-0266(02)00055-4.

Suva, L.J., Winslow, G.A., Wettenhall, R.E., Hammonds, R.G., Moseley, J.M. *et al.* (1987) A parathyroid hormone-related protein implicated in malignant hypercalcemia: cloning and expression. *Science* 237(4817), 893–896. DOI: 10.1126/science.3616618.

Swartzman, J.A., Hintz, H.F. and Schryver, H.F. (1978) Inhibition of calcium absorption in ponies fed diets containing oxalic acid. *American Journal of Veterinary Research* 39(10), 1621–1623.

Tomlinson, J.E., Johnson, A.L., Ross, M.W., Engiles, J.B., Levine, D.G. *et al.* (2014) Successful detection and removal of a functional parathyroid adenoma in a pony using technetium Tc 99m sestamibi scintigraphy. *Journal of Veterinary Internal Medicine* 28(2), 687–692. DOI: 10.1111/jvim.12285.

Toribio, R.E. (2011) Disorders of calcium and phosphate metabolism in horses. *Veterinary Clinics of North America: Equine Practice* 27(1), 129–147. DOI: 10.1016/j.cveq.2010.12.010.

Toribio, R.E., Kohn, C.W., Chew, D.J., Sams, R.A. and Rosol, T.J. (2001) Comparison of serum parathyroid hormone and ionized calcium and magnesium concentrations and fractional urinary clearance of calcium and phosphorus in healthy horses and horses with enterocolitis. *American Journal of Veterinary Research* 62(6), 938–947. DOI: 10.2460/ajvr.2001.62.938.

Toribio, R.E., Kohn, C.W., Capen, C.C. and Rosol, T.J. (2003a) Parathyroid hormone (PTH) secretion, PTH mRNA and calcium-sensing receptor mRNA expression in equine parathyroid cells, and effects of interleukin (IL)-1, IL-6, and tumor necrosis factor-alpha on equine parathyroid cell function. *Journal of Molecular Endocrinology* 31, 609–620. DOI: 10.1677/jme.0.0310609.

Toribio, R.E., Kohn, C.W., Capen, C.C. and Rosol, T.J. (2003b) Parathyroid hormone (PTH) secretion, PTH mRNA and calcium-sensing receptor mRNA expression in equine parathyroid cells, and effects of interleukin (IL)-1, IL-6, and tumor necrosis factor-alpha on equine parathyroid cell function. *Journal of Molecular Endocrinology* 31(3), 609–620. DOI: 10.1677/jme.0.0310609.

Toribio, R.E., Kohn, C.W., Sams, R.A., Capen, C.C. and Rosol, T.J. (2003c) Hysteresis and calcium set-point for the calcium parathyroid hormone relationship in healthy horses. *General and Comparative Endocrinology* 130(3), 279–288. DOI: 10.1016/S0016-6480(02)00621-4.

Toribio, R.E., Kohn, C.W., Hardy, J. and Rosol, T.J. (2005) Alterations in serum parathyroid hormone and electrolyte concentrations and urinary excretion of electrolytes in horses with induced endotoxemia. *Journal of Veterinary Internal Medicine* 19(2), 223–231. DOI: 10.1111/j.1939-1676.2005.tb02686.x.

Wasserman, R.H. and Fullmer, C.S. (1995) Vitamin D and intestinal calcium transport: facts, speculations and hypotheses. *The Journal of Nutrition* 125(Suppl 7), 1971S–1979S. DOI: 10.1093/jn/125.suppl_7.1971S.

Wilkens, M.R., Marholt, L., Eigendorf, N., Muscher-Banse, A.S., Feige, K. *et al*. (2017) Trans- and paracellular calcium transport along the small and large intestine in horses. *Comparative Biochemistry and Physiology Part A: Molecular & Integrative Physiology* 204, 157–163. DOI: 10.1016/j.cbpa.2016.11.020.

Wong, D., Sponseller, B., Miles, K., Butt, T., Kersh, K. *et al*. (2004) Failure of technetium Tc 99m sestamibi scanning to detect abnormal parathyroid tissue in a horse and a mule with primary hyperparathyroidism. *Journal of Veterinary Internal Medicine* 18(4), 589–593. DOI: 10.1111/j.1939-1676.2004.tb02591.x.

Woodrow, J.P., Sharpe, C.J., Fudge, N.J., Hoff, A.O., Gagel, R.F. *et al*. (2006) Calcitonin plays a critical role in regulating skeletal mineral metabolism during lactation. *Endocrinology* 147(9), 4010–4021. DOI: 10.1210/en.2005-1616.

Wysolmerski, J.J. and Stewart, A.F. (1998) The physiology of parathyroid hormone-related protein: an emerging role as a developmental factor. *Annual Review of Physiology* 60, 431–460. DOI: 10.1146/annurev.physiol.60.1.431.

Zaloga, G.P. (2000) Ionized hypocalcemia during sepsis. *Critical Care Medicine* 28(1), 266–268. DOI: 10.1097/00003246-200001000-00054.

4 Diseases of the Hypothalamo–Pituitary–Adrenocortical Axis

The hypothalamo–pituitary–adrenocortical axis is a major neuroendocrine system that involves the paraventricular nucleus of the hypothalamus, the anterior lobe of the pituitary gland and the cortex of the adrenal gland. This axis, tightly regulated by stimulating hormones and loops of negative feedback, is responsible for the secretion of hormones involved in many physiological processes such as circadian rhythm, fluid and electrolyte balance, stress response, protein, carbohydrate and lipid metabolism, reproductive function, as well as immune response.

Diseases of the hypothalamo–pituitary–adrenocortical axis are caused by excessive or insufficient hormone secretion that can originate from any element of the axis and result in a variety of clinical signs. In horses, the most common disorders of the hypothalamo–pituitary–adrenocortical axis are pituitary pars intermedia dysfunction (PPID) and relative adrenocortical insufficiency.

Hypothalamo–Pituitary–Adrenocortical Axis Physiology

The paraventricular nucleus of the anterior hypothalamus is the first step of the hypothalamo–pituitary–adrenocortical axis. By secreting releasing hormones, the hypothalamus activates a collection of cells or a single cell type in the pituitary gland. The pituitary gland is composed of the adenohypophysis (or pars anterior) and the neurohypophysis (or pars nervosa). The adenohypophysis can be further divided into the pars distalis, composed of five cell types (corticotropes, somatotropes, gonadotropes, lactotropes and thyrotropes), the pars tuberalis (rich in melatonin receptors) and the pars intermedia (exclusively composed of melanotropes) (Saland, 2001). The neurohypophysis, on the other hand, is a cluster of axons originating from paraventricular and optic neurons that secrete oxytocin and vasopressin (or anti-diuretic hormone). The two cell types of major clinical relevance in equine endocrinology are the corticotrope of the pars distalis of the pituitary gland and the melanotrope of the pars intermedia of the pituitary gland.

The corticotropin-releasing hormone (CRH), a peptide hormone released in response to stress, is the corticotrope stimulator. Secreted in the hypophyseal portal system in a pulsatile fashion, CRH stimulates type-1 CRH receptors located on corticotropes of the pars distalis of the pituitary gland, resulting in the production of proopiomelanocortin-derived peptides (De Souza and Battaglia, 1988). Systemic effects of CRH secretion are mild and include appetite and inflammation modulation. Proopiomelanocortin (POMC) is a polypeptide that undergoes multiple post-transcriptional modifications and cleavages, yielding a wide variety of polypeptide fragments such as gamma-melanocyte-stimulating hormone (γ-MSH), adrenocorticotropic hormone (ACTH), alpha-melanocyte-stimulating hormone (α-MSH), corticotropin-like intermediate peptide (CLIP), beta-melanocyte-stimulating hormone (β-MSH) and beta-endorphin. Each POMC fragment is reported to have different yet overlapping functions; however, limited data are available in horses and, as corticotropes mainly express prohormone convertase 1, ACTH is the principal product of successive POMC cleavages (Fig. 4.1(A)) (Lo, 1962; Altmeyer *et al.*, 1984; Donaldson *et al.*, 2004a, b).

In the main circulation, ACTH primarily stimulates the cortex of adrenal glands. The adrenal cortex is divided into three layers each containing a particular type of cell responsible for the secretion of a specific hormone type (Alesci *et al.*, 2001; Arlt and Stewart, 2005):

- The *zona glomerulosa* is the peripheral zone of the adrenal cortex and is responsible for the secretion of mineralocorticoids such as aldosterone.

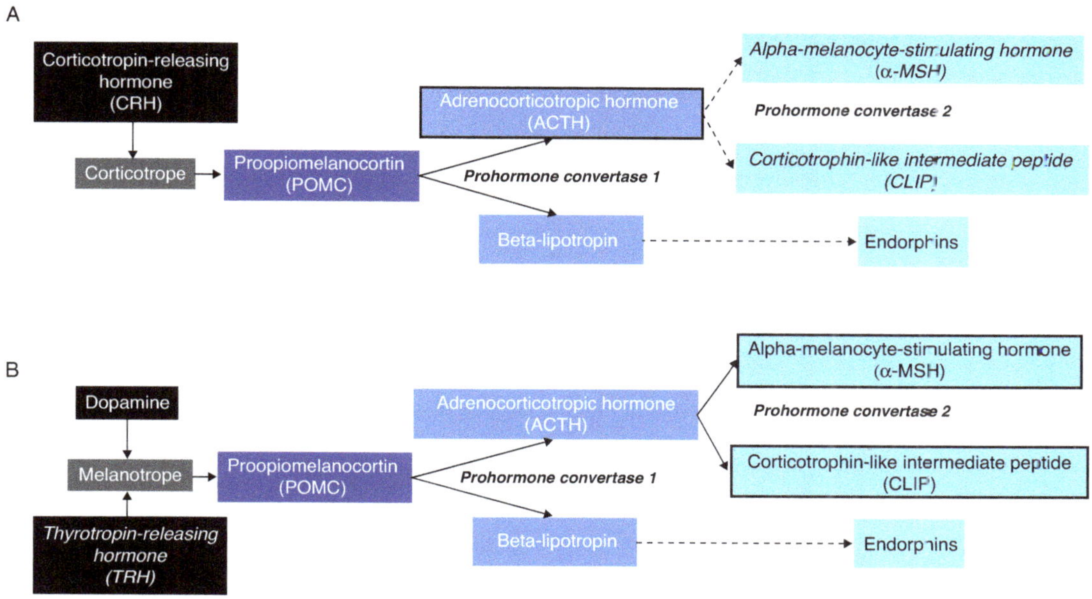

Fig. 4.1. Simplified corticotrope (A) and melanotrope (B) physiology. The difference in prohormone convertase expression between the pars distalis corticotrope and the pars intermedia melanotrope changes the proportions of proopiomelanocortin-derived peptides (Author's own diagram).

- The *zona fasciculata* is the intermediate and larger zone of the adrenal cortex representing about 75% of the gland and is responsible for the secretion of glucocorticoids such as cortisol.
- The *zona reticularis* is the inner zone of the adrenal cortex and is responsible for the secretion of androgens such as androstenedione.

Mineralocorticoids, glucocorticoids and androgens are lipidic hormones all originating from cholesterol after multiple steps of enzymatic cleavage, hydroxylation and dehydrogenization (Arlt and Stewart, 2005). In plasma, these hormones are transported when bound to proteins such as albumin and steroid-binding globulins (cortisol-binding protein and sex hormone-binding protein) but only the free fraction is metabolically active. Being lipophilic, these hormones cross the cellular plasma membrane by simple diffusion and reach their cytosolic receptor. Once formed, the ligand–receptor complex enters the nucleus and regulates the expression of steroid-responsive genes.

Although they are secreted in small quantities, mineralocorticoids, and mainly aldosterone, play a key role in the regulation of blood pressure through the renin–angiotensin–aldosterone system (Dembek *et al.*, 2013). Angiotensin, hypotension, plasma osmolality and plasma potassium are the main triggers for aldosterone production and secretion, but ACTH is another important regulator of aldosterone release (Guthrie *et al.*, 1982; Hart and Barton, 2011). As aldosterone mainly increases the activity of sodium channels, mineralocorticoid receptors are predominantly located on the renal tubular cells and the colon (Hart and Barton, 2011).

Glucocorticoids, and mainly cortisol, are the main hormones of the hypothalamo–pituitary–adrenocortical axis and are synthesized and released in large amounts after ACTH stimulation of melanocortin receptor 2 (MC2R) (Arlt and Stewart, 2005). Cortisol is not stored in adrenocortical cells and its synthesis and release is dependent on ACTH stimulation. As cortisol is a lipidic hormone, it is transported when bound to plasma protein and only 10% of circulating cortisol is present in its free and active form (Irvine and Alexander, 1987; Meyer and Rothuizen, 1993; Lewis *et al.*, 2005). Many types of cell express glucocorticoid receptors and cortisol plays a paramount role in the response to stress, increasing blood pressure, improving tissue perfusion and regulating inflammation (Hurcombe *et al.*,

2008; Hoffman *et al.*, 2015; Stewart *et al.*, 2019b). Another key role of cortisol is the regulation of the hypothalamo–pituitary–adrenocortical axis itself as cortisol is a potent down regulator of CRH secretion by the hypothalamus, of ACTH secretion by the pituitary gland and of mineralocorticoids, glucocorticoids and androgens secretion by the adrenal cortex.

Androgens are mainly secreted by testicles in males but in females they are predominantly secreted by the zona reticularis of the adrenal gland under ACTH stimulation. Androstenedione is metabolized into oestrogen and testosterone, which play a role in sexual development during puberty (Hart and Barton, 2011).

Dopamine, a peptide hormone of the catecholamine family, is the main melanotrope regulator. Released by hypothalamic nerves, dopamine interacts with dopamine D2 receptors on melanotropes located in the pars intermedia of the pituitary gland, to limit their proliferation and the synthesis and secretion of POMC (Saiardi and Borrelli, 1998). Another regulator of POMC secretion by melanotropes of clinical interest is the thyrotropin-releasing hormone (TRH) (McFarlane *et al.*, 2006). Although both corticotropes and melanotropes secrete POMC, post-translational processing of the peptide differs. While corticotropes mainly express prohormone convertase 1 leading to the secretion of a large amount of ACTH, melanotropes express prohormone convertase 1 and prohormone convertase 2 leading to the secretion of smaller amounts of ACTH and a larger amount of α-MSH and CLIP (Fig. 4.1(B)) (McFarlane, 2011).

The physiological role of α-MSH and CLIP is unclear. Melanocortin receptor 1 (MC1R) is found in the skin and is associated with skin and coat colour: receptor mutation in chestnut horses and high receptor density in grey horses (Altmeyer *et al.*, 1984; Marklund *et al.*, 1996). Melanocortin receptors 3 and 4 (MC3R and MC4R) are present in the central nervous system and are involved in the leptin–melanocortin pathway responsible for appetite regulation and fat metabolism (Nahon, 2006). Subjects with receptor 3 or 4 mutation are more likely to be obese (Donaldson *et al.*, 2004b; Clément, 2006). Another alpha-melanocyte function is modulation of the inflammatory and innate immune response with a decreased activation of nuclear factor kappa-light-chain-enhancer of activated B-cells (NFKB), a potent proinflammatory transcription factor, and a decreased neutrophilic function (Catania and Lipton, 1993; McFarlane *et al.*, 2015). One of the functions of clinical relevance for CLIP is its role as a direct stimulator of pancreatic beta cells leading to insulin secretion (Frank and Tadros, 2014). A strong, yet poorly understood, effect of seasons on the activity of pituitary pars intermedia is demonstrated with higher secretion of POMC-derived peptides in autumn (McFarlane, 2011; Copas and Durham, 2012; Cordero *et al.*, 2012; Diez de Castro *et al.*, 2014; Rendle *et al.*, 2014). This seasonality might be related to changes in metabolic needs with adaptation to seasons of food abundance and seasons of food scarcity.

Pituitary Pars Intermedia Dysfunction

PPID, previously known as equine Cushing's disease, is a common geriatric endocrinopathy of the equine population worldwide (Karikoski *et al.*, 2011; McGowan *et al.*, 2013a; Menzies-Gow, 2018). The disease has been the focus of extensive research and recent studies have allowed a better understanding of the disease; however, the fine details of the pathophysiology of this disorder and the association with its clinical signs are still to be unravelled. The more recent description of equine metabolic syndrome (EMS) and insulin dysregulation (ID) has allowed a better definition of the disorder and its association with laminitis, but more research is still required in this field (McGowan *et al.*, 2004; Asplin *et al.*, 2007; Frank and Tadros, 2014).

Epidemiology of pituitary pars intermedia dysfunction

PPID is a disease of old horses and is rarely reported in horses younger than 10 years of age (Orth *et al.*, 1982). Therefore, it is virtually impossible to dissociate the epidemiology of this disease from the demographic analysis of the equine population. Although there is no consensus on the definition of an old horse, the proportion of horses considered old increases worldwide (Miller *et al.*, 2016). Recent studies have described that between 25% and 30% of horses were older than 15 years of age and that, in some regions, the proportion of horses considered old increased from less than 20% in 2005 to more than 30% in 2018 (Cole *et al.*, 2005; McGowan *et al.*, 2010; Ireland *et al.*, 2011). As a consequence of this ageing population and also as a result of expanded interest about this condition in recent years, the prevalence of PPID has increased, making it one of the most common equine endocrinopathies (Rohrbach *et al.*, 2012; McGowan *et al.*, 2013a; Horn *et al.*, 2019a). In the general hospitalized population, PPID is around 10% while in some specific groups in which older horses are more common, the prevalence of the disease can reach 20% to 40% (Brosnahan and Paradis, 2003; McGowan *et al.*, 2013b) It is assumed that the actual prevalence of the disease could be even higher as many of these studies are based on owner questionnaires; some of the horses in the early stages of the disease and appearing normal without any obvious clinical sign could be missed (Couëtil *et al.*, 1996; Couëtil and Hoffman, 1998; Perkins *et al.*, 2002). The breed predisposition of PPID is unclear with some studies describing a possible predisposition in ponies and Quarter Horses; however, most studies have failed to confirm these findings, suggesting a possible bias (Donaldson *et al.*, 2002, 2004a; Rohrbach *et al.*, 2012). Similarly, the sex predisposition in PPID seems controversial (Miller *et al.*, 2016). On one hand, most studies have failed to find any gender predisposition while on the other, a few studies have identified some association in either the gelding or the female sex (Heinrichs *et al.*, 1990; van der Kolk *et al.*, 1993; Couëtil *et al.*, 1996; Rohrbach *et al.*, 2012; McGowan *et al.*, 2013b). In one study, the apparent predisposition of females was explained by the confounding effect of longer female survival rather than actual predisposition, but the small sample size of this study prevents further interpretation (Rohrbach *et al.*, 2012). In human medicine, however, there is a clear predisposition for women to develop Cushing's disease, presumably due to the involvement of sex hormones in the pathogenesis of the human disease (Clayton *et al.*, 2011; Tjörnstrand *et al.*, 2014; Carluccio *et al.*, 2015).

Pathophysiology of pituitary pars intermedia dysfunction

PPID is very different from the canine and human counterparts and the use of the term 'equine Cushing's disease' is therefore strongly discouraged to prevent confusion. Unlike Cushing's disease in humans and dogs, where the condition results from hyperplasia or benign neoplasia of the pituitary pars anterior or adrenal gland, PPID in horses results from a micro- or macroadenoma or hyperplasia of the pars intermedia of the pituitary gland (Halmi *et al.*, 1981; Orth *et al.*, 1982; Wilson *et al.*, 1982; Leroux and Pelletier, 1984; Doniach, 1985; Ikeda *et al.*, 1988). Degeneration of hypothalamic dopaminergic neurons is thought to result in a loss of tonic inhibition of melanotropes located in the pars intermedia of the pituitary gland and, in the absence of inhibition, melanotrope activity increases resulting in adenoma formation (Fig. 4.2) (Millington *et al.*, 1988; McFarlane *et al.*, 2005a). In these horses, the pars intermedia dopamine concentration is decreased by a factor of 8 (Millington *et al.*, 1988). The reason for the loss of hypothalamic dopaminergic inhibition is unclear; some of the pathophysiology of this disease is shared with Parkinson's disease in humans, with oxidative stress and accumulation of misfolded alpha-synuclein leading to neurodegeneration (McFarlane *et al.*, 2005a; McFarlane, 2011).

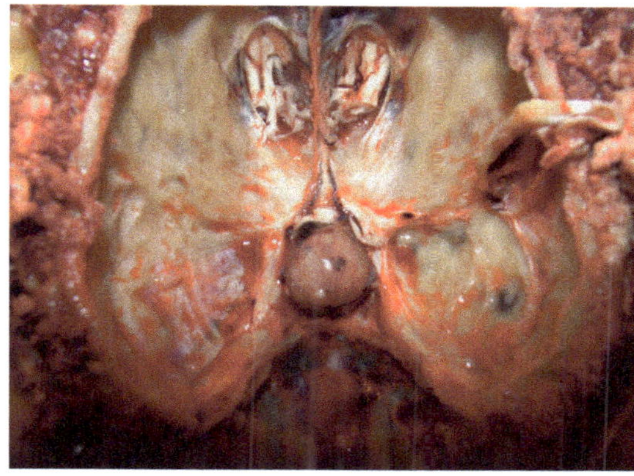

Fig. 4.2. Pituitary adenoma in a 22-year-old Stockhorse mare with pituitary pars intermedia dysfunction (PPID) (Author's own diagram).

At the level of the pituitary gland, both corticotropes located in the pars distalis and melanotropes located in the pars intermedia produce POMC which is then cleaved into ACTH and beta-lipotropin by the prohormone convertase 1 (Fig. 4.1). The production and secretion of ACTH from corticotropes in the pars distalis are under the glucocorticoid negative feedback loop, while the production and secretion of ACTH from melanotropes in the pars intermedia are entirely under hypothalamic dopaminergic regulation (McFarlane *et al.*, 2004; Beech *et al.*, 2009; Schreiber *et al.*, 2012). As stated previously, in healthy horses the majority of ACTH originates from the pars distalis and, due to hypothalamic inhibition, only small amounts originate from the pars intermedia (McFarlane, 2011). In horses with PPID, however, due to the decreased hypothalamic inhibition of the pars intermedia, a dysregulated POMC secretion is observed and excessive amounts of ACTH originating from the pars intermedia are released (McFarlane, 2011). Once released, ACTH is cleaved into α-MSH and CLIP by prohormone convertase 2 (Fig. 4.1); however, in horses with PPID, a mutation in the prohormone convertase 2 sequence reduces conversion of ACTH into α-MSH, resulting in excessive plasma concentrations of an ACTH peptide with low bioactivity (McFarlane *et al.*, 2005a; Haritou *et al.*, 2008; Beech *et al.*, 2009; Cordero *et al.*, 2011; Copas and Durham, 2012; Carmalt *et al.*, 2018). This mutation, resulting in a decreased ACTH bioactivity in horses with PPID, would explain the variable and unreliable increases in cortisol concentration in these horses (Cordero *et al.*, 2011). The exact consequences of increased concentrations of POMC by-products are still poorly understood (Haritou *et al.*, 2008; Beech *et al.*, 2009; Copas and Durham, 2012). CLIP and α-MSH, as stimulators of insulin secretion, could link PPID and ID, while α-MSH, as an immunomodulator, could explain the impaired neutrophilic function and the increased rate of infections in horses with PPID (Marshall *et al.*, 1984; McFarlane and Holbrook, 2008; Frank and Tadros, 2014; McFarlane *et al.*, 2015).

Clinical signs of pituitary pars intermedia dysfunction

The clinical signs of advanced PPID are well described and easily recognized by owners and veterinarians (Fig. 4.3). They include hypertrichosis (or delayed and incomplete shedding), lameness (associated or not with laminitis), tachypnoea, muscle atrophy (characterized by the loss of type-2 myofibres), lethargy, abnormal fat distribution (including in the supraorbital fossa), weight loss, pendulous abdomen, abnormal perspiration including hyperhidrosis or anhidrosis and polyuria/polydipsia (Couëtil *et al.*, 1996; Perkins *et al.*, 2002; Frank *et al.*, 2006; Rohrbach *et al.*, 2012; McGowan *et al.*, 2013b; Horn *et al.*, 2019b). The clinical picture of PPID has been reported to vary depending on season, latitude, hours of daylight, percentage of humidity, ambient temperature and rainfalls (Horn *et al.*, 2019b). Additional clinical signs can be present, as PPID is associated with a higher rate of infections mainly involving the respiratory, gastrointestinal, ocular and integumentary systems (Sgorbini *et al.*, 2004; Horn *et al.*, 2019b). Therefore, in such cases, a history of recurrent sinusitis, chronic tooth disease, endoparasitism or non-healing corneal ulcers is common (McFarlane *et al.*, 2010; Miller *et al.*, 2013; Berryhill *et al.*, 2017). Less commonly, severe neurological impairment with ataxia, blindness or seizures is reported but these signs are limited to an advanced stage of the disease, with large pituitary adenomas pressing on other parts of the nervous system (McFarlane, 2011).

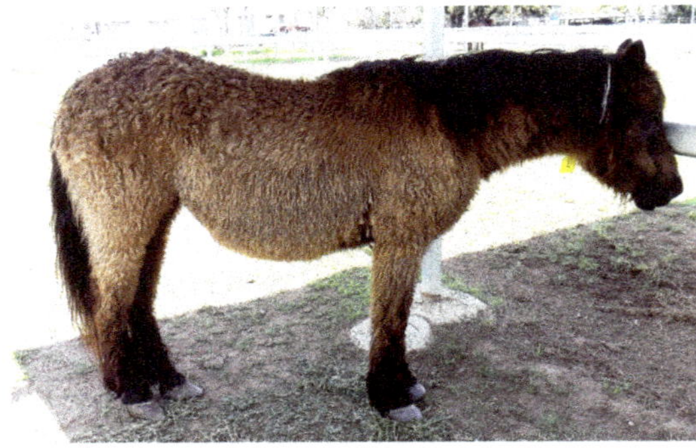

Fig. 4.3. Pathognomonic presentation of pituitary pars intermedia dysfunction (PPID) in a 24-year-old Australian Stockhorse mare. Note the severe hypertrichosis and the muscle atrophy (Author's own photograph).

Diagnosis of pituitary pars intermedia dysfunction

A clinical diagnosis based on the presence of hypertrichosis and another one of the most common clinical signs of PPID is common practice; however, a clinical diagnosis is considered a late diagnostic tool with high specificity but low sensitivity (Couëtil *et al.*, 1996; Perkins *et al.*, 2002; Frank *et al.*, 2006; Miller *et al.*, 2008). Complete blood count is a poor indicator of PPID with inconsistent lymphopoenia, neutrophilia and hyperfibrinogenaemia (McGowan *et al.*, 2013b; Horn *et al.*, 2019a). Serum chemistry is also poorly specific with hyperglycaemia, increased gamma-glutamyl transferase and aspartate aminotransferase activities, as well as hyperproteinaemia, being the most common parameters outside reference intervals (Rohrbach *et al.*, 2012; McGowan *et al.*, 2013b; Horn *et al.*, 2019a).

Gross examination of the pituitary gland and histopathology are considered as a confirmative

Table 4.1. Histological grading of pituitary pars intermedia lesions in horses. Adapted from Miller *et al.*, 2008.

Grade	Description
1	Within normal limit, no hypertrophy, no hyperplasia
2	Focal or multifocal pituitary pars intermedia hypertrophy or hyperplasia
3	Diffuse pituitary pars intermedia adenomatous hyperplasia
4	Pituitary pars intermedia adenomatous hyperplasia with microadenomas ranging from 1 to 5 mm in diameter
5	Adenoma of the pituitary pars intermedia larger than 5 mm in diameter

'gold standard' for a diagnosis of PPID with identification of the adenomatous hyperplasia or adenoma of the pituitary pars intermedia; however, the size and internal architecture of the pituitary gland experience physiological seasonal changes and need to be taken into account to properly establish a diagnosis (Dybdal *et al.*, 1994; McFarlane *et al.*, 2005a, b; Cordero *et al.*, 2012; Miller *et al.*, 2008, 2016). A five-grade histological scale has been developed to assess the severity of pituitary pars intermedia lesions (Table 4.1) (Miller *et al.*, 2008). Although there may only be a mild agreement between pathologists when grading pituitary lesions, this grading system correlates well with ACTH concentrations after dynamic testing (McFarlane *et al.*, 2005b; Frank *et al.*, 2006; Miller *et al.*, 2008).

Additional extrapituitary lesions identified during necropsy of PPID include laminitis, osteoarthritis, hoof abscesses and deformations, bone fracture, fetlock hyperextension and muscle atrophy (Boujon *et al.*, 1993; Aleman *et al.*, 2006; Spelta and Axon, 2012; Wylie *et al.*, 2013; Hofberger *et al.*, 2015; Mastro *et al.*, 2015; Shepard *et al.*, 2015).

Contrast-enhanced computed tomography and magnetic resonance imaging have been shown to be potentially helpful in the diagnosis of PPID as these techniques can identify pars intermedia enlargements in a manner comparable to gross postmortem examination; however, similar adjustments for seasonal changes are also required (Pease *et al.*, 2011).

Specific endocrine testing for PPID can be historically divided into three categories: the tests using ACTH as an end point; the tests using cortisol as an end point; and the tests using another end point. The interpretation of these tests is always challenging as PPID is a slowly progressive disease; however, the understanding of the disease has improved in the last few decades, and with it our ability to interpret testing results. For example, the strong effect of season on the equine hypothalamo–pituitary–adrenocortical axis has only been demonstrated in the early 2000s, and the changes in endocrine assays have limited the ability to compare studies from different research groups (Donaldson *et al.*, 2005; Beech *et al.*, 2009). In all cases, when the results of diagnostic testing are unclear or do not match the clinical picture, repeat testing is warranted.

Tests using adrenocorticotropic hormone as an end point

Considering the pathophysiology of PPID, determination of ACTH concentration is an attractive diagnostic tool and is the most commonly measured analyte to establish a diagnosis (McGowan *et al.*, 2013b; Horn *et al.*, 2019a).

ENDOGENOUS OR BASELINE ADRENOCORTICOTROPIC HORMONE. Measurement of plasma ACTH in horses suspected of PPID is the most common screening and diagnostic test (Horn *et al.*, 2019a). As mentioned above, in control horses, most of the ACTH is secreted from the pars distalis under glucocorticoid negative feedback, whereas in horses with PPID, most of the ACTH is secreted from the pars intermedia in an unregulated fashion and at high concentrations; therefore, an increased ACTH concentration is diagnostic for PPID and is a good estimation of the pars intermedia function (Couëtil *et al.*, 1996; Miller *et al.*, 2008; Beech *et al.*, 2009). The definition of an increased concentration of ACTH has been controversial and a wide range of reference intervals and diagnostic cut-off values have been published (McGowan *et al.*, 2013a; Secombe *et al.*, 2017; McGowan, 2018). The limitation of some of these studies is the lack of inclusion of both positive and negative horses, as well as the absence of age-matched controls to properly determine reference intervals and diagnostic cut-off values in a relevant population (Jacob *et al.*, 2018; McGowan, 2018; Horn *et al.*, 2019b). This interpretation is further complicated by the physiological circannual variation in ACTH concentration (Beech *et al.*, 2009; Schreiber *et al.*, 2012). Changes in photoperiod have a direct impact on hypothalamo–pituitary–adrenocortical activity resulting in physiologically higher concentrations of ACTH in autumn (McFarlane, 2011; Copas and Durham, 2012; Cordero *et al.*, 2012; Diez de Castro *et al.*, 2014; Rendle *et al.*, 2014). This effect would also be amplified by geographic location, latitude and climate (McFarlane *et al.*, 2011; Copas and Durham, 2012; Secombe *et al.*, 2017; Byrne *et al.*, 2018). The physiological increase in ACTH concentration has been shown to be even greater in horses with PPID and autumn had previously been proposed to be the optimal season to test horses (Beech *et al.*, 2009). However, more recent data in a larger sample suggest that there is more variability in ACTH concentrations in autumn, potentially limiting the accuracy of endogenous ACTH as a diagnostic tool during this season (Jacob *et al.*, 2018; Horn *et al.*, 2019a). In addition to this physiological variation, many factors such as stress, inflammation and exercise have been shown to increase ACTH concentration and could confound the interpretation of the concentration of this hormone (Alexander *et al.*, 1988, 1991; Nagata *et al.*, 1999; Fazio *et al.*, 2008; Stewart *et al.*, 2019a). Another important factor to be considered when interpreting an ACTH concentration is the poor stability of the compound. As a peptide, ACTH is prone to proteolytic degradation; therefore, close attention must be paid when handling samples (Evans *et al.*, 2001; Jane Ellis *et al.*, 2003). Delayed centrifugation, storage at room temperature, multiple freeze–thaw cycles, presence of haemolysis and collection in glass tubes have all been shown to modify ACTH concentrations in unpredictable manners, with some spurious increases or decreases limiting the interpretation of a single value (Talbot *et al.*, 2003; Rendle *et al.*, 2009, 2015; Oddoze *et al.*, 2012; Prutton *et al.*, 2015; Hillebrand *et al.*, 2017; Hinrichsen *et al.*, 2019; Stewart *et al.*, 2019a; Hu *et al.*, 2020). Finally, different laboratories use various assays and different assays do not provide similar results. As most assays are immunoassays, the antibodies used to detect ACTH will vary, leading to different concentrations of immunoreactive ACTH (Schreiber *et al.*, 2012; Knowles *et al.*, 2018). For example, the radioimmunoassay used in most earlier studies provided lower results than the immunochemiluminescent assay currently used in most laboratories, limiting the use of historical data (Schreiber *et al.*, 2012; Banse *et al.*, 2018). Overall, the recommendation to optimize the test is to collect a blood sample from a quiet horse in a plastic ethylenediaminetetraacetic acid tube, chill the sample at 4°C (never frozen), centrifuge it within 1 h, and analyse it within 8 h at a local laboratory that has developed its own diagnostic cut-off values.

Thyrotropin-releasing hormone stimulation test. TRH physiologically stimulates the production of POMC-derived peptides, including ACTH and α-MSH, from the melanotropes located in the pars intermedia, as well as cortisol from the adrenal glands (Beech and Garcia, 1985; Danger *et al.*, 1989; Frank *et al.*, 2006; McFarlane *et al.*, 2006; Beech *et al.*, 2007, 2011a, b). After intravenous administration of 1 mg of TRH in horses and 0.5 mg in ponies, plasma ACTH concentration peaks at 10 min and slowly returns to baseline within approximately 1 h; therefore, blood samples can be taken at 10 and/or 30 min after TRH injection to measure ACTH concentration (Beech *et al.*, 2007, 2011a, b; Funk *et al.*, 2011; Horn and Bertin, 2019). Although ACTH concentration increases in both control and PPID horses, the increase of the hormone in the latter group of horses is larger and used for diagnosis (Beech *et al.*, 2007, 2011a, b). This test is safe with only minor side effects (yawning, flehmen, muscle trembling and coughing), is more sensitive than baseline endogenous ACTH concentration and is therefore recommended, especially for an early diagnosis of PPID (Beech *et al.*, 2007). As ACTH is the end point of this test, the same precautions regarding ACTH interpretation should be applied. After TRH, ACTH also follows a circannual variability and has a similar stability to baseline endogenous ACTH (Abraham *et al.*, 2011; Funk *et al.*, 2011; Byrne *et al.*, 2018; Hinrichsen *et al.*, 2019; Stewart *et al.*, 2019b).

Domperidone response test. Domperidone is a dopamine D2-receptor antagonist that blocks dopamine receptors on the pituitary pars intermedia melanotropes. Since most of the ACTH secreted by control horses originates from the corticotropes of the pars distalis and most of the ACTH secreted by PPID horses originates from the melanotropes of the pars intermedia, using a dopamine antagonist would only result in increases in ACTH in PPID horses (Miller *et al.*, 2008; Beech *et al.*, 2011b). ACTH concentration 8 h after oral administration of 3.3 mg/kg of domperidone correlates well with histological grades of the pituitary gland (Miller *et al.*, 2008). Although this test is physiologically sound, the time required to perform it has limited its use and only limited data are available. In addition, in one study, the TRH stimulation test appeared to diagnose PPID more accurately (Beech *et al.*, 2011b).

Tests using cortisol as an end point

Cortisol was a commonly measured hormone before the pathophysiology of PPID was better understood; however, as PPID differs from Cushing's syndrome as described in other species, the use of cortisol in the diagnosis of PPID is limited to a few tests.

Endogenous or baseline serum cortisol. Despite an increase in plasma ACTH in PPID horses, no consistent increase in serum cortisol is observed, limiting the value of determining cortisol concentration to diagnose PPID (Orth *et al.*, 1982; McFarlane *et al.*, 2006; McFarlane, 2011; Cordero *et al.*, 2012). The absence of a correlation between ACTH and cortisol in PPID horses is explained by the decreased bioactivity of ACTH originating from the pars intermedia of the pituitary gland (Cordero *et al.*, 2011). Similar to other hormones of the hypothalamo–pituitary–adrenocortical axis, cortisol has a circadian rhythm that has been explored as a diagnostic tool for PPID (Dybdal *et al.*, 1994; Cordero *et al.*, 2012). In PPID horses, the cortisol circadian rhythm would be disrupted in about 64% of these horses with erratic cortisol rhythms. This diagnostic test is therefore poorly appealing as it has limited specificity, requires multiple blood samples during a day and should be interpreted cautiously as age and stress alter cortisol variability (Alexander and Irvine, 1998; Cordero *et al.*, 2012). Determination of the free cortisol fraction would be more relevant than total cortisol as horses with PPID have a higher free cortisol fraction than control horses, despite a normal total cortisol fraction (Hart *et al.*, 2016).

Overnight dexamethasone suppression test. Dexamethasone is an exogenous glucocorticoid that triggers a negative feedback loop to inhibit ACTH secretion by the pituitary pars distalis corticotropes. In control horses, most of the secreted ACTH originates from the pars distalis and is inhibited by dexamethasone administration, while in PPID horses, most of the secreted ACTH originates from the pars intermedia and is not inhibited by dexamethasone administration. The dexamethasone-induced decrease in ACTH secretion in control horses results, a few hours later, in a suppression of cortisol secretion by the adrenal glands; a cortisol concentration of over 276 nmol/l indicates an absence of suppression and gives a diagnosis of PPID (Antakly and Eisen, 1984; Dybdal *et al.*, 1994). This test was previously the test of reference to diagnose PPID with a reported perfect sensitivity (Dybdal *et al.*, 1994; Bertin *et al.*, 2013). However, more recent data regarding the poor bioactivity of ACTH in PPID horses, the seasonality of the cortisol response, the possible risk of inducing iatrogenic laminitis and the necessity of a second visit at the farm by a veterinarian, 15 to 19 h after dexamethasone injection, have limited enthusiasm for the test (Schott, 2002; Donaldson *et al.*, 2005; Borer-Weir *et al.*, 2013). In addition, the sensitivity of the test has been shown to be lower than expected, based on combining necropsy findings with clinical appearance (Frank *et al.*, 2006). The combination of the overnight dexamethasone suppression test and the TRH stimulation test was proposed to improve the sensitivity and specificity of the test and provide a standard cortisol baseline; however, this combination only mildly improved the test characteristics despite requiring multiple injections and sampling (Frank *et al.*, 2006).

Adrenocorticotropic hormone stimulation test. This test is mentioned in earlier studies but considering the differences between PPID and Cushing's syndrome in other species, it has been shown to be of no value in diagnosis of PPID (Boujon *et al.*, 1993; Dybdal *et al.*, 1994).

Urinary cortisol/creatinine ratio. This test, useful in the diagnosis of canine hyperadrenocorticism, has been investigated in horses; however, no significant difference between control and PPID horses has been found and no satisfactory diagnostic cut-off values have been established (van der Kolk *et al.*, 1994, 1995; Chandler and Dixon, 2002; Zeugswetter *et al.*, 2017), Salivary cortisol concentration has also been investigated but further studies are necessary (van der Kolk *et al.*, 2001).

Tests using other end points

As the testing protocols described above have all shown limitations, newer targets have been explored; however, as PPID is a complex disease, it is unlikely that a single test will prove to have a perfect sensitivity and specificity.

Plasma alpha-melanocyte-stimulating hormone. Concentration of α-MSH is a direct expression of melanotrope activity and therefore an attractive proxy to assess pars intermedia function. Although more data are required, increased endogenous α-MSH is highly indicative of PPID, and the sensitivity and specificity of increased α-MSH, either endogenous or after TRH stimulation, are high (McFarlane *et al.*, 2006, 2011; Beech *et al.*, 2009, 2011b; Funk *et al.*, 2011; McGowan *et al.*, 2013a). Unfortunately, this assay is not commercially available and is only used in research settings; however, it would appear to be a promising tool.

Serum insulin. Serum insulin is commonly increased in horses with PPID (van der Kolk *et al.*, 1995; Schott, 2002; Keen *et al.*, 2004; McGowan *et al.*, 2004; Beech *et al.*, 2009; Horn *et al.*, 2019a). However, rather than being an indicator of PPID, hyperinsulinaemia is an indicator of ID, associated or not with EMS (Bertin and de Laat, 2017). As both conditions can coexist in the same animal, it is good practice to monitor insulin concentration when assessing a case for PPID, but this has a prognostic value rather than a diagnostic value (McGowan *et al.*, 2004; Horn *et al.*, 2019a). Cortisol is an insulin antagonist and erratic cortisol secretion would result in hyperinsulinaemia; CLIP is an insulin secretagogue (Frank and Tadros, 2014). The association between PPID and ID needs further exploration.

Overall, the diagnosis of PPID is performed by determination of endogenous basal ACTH concentration and can be improved by performing a TRH stimulation test. Although there are some limitations to measuring ACTH, it is the best analyte currently available to establish a diagnosis.

Treatment of pituitary pars intermedia dysfunction

Pergolide mesylate is the most commonly prescribed drug to manage PPID (Rohrbach *et al.*, 2012; Horn *et al.*, 2019a). Pergolide is a dopamine D2-receptor agonist that restores the dopaminergic inhibition of the hypothalamus on the pituitary pars intermedia (Muñoz *et al.*, 1996; Donaldson *et al.*, 2002). Treatment is usually started at 2 µg/kg (1 mg for a 500 kg horse) once a day orally and the dose is increased by a 1 µg/kg increment depending on clinical response and retesting results (Horn *et al.*, 2019a). Data regarding the pharmacokinetics of pergolide would indicate that an administration twice daily could provide a more consistent dopaminergic inhibition, but further research is warranted (Rendle *et al.*, 2019). After initiating treatment, improvement is expected after 4 to 8 weeks, so the dose of pergolide should not be re-evaluated before 6 to 8 weeks of treatment (Durham, 2017). At that time, clinical evaluation is recommended, and a basal endogenous ACTH or TRH stimulation test can be used to evaluate the degree of pars intermedia inhibition. As pergolide does not cure PPID but only restores dopaminergic inhibition, there is no need to stop treatment before retesting horses to assess response to treatment. The maximum recommended dose of pergolide is 14 µg/kg (7 mg for a 500 kg horse); however, doses of 16 µg/kg have been used in severe cases (Horn *et al.*, 2019a). At high doses, some minor side effects have been reported with anorexia being the most frequent (Durham, 2017). These side effects are uncommon and can be managed by reducing the dose or administering half the dose, twice a day. As the disease is progressive, more than a third of horses will require some dose increases during their lives and lifelong treatment is recommended (McFarlane, 2011; Horn *et al.*, 2019a). In a retrospective study, 44% of the horses receiving pergolide had ACTH concentrations within reference intervals and horses receiving pergolide were 3.8 times more likely to survive (Horn *et al.*, 2019a). Due to the seasonal variations in ACTH concentrations, some clinicians have elected to only treat mild cases of PPID during autumnal months; however, there is no data to support this approach. Depending on the country of practice, different forms of pergolide are available. It should be noted that pergolide is poorly stable in aqueous solutions and needs to be stored in the dark at 4°C and used within 30 days (Davis *et al.*, 2009; Shank and Ofner, 2009, 2010). This could be an issue with compounded pergolide when large amounts are bought at once and stored in a barn.

Other dopamine agonists such as bromocriptine and cabergoline have been used but limited data are available (Durham, 2017).

Cyproheptadine is another drug that has been used in the treatment of PPID. Cyproheptadine is a serotonin antagonist with antihistamine and anti-muscarinic effects that decreases ACTH secretion from the corticotropes (Ishibashi and Yamaji, 1981). Used alone, it has very little action but used in combination with pergolide, when maximal doses of pergolide have been reached, it can provide some beneficial effects (Donaldson *et al.*, 2002; Perkins *et al.*, 2002).

Trilostane has also been used to manage PPID. Trilostane is a competitive inhibitor of the 3β-hydroxysteroid dehydrogenase resulting in a decreased conversion of cholesterol into cortisol (Singh-Asa *et al.*, 1982). This drug has no effect on the pituitary gland and only a few horses with PPID develop some degree of adrenal hyperplasia; therefore, this drug has very limited relevance in the treatment of PPID (McGowan and Neiger, 2003; McGowan *et al.*, 2004).

Geriatric care is paramount in the management of PPID. Specifically, these horses need excellent hoof care, dental care and endoparasite control (McFarlane *et al.*, 2010; Horn *et al.*, 2019a). Due to decreased neutrophilic function, close attention to infections can help limit secondary illnesses (McFarlane *et al.*, 2015). Proper nutrition is also crucial in these horses as maintaining a good body condition score has been shown to be associated with survival (Horn *et al.*, 2019a). Investigation of ID is a key element when deciding on a diet for a geriatric horse in order to limit the risk of laminitis, but commercial 'senior' diets are usually well balanced. Excessive haircoat might require clipping to help with thermoregulation and limit the risk of skin infections.

Although PPID can be managed with lifelong medication, it is currently an incurable disease that carries a guarded prognosis, as half of the horses diagnosed with this disease are euthanized within 5 years of detection. However, better diagnostic tools, availability of pergolide and proper geriatric care would improve the prognosis of this condition (Rohrbach *et al.*, 2012; Spelta and Axon, 2012).

Adrenocortical Insufficiency

Permanent adrenocortical insufficiency is rare in horses, with only a few case reports of sustained hypoadrenocorticism, and Addison's disease is not recognized as an equine disorder (Dowling *et al.*, 1993; Couëtil and Hoffman, 1998; Hart and Barton, 2011). Rare cases of transient adrenal insufficiency following discontinuation of long-term corticosteroid therapy and chronic stress have been reported in racehorses; however, the evidence for real insufficiency is weak overall (Dybdal *et al.*, 1980; Baker *et al.*, 1982; Dowling *et al.*, 1993). On the other hand, in horses with systemic inflammation, a relative, transient and reversible adrenocortical insufficiency is becoming an emerging syndrome of clinical relevance (Stewart *et al.*, 2019a).

Pathogenesis of adrenocortical insufficiency

Transient and reversible adrenocortical insufficiency, or relative adrenal insufficiency (RAI) or critical illness-related corticosteroid insufficiency (CIRCI), would result from one or a combination of the following mechanisms: suppression of the hypothalamo–pituitary–adrenocortical axis by inhibition of CRH secretion from the hypothalamus; inhibition of ACTH secretion by the pituitary gland; decreased sensitivity to CRH or ACTH; exhaustion of cortisol secretion capacity; and decreased sensitivity to cortisol (Marik and Zaloga, 2002; Marik, 2007, 2009). The specific mechanisms by which RAI develops are unknown but presence of a critical illness and development of sepsis would be the main predisposing factors in both humans and horses (Soni *et al.*, 1995; Kenyon, 2003; Marik and Zaloga, 2003; Annane *et al.*, 2006; Spurzem, 2007; Hart *et al.*, 2009, 2011; Vila-Pérez and Jordan-García, 2015). The use of specific drugs such as ketoconazole, rifampicin or etomidate have been shown to inhibit cortisol synthesis in septic patients and could exacerbate adrenocortical insufficiency (Mohammad *et al.*, 2006; Marik, 2009; Mosier *et al.*, 2015). In addition, the release of proinflammatory cytokine during severe sepsis such as tumour necrosis factor α or interleukin 1 beta, as well as endotoxaemia have also been shown to decrease both ACTH and cortisol release (Marik *et al.*, 2002; Marik, 2009).

Diagnosis of adrenocortical insufficiency

In the absence of a clear definition of adrenocortical insufficiency, the diagnosis of the condition is challenging. Two types of test have been developed: static tests investigating ACTH and cortisol concentrations and dynamic tests investigating the cortisol response after ACTH stimulation (Wong *et al.*, 2009).

As hormones of the hypothalamo–pituitary–adrenocortical axis are secreted in a pulsatile fashion, caution is warranted when establishing a diagnosis of adrenocortical insufficiency based on a single value obtained at one timepoint (Mair *et al.*, 2014; Stewart *et al.*, 2019a). In order to improve the diagnostic value of a baseline, ACTH and cortisol ratios have been investigated; however, no clear diagnostic cut-off values have been described (Hart *et al.*, 2007; Dembek *et al.*, 2017; Stewart *et al.*, 2019a). It is also important to note that, in addition to the physiological changes of the hypothalamo–pituitary–adrenocortical axis, horses with systemic inflammation are in a dynamic state with changes in their disease status and response; therefore, endocrine testing might need to be repeated as the patient progresses (Hassan-Smith and Cooper, 2011).

The most common test to diagnose adrenocortical insufficiency is the ACTH stimulation test with serum cortisol measured 20–30 min after intravenous or intramuscular injection of ACTH. Several doses have been used to diagnose the condition, depending on the severity of the disorder anticipated. The use of a high-dose test (1–2 μg/kg) is indicated when a severe disease is suspected with complete disruption of the axis, while the use of a low-dose test (0.01–0.20 μg/kg) is more accurate to diagnose milder cases and would be more relevant in the diagnosis of transient and reversible adrenocortical insufficiency (Wong *et al.*, 2009; Stewart *et al.*, 2013). The main limitation of this test, regardless of the dose of ACTH used, is the partial investigation of the hypothalamo–pituitary–adrenocortical axis in the context of adrenocortical insufficiency. As the origin of the disorder can stem from anywhere between the hypothalamus and the cortisol target tissues, investigation of the zone fasciculata response to exogenous ACTH only offers a limited diagnostic ability.

Additional hormones such as aldosterone, progesterone and arginine vasopressin (AVP) have been investigated to diagnose adrenocortical insufficiency. The combination of baseline concentrations, concentrations after ACTH stimulation or ratios between different hormone concentrations, has been reported as a diagnostic tool; however, measurement of these analytes in critical cases appears limited to specific centres (Dembek *et al.*, 2017, 2019; Stewart *et al.*, 2019a).

Considering the absence of a clear definition of the disorder limiting the interpretation of the diagnostic tests, clinical judgement is paramount in the diagnosis and management of these cases.

Adrenocortical insufficiency in foals

Unlike other species, the maturation of the equine hypothalamo–pituitary–adrenocortical axis occurs in the final days of gestation and continues for a few weeks after parturition; therefore, foals have a physiological adrenocortical insufficiency at birth with low cortisol concentrations and high ACTH concentrations (Silver *et al.*, 1984; Wong *et al.*, 2009; Hart *et al.*, 2011). This low zona fasciculata activity in foals is caused by a paucity in enzymes necessary for cortisol synthesis in the early days of life (Han *et al.*, 1995). The immaturity of the hypothalamo–pituitary–adrenocortical axis in foals complicates the interpretation of the ACTH stimulation test, with a possible overestimation of cases. Potentially up to 50% of all hospitalized foals may show some degree of adrenocortical insufficiency (Hart *et al.*, 2009). Although a diagnostic cut-off value is not defined, a low cortisol response to exogenous ACTH administration has been shown to be associated with poorer survival and increased odds of developing shock and multi-organ dysfunction syndrome (Hart *et al.*, 2009). Another point of difference between foals and adults is the proportion between bound and free cortisol. In foals, the proportion of free cortisol is between 3 and 12 times higher than in adults, and as free cortisol is more rapidly excreted and metabolized than bound cortisol, foals have a higher cortisol clearance rate than adults (Bright, 1995; Hart *et al.*, 2011).

Clinically, foals with adrenocortical insufficiency present with similar signs as septic neonates; however, the severity of the clinical signs would be more severe with serum electrolyte abnormalities characterized by hyponatraemia (Couëtil and Hoffman, 1998).

Aggressive management of the initiating condition is recommended and cortisol replacement therapy with hydrocortisone at 1–4 mg/kg/day administered in 4 to 6 treatments is suggested;

however, there has not been any critical evaluation of such a treatment (Hart and Barton, 2011).

Adrenocortical insufficiency in adult horses

In healthy adult horses, the hypothalamo–pituitary–adrenocortical axis is fully functional and resting cortisol concentrations are similar to what has been described in other species with a larger effect of season (Lefcourt *et al.*, 1993; Martin *et al.*, 2007; Place *et al.*, 2010). Similar to what is described in foals, sick adult horses with low cortisol concentration despite a high ACTH concentration suggestive of adrenocortical insufficiency, are less likely to survive (Stewart *et al.*, 2019b). In more mature adults, the interpretation of baseline ACTH and cortisol concentrations is however complicated by the possible presence of subclinical PPID resulting in higher ACTH concentrations without changes in cortisol concentrations (Orth *et al.*, 1982; McFarlane *et al.*, 2006; McFarlane, 2011; Cordero *et al.*, 2012).

The clinical description of adult horses with adrenocortical insufficiency is limited and, similar to that described in foals, signs of severe sepsis are reported (Stewart *et al.*, 2019a). Anecdotal reports of iatrogenic adrenocortical insufficiency subsequent to prolonged administration of exogenous glucocorticoids have described horses with poor performance, lethargy, anorexia or oestral disorders (Dowling *et al.*, 1993; Hedberg *et al.*, 2007).

Management of the underlying condition is recommended and replacement therapy with hydrocortisone would be indicated; however, there is no evidence to support this statement.

References

Abraham, G., Allersmeier, M., Schusser, G.F. and Ungemach, F.R. (2011) Serum thyroid hormone, insulin, glucose, triglycerides and protein concentrations in normal horses: association with topical dexamethasone usage. *The Veterinary Journal* 188(3), 307–312. DOI: 10.1016/j.tvjl.2010.05.033.

Aleman, M., Watson, J.L., Williams, D.C., LeCouteur, R.A., Nieto, J.E. *et al.* (2006) Myopathy in horses with pituitary pars intermedia dysfunction (Cushing's disease). *Neuromuscular Disorders* 16(11), 737–744. DOI: 10.1016/j.nmd.2006.07.019.

Alesci, S., Koch, C.A., Bornstein, S.R. and Pacak, K. (2001) Adrenal androgens regulation and adrenopause. *Endocrine Regulations* 35(2), 95–100.

Alexander, S.L. and Irvine, C.H. (1998) The effect of social stress on adrenal axis activity in horses: the importance of monitoring corticosteroid-binding globulin capacity. *Journal of Endocrinology* 157(3), 425–432. DOI: 10.1677/joe.0.1570425.

Alexander, S.L., Irvine, C.H.G., Livesey, J.H. and Donald, R.A. (1988) Effect of isolation stress on concentrations of arginine vasopressin, α-melanocyte-stimulating hormone and ACTH in the pituitary venous effluent of the normal horse. *Journal of Endocrinology* 116(3), 325–334. DOI: 10.1677/joe.0.1160325.

Alexander, S.L., Irvine, C.H.G., Ellis, M.J. and Donald, R.A. (1991) The effect of acute exercise on the secretion of corticotropin-releasing factor, arginine vasopressin, and adrenocorticotropin as measured in pituitary venous blood from the horse. *Endocrinology* 128(1), 65–72. DOI: 10.1210/endo-128-1-65.

Altmeyer, P., Holzmann, H., Stöhr, L. and Koch, H.-J. (1984) The relationship between α-MSH level and coat color in white Camarque horses. *Journal of Investigative Dermatology* 82(2), 199–201. DOI: 10.1111/1523-1747.ep12259846.

Annane, D., Maxime, V., Ibrahim, F., Alvarez, J.C., Abe, E. *et al.* (2006) Diagnosis of adrenal insufficiency in severe sepsis and septic shock. *American Journal of Respiratory and Critical Care Medicine* 174(12), 1319–1326. DOI: 10.1164/rccm.200509-1369OC.

Antakly, T. and Eisen, H.J. (1984) Immunocytochemical localization of glucocorticoid receptor in target cells. *Endocrinology* 115(5), 1984–1989. DOI: 10.1210/endo-115-5-1984.

Arlt, W. and Stewart, P.M. (2005) Adrenal corticosteroid biosynthesis, metabolism, and action. *Endocrinology and Metabolism Clinics of North America* 34(2), 293–313. DOI: 10.1016/j.ecl.2005.01.002.

Asplin, K.E., Sillence, M.N., Pollitt, C.C. and McGowan, C.M. (2007) Induction of laminitis by prolonged hyperinsulinaemia in clinically normal ponies. *The Veterinary Journal* 174(3), 530–535. DOI: 10.1016/j.tvjl.2007.07.003.

Baker, H.W.G., Baker, I.D.C., Epstein, V.M. and Hudson, B. (1982) Effect of stress on steroid hormone levels in racehorses. *Australian Veterinary Journal* 58(2), 70–71. DOI: 10.1111/j.1751-0813.1982.tb02692.x.

Banse, H.E., Schultz, N., McCue, M., Geor, R. and McFarlane, D. (2018) Comparison of two methods for measurement of equine adrenocorticotropin. *Journal of Veterinary Diagnostic Investigation* 30(2), 233–237. DOI: 10.1177/1040638717752216.

Beech, J. and Garcia, M. (1985) Hormonal response to thyrotropin-releasing hormone in healthy horses and in horses with pituitary adenoma. *American Journal of Veterinary Research* 46(9), 1941–1943.

Beech, J., Boston, R., Lindborg, S. and Russell, G.E. (2007) Adrenocorticotropin concentration following administration of thyrotropin-releasing hormone in healthy horses and those with pituitary pars intermedia dysfunction and pituitary gland hyperplasia. *Journal of the American Veterinary Medical*

Association 231(3), 417–426. DOI: 10.2460/javma.231.3.417.

Beech, J., Boston, R.C., McFarlane, D. and Lindborg, S. (2009) Evaluation of plasma ACTH, α-melanocyte–stimulating hormone, and insulin concentrations during various photoperiods in clinically normal horses and ponies and those with pituitary pars intermedia dysfunction. *Journal of the American Veterinary Medical Association* 235(6), 715–722. DOI: 10.2460/javma.235.6.715.

Beech, J., Boston, R. and Lindborg, S. (2011a) Comparison of cortisol and ACTH responses after administration of thyrotropin releasing hormone in normal horses and those with pituitary pars intermedia dysfunction. *Journal of Veterinary Internal Medicine* 25(6), 1431–1438. DOI: 10.1111/j.1939-1676.2011.00810.x.

Beech, J., McFarlane, D., Lindborg, S., Sojka, J.E. and Boston, R.C. (2011b) α-Melanocyte—stimulating hormone and adrenocorticotropin concentrations in response to thyrotropin-releasing hormone and comparison with adrenocorticotropin concentration after domperidone administration in healthy horses and horses with pituitary pars intermedia dysfunction. *Journal of the American Veterinary Medical Association* 238(10), 1305–1315. DOI: 10.2460/javma.238.10.1305.

Berryhill, E.H., Thomasy, S.M., Kass, P.H., Reilly, C.M., Good, K.L. *et al.* (2017) Comparison of corneal degeneration and calcific band keratopathy from 2000 to 2013 in 69 horses. *Veterinary Ophthalmology* 20(1), 16–26. DOI: 10.1111/vop.12338.

Bertin, F.R. and de Laat, M.A. (2017) The diagnosis of equine insulin dysregulation. *Equine Veterinary Journal* 49(5), 570–576. DOI: 10.1111/evj.12703.

Bertin, F.R., Pader, K.S., Lescun, T.B. and Sojka-Kritchevsky, J.E. (2013) Short-term effect of ovariectomy on measures of insulin sensitivity and response to dexamethasone administration in horses. *American Journal of Veterinary Research* 74(12), 1506–1513. DOI: 10.2460/ajvr.74.12.1506.

Borer-Weir, K.E., Menzies-Gow, N.J., Bailey, S.R., Harris, P.A. and Elliott, J. (2013) Seasonal and annual influence on insulin and cortisol results from overnight dexamethasone suppression tests in normal ponies and ponies predisposed to laminitis. *Equine Veterinary Journal* 45(6), 688–693. DOI: 10.1111/evj.12053.

Boujon, C.E., Bestetti, G.E., Meier, H.P., Straub, R., Junker, U. *et al.* (1993) Equine pituitary adenoma: a functional and morphological study. *Journal of Comparative Pathology* 109(2), 163–178. DOI: 10.1016/S0021-9975(08)80260-5.

Bright, G.M. (1995) Corticosteroid-binding globulin influences kinetic parameters of plasma cortisol transport and clearance. *The Journal of Clinical Endocrinology and Metabolism* 80(3), 770–775. DOI: 10.1210/jcem.80.3.7883829.

Brosnahan, M.M. and Paradis, M.R. (2003) emographic and clinical characteristics of geriatric horses: 467 cases (1989–1999). *Journal of the American Veterinary Medical Association* 223(1), 93–98. DOI: 10.2460/javma.2003.223.93.

Byrne, D.P., Secombe, C.J., Tan, R.H.H., Perera, D.I., Watts, S.P. *et al.* (2018) Circannual variability in adrenocorticotropic hormone responses to administration of thyrotropin-releasing hormone in clinically normal horses in Australia. *The Veterinary Journal* 238, 58–62. DOI: 10.1016/j.tvjl.2018.07.008.

Carluccio, A., Sundaram, N.K., Chablani, S., Amrock, L.G., Lambert, J.K. *et al.* (2015) Predictors of quality of life in 102 patients with treated Cushing's disease. *Clinical Endocrinology* 82(3), 404–411. DOI: 10.1111/cen.12521.

Carmalt, J.L., Mortazavi, S., Maconie, R.C., Allen, A.L. and Unniappan, S. (2018) Profiles of pro-opiomelanocortin and encoded peptides, and their processing enzymes in equine pituitary pars intermedia dysfunction. *PLoS One* 13(1), e0190796. DOI: 10.1371/journal.pone.0190796.

Catania, A. and Lipton, J.M. (1993) Alpha-Melanocyte stimulating hormone in the modulation of host reactions. *Endocrine Reviews* 14(5), 564–576. DOI: 10.1210/er.14.5.564.

Chandler, K.J. and Dixon, R.M. (2002) Urinary cortisol:creatinine ratios in healthy horses and horses with hyperadrenocorticism and non.adrenal disease. *Veterinary Record* 150(25), 773–776. DOI: 10.1136/vr.150.25.773.

Clayton, R.N., Raskauskiene, D., Reulen, R.C. and Jones, P.W. (2011) Mortality and morbidity in Cushing's disease over 50 years in Stoke-on-Trent, UK: audit and meta-analysis of literature. *The Journal of Clinical Endocrinology & Metabolism* 96(3), 632–642. DOI: 10.1210/jc.2010-1942.

Clément, K. (2006) Genetics of human obesity. *Comptes Rendus Biologies* 329(8), 608–622 DOI: 10.1016/j.crvi.2005.10.009.

Cole, F.L., Hodgson, D.R., Reid, S.W.J. and Mellor, D.J. (2005) Owner-reported equine health disorders: results of an Australia-wide postal survey. *Australian Veterinary Journal* 83(8), 490–495. DOI: 10.1111/j.1751-0813.2005.tb13301.x.

Copas, V.E.N. and Durham, A.E. (2012) Circannual variation in plasma adrenocorticotropic hormone concentrations in the UK in normal horses and ponies, and those with pituitary *pars intermedia* dysfunction. *Equine Veterinary Journal* 44(4), 440–443. DOI: 10.1111/j.2042-3306.2011.00444.x.

Cordero, M., Shrauner, B. and McFarlane, D. (2011) Bioactivity of plasma ACTH from horses with PPID compared to normal horses. *Journal of Veterinary Internal Medicine* 25, 664–664.

Cordero, M., Brorsen, B.W. and McFarlane, D. (2012) Circadian and circannual rhythms of cortisol, ACTH, and α-melanocyte-stimulating hormone in healthy horses. *Domestic Animal Endocrinology* 43(4), 317–324. DOI: 10.1016/j.domaniend.2012.05.005.

Couëtil, L.L. and Hoffman, A.M. (1998) Adrenal insufficiency in a neonatal foal. *Journal of the American Veterinary Medical Association* 212(10), 1594–1596.

Couëtil, L., Paradis, M.R. and Knoll, J. (1996) Plasma adrenocorticotropin concentration in healthy horses and in horses with clinical signs of hyperadrenocorticism. *Journal of Veterinary Internal Medicine* 10(1), 1–6. DOI: 10.1111/j.1939-1676.1996.tb02016.x.

Danger, J.-M., Perroteau, I., Franzoni, M.F., Saint-Pierre, S., Fasolo, A. *et al.* (1989) Innervation of the pars intermedia and control of alpha-melanotropin secretion in the newt. *Neuroendocrinology* 50(5), 543–549. DOI: 10.1159/000125278.

Davis, J.L., Kirk, L.M., Davidson, G.S. and Papich, M.G. (2009) Effects of compounding and storage conditions on stability of pergolide mesylate. *Journal of the American Veterinary Medical Association* 234(3), 385–389. DOI: 10.2460/javma.234.3.385.

De Souza, E.B. and Battaglia, G. (1988) Corticotropin-releasing hormone (CRH) receptors in brain. *Advances in Experimental Medicine and Biology* 245, 123–136. DOI: 10.1007/978-1-4899-2064-5_9.

Dembek, K.A., Onasch, K., Hurcombe, S.D.A., MacGillivray, K.C., Slovis, N.M. *et al.* (2013) Renin-Angiotensin-Aldosterone system and hypothalamic-pituitary-adrenal axis in hospitalized newborn foals. *Journal of Veterinary Internal Medicine* 27(2), 331–338. DOI: 10.1111/jvim.12043.

Dembek, K.A., Timko, K.J., Johnson, L.M., Hart, K.A., Barr, B.S. *et al.* (2017) Steroids, steroid precursors, and neuroactive steroids in critically ill equine neonates. *The Veterinary Journal* 225, 42–49. DOI: 10.1016/j.tvjl.2017.05.009.

Dembek, K.A., Johnson, L.M., Timko, K.J., Minuto, J.S., Hart, K.A. *et al.* (2019) Multiple adrenocortical steroid response to administration of exogenous adrenocorticotropic hormone to hospitalized foals. *Journal of Veterinary Internal Medicine* 33(4), 1766–1774. DOI: 10.1111/jvim.15527.

Diez de Castro, E., Lopez, I., Cortes, B., Pineda, C., Garfia, B. *et al.* (2014) Influence of feeding status, time of the day, and season on baseline adrenocorticotropic hormone and the response to thyrotropin releasing hormone-stimulation test in healthy horses. *Domestic Animal Endocrinology* 48, 77–83. DOI: 10.1016/j.domaniend.2014.02.004.

Donaldson, M.T., LaMonte, B.H., Morresey, P., Smith, G. and Beech, J. (2002) Treatment with pergolide or cyproheptadine of pituitary pars intermedia dysfunction (equine Cushing's disease). *Journal of Veterinary Internal Medicine* 16(6), 742–746. DOI: 10.1892/0891-6640(2002)016<0742:twpoco>2.3.co;2.

Donaldson, M.T., Jorgensen, A.J.R. and Beech, J. (2004a) Evaluation of suspected pituitary pars intermedia dysfunction in horses with laminitis. *Journal of the American Veterinary Medical Association* 224(7), 1123–1127. DOI: 10.2460/javma.2004.224.1123.

Donaldson, M.T., McFarlane, D., Jorgensen, A.J.R. and Beech, J. (2004b) Correlation between plasma -melanocyte-stimulating hormone concentration and body mass index in healthy horses. *American Journal of Veterinary Research* 65(11), 1469–1473. DOI: 10.2460/ajvr.2004.65.1469.

Donaldson, M.T., McDonnell, S.M., Schanbacher, B.J., Lamb, S.V., McFarlane, D. *et al.* (2005) Variation in plasma adrenocorticotropic hormone concentration and dexamethasone suppression test results with season, age, and sex in healthy ponies and horses. *Journal of Veterinary Internal Medicine* 19(2), 217–222. DOI: 10.1111/j.1939-1676.2005.tb02685.x.

Doniach, I. (1985) Histopathology of the pituitary. *Clinics in Endocrinology and Metabolism* 14(4), 765–789. DOI: 10.1016/S0300-595X(85)80077-3.

Dowling, P.M., Williams, M.A. and Clark, T.P. (1993) Adrenal insufficiency associated with long-term anabolic steroid administration in a horse. *Journal of the American Veterinary Medical Association* 203(8), 1166–1169.

Durham, A.E. (2017) Therapeutics for equine endocrine disorders. *Veterinary Clinics of North America: Equine Practice* 33(1), 127–139. DOI: 10.1016/j.cveq.2016.11.003.

Dybdal, N.O., Gribble, D., Madigan, J.E. and Stabenfelt, G.H. (1980) Alterations in plasma corticosteroids, insulin and selected metabolites in horses used in endurance rides. *Equine Veterinary Journal* 12(3), 137–140. DOI: 10.1111/j.2042-3306.1980.tb03403.x.

Dybdal, N.O., Hargreaves, K.M., Madigan, J.E., Gribble, D.H., Kennedy, P.C. *et al.* (1994) Diagnostic testing for pituitary pars intermedia dysfunction in horses. *Journal of the American Veterinary Medical Association* 204(4), 627–632.

Evans, M.J., Livesey, J.H., Ellis, M.J. and Yandle, T.G. (2001) Effect of anticoagulants and storage temperatures on stability of plasma and serum hormones. *Clinical Biochemistry* 34(2), 107–112. DOI: 10.1016/S0009-9120(01)00196-5.

Fazio, E., Medica, P., Aronica V., Grasso, L. and Ferlazzo, A. (2008) Circulating β-endorphin, adrenocorticotrophic hormone and cortisol levels of stallions before and after short road transport: stress effect of different distances. *Acta Veterinaria Scandinavica* 50(1), 6. DOI: 10.1186/1751-0147-50-6.

Frank, N. and Tadros, E.M. (2014) Insulin dysregulation. *Equine Veterinary Journal* 46(1), 103–112. DOI: 10.1111/evj.12169.

Frank, N., Andrews, F.M., Sommardahl, C.S., Eiler, H., Rohrbach, B.W. *et al.* (2006) Evaluation of the combined dexamethasone suppression/

thyrotropin-releasing hormone stimulation test for detection of pars intermedia pituitary adenomas in horses. *Journal of Veterinary Internal Medicine* 20(4), 987–993. DOI: 10.1111/j.1939-1676.2006.tb01816.x.

Funk, R.A., Stewart, A.J., Wooldridge, A.A., Kwessi, E., Kemppainen, R.J. *et al.* (2011) Seasonal changes in plasma adrenocorticotropic hormone and α-melanocyte-stimulating hormone in response to thyrotropin-releasing hormone in normal, aged horses. *Journal of Veterinary Internal Medicine* 25(3), 579–585. DOI: 10.1111/j.1939-1676.2011.0712.x.

Guthrie, G.P., Cecil, S.G., Darden, E.D. and Kotchen, T.A. (1982) Dynamics of renin and aldosterone in the thoroughbred horse. *General and Comparative Endocrinology* 48(3), 296–299. DOI: 10.1016/0016-6480(82)90140-X.

Halmi, N., Peterson, M., Colurso, G., Liotta, A. and Krieger, D. (1981) Pituitary intermediate lobe in dog: two cell types and high bioactive adrenocorticotropin content. *Science* 211(4477), 72–74. DOI: 10.1126/science.6255564.

Han, X., Fowden, A.L., Silver, M., Holdstock, N., Mcgladdery, A.J. *et al.* (1995) Immunohistochemical localisation of steroidogenic enzymes and phenylethanolamine-N-methyl-transferase (PNMT) in the adrenal gland of the fetal and newborn foal. *Equine Veterinary Journal* 27(2), 140–146. DOI: 10.1111/j.2042-3306.1995.tb03051.x.

Haritou, S.J.A., Zylstra, R., Ralli, C., Turner, S. and Tortonese, D.J. (2008) Seasonal changes in circadian peripheral plasma concentrations of melatonin, serotonin, dopamine and cortisol in aged horses with Cushing's disease under natural photoperiod. *Journal of Neuroendocrinology* 20(8), 988–996. DOI: 10.1111/j.1365-2826.2008.01751.x.

Hart, K.A., Barton, M.H., Ferguson, D.C., Berghaus, R., Slovis, N.M. *et al.* (2011) Serum free cortisol fraction in healthy and septic neonatal foals. *Journal of Veterinary Internal Medicine* 25(2), 345–355. DOI: 10.1111/j.1939-1676.2010.0667.x.

Hart, K.A., Ferguson, D.C., Heusner, G.L. and Barton, M.H. (2007) Synthetic adrenocorticotropic hormone stimulation tests in healthy neonatal foals. *Journal of Veterinary Internal Medicine* 21(2), 314–321. DOI: 10.1111/j.1939-1676.2007.tb02966.x.

Hart, K.A., Slovis, N.M. and Barton, M.H. (2009) Hypothalamic-pituitary-adrenal axis dysfunction in hospitalized neonatal foals. *Journal of Veterinary Internal Medicine* 23(4), 901–912. DOI: 10.1111/j.1939-1676.2009.0323.x.

Hart, K.A., Wochele, D.M., Norton, N.A., McFarlane, D., Wooldridge, A.A. *et al.* (2016) Effect of age, season, body condition, and endocrine status on serum free cortisol fraction and insulin concentration in horses. *Journal of Veterinary Internal Medicine* 30(2), 653–663. DOI: 10.1111/jvim.13839.

Hart, K.A. and Barton, M.H. (2011) Adrenocortical insufficiency in horses and foals. *Veterinary Clinics of North America: Equine Practice* 27(1), 19–34. DOI: 10.1016/j.cveq.2010.12.005.

Hassan-Smith, Z. and Cooper, M.S. (2011) Overview of the endocrine response to critical illness: how to measure it and when to treat. *Best Practice & Research Clinical Endocrinology & Metabolism* 25(5), 705–717. DOI: 10.1016/j.beem.2011.04.002.

Hedberg, Y., Dalin, A.-M., Forsberg, M., Lundeheim, N., Hoffmann, B. *et al.* (2007) Effect of ACTH (tetracosactide) on steroid hormone levels in the mare. Part A: effect in intact normal mares and mares with possible estrous related behavioral abnormalities. *Animal Reproduction Science* 100(1–2), 73–91. DOI: 10.1016/j.anireprosci.2006.06.008.

Heinrichs, M., Baumgärtner, W. and Capen, C.C. (1990) Immunocytochemical demonstration of proopiomelanocortin-derived peptides in pituitary adenomas of the pars intermedia in horses. *Veterinary Pathology* 27(6), 419–425. DOI: 10.1177/030098589902700606.

Hillebrand, J.J., Heijboer, A.C. and Endert, E. (2017) Effects of repeated freeze–thaw cycles on endocrine parameters in plasma and serum. *Annals of Clinical Biochemistry* 54(2), 289–292. DOI: 10.1177/0004563216657361.

Hinrichsen, S., Stewart, A.J., Yuen, K.Y. and Bertin, F.R. (2019) Effect of various ambient temperatures on the determination of immunoreactive ACTH concentrations in aged horses. *Journal of Veterinary Internal Medicine* 33, 2431–2432.

Hofberger, S., Gauff, F. and Licka, T. (2015) Suspensory ligament degeneration associated with pituitary pars intermedia dysfunction in horses. *The Veterinary Journal* 203(3), 348–350. DOI: 10.1016/j.tvjl.2014.12.037.

Hoffman, C.J., McKenzie, H.C., Furr, M.O. and Desrochers, A. (2015) Glucocorticoid receptor density and binding affinity in healthy horses and horses with systemic inflammatory response syndrome. *Journal of Veterinary Internal Medicine* 29(2), 626–635. DOI: 10.1111/jvim.12558.

Horn, R. and Bertin, F.-R. (2019) Evaluation of combined testing to simultaneously diagnose pituitary pars intermedia dysfunction and insulin dysregulation in horses. *Journal of Veterinary Internal Medicine* 33(5), 2249–2256. DOI: 10.1111/jvim.15617.

Horn, R., Bamford, N.J., Afonso, T., Sutherland, M., Buckerfield, J. *et al.* (2019a) Factors associated with survival, laminitis and insulin dysregulation in horses diagnosed with equine pituitary pars intermedia dysfunction. *Equine Veterinary Journal* 51(4), 440–445. DOI: 10.1111/evj.13041.

Horn, R., Stewart, A.J., Medina-Torres, C.E., Jackson, K.V. and Bertin, F.R. (2019b) Clinical implications of the use of different methods to determine ACTH reference intervals in horses. *Journal of Veterinary Internal Medicine* 33, 2432–2432.

Hu, K., Stewart, A.J., Yuen, K.Y., Hinrichsen, S., Dryburgh, E.L. *et al.* (2020) The effect of freeze-thaw cycles on determination of immunoreactive plasma adrenocorticotrophic hormone concentrations in horses. *Journal of veterinary internal medicine* 34(3), 1350–1356.

Hurcombe, S.D.A., Toribio, R.E., Slovis, N., Kohn, C.W., Refsal, K. *et al.* (2008) Blood arginine vasopressin, adrenocorticotropin hormone, and cortisol concentrations at admission in septic and critically ill foals and their association with survival. *Journal of Veterinary Internal Medicine* 22(3), 639–647. DOI: 10.1111/j.1939-1676.2008.0090.x.

Ikeda, H., Suzuki, J., Sasano, N. and Niizuma, H. (1988) The development and morphogenesis of the human pituitary gland. *Anatomy and Embryology* 178(4), 327–336. DOI: 10.1007/BF00698663.

Ireland, J.L., Clegg, P.D., McGowan, C.M., McKane, S.A. and Pinchbeck, G.L. (2011) A cross-sectional study of geriatric horses in the United Kingdom. Part 1: demographics and management practices. *Equine Veterinary Journal* 43(1), 30–36. DOI: 10.1111/j.2042-3306.2010.00145.x.

Irvine, C.H. and Alexander, S.L. (1987) Measurement of free cortisol and the capacity and association constant of cortisol-binding proteins in plasma of foals and adult horses. *Journal of Reproduction and Fertility. Supplement* 35, 19–24.

Ishibashi, M. and Yamaji, T. (1981) Direct effects of thyrotropin-releasing hormone, cyproheptadine, and dopamine on adrenocorticotropin secretion from human corticotroph adenoma cells in vitro. *Journal of Clinical Investigation* 68(4), 1018–1027. DOI: 10.1172/JCI110324.

Jacob, S.I., Geor, R.J., Weber, P.S.D., Harris, P.A. and McCue, M.E. (2018) Effect of dietary carbohydrates and time of year on ACTH and cortisol concentrations in adult and aged horses. *Domestic Animal Endocrinology* 63, 15–22. DOI: 10.1016/j.domaniend.2017.10.005.

Jane Ellis, M., Livesey, J.H. and Evans, M.J. (2003) Hormone stability in human whole blood. *Clinical Biochemistry* 36(2), 109–112. DOI: 10.1016/S0009-9120(02)00440-X.

Karikoski, N.P., Horn, I., McGowan, T.W. and McGowan, C.M. (2011) The prevalence of endocrinopathic laminitis among horses presented for laminitis at a first-opinion/referral equine Hospital. *Domestic Animal Endocrinology* 41(3), 111–117. DOI: 10.1016/j.domaniend.2011.05.004.

Keen, J.A., Mclaren, M., Chandler, K.J. and Mcgorum, B.C. (2004) Biochemical indices of vascular function, glucose metabolism and oxidative stress in horses with equine Cushing's disease. *Equine Veterinary Journal* 36(3), 226–229. DOI: 10.2746/0425164044877215.

Kenyon, N. (2003) Defining adrenal insufficiency in septic shock. *Critical Care Medicine* 31(1), 321–323. DOI: 10.1097/00003246-200301000-00059.

Knowles, E.J., Moreton-Clack, M.C., Shaw, S., Harris, P.A., Elliott, J. *et al.* (2018) Plasma adrenocorticotropic hormone (ACTH) concentrations in ponies measured by two different assays suggests seasonal cross-reactivity or interference. *Equine Veterinary Journal* 50(5), 672–677. DOI: 10.1111/evj.12797.

Lefcourt, A.M., Bitman, J., Kahl, S. and Wood, D.L. (1993) Circadian and ultradian rhythms of peripheral cortisol concentrations in lactating dairy cows. *Journal of Dairy Science* 76(9), 2607–2612. DOI: 10.3168/jds.S0022-0302(93)77595-5.

Leroux, P. and Pelletier, G. (1984) Radioautographic study of binding and internalization of corticotropin-releasing factor by rat anterior pituitary corticotrophs. *Endocrinology* 114(1), 14–21. DOI: 10.1210/endo-114-1-14.

Lewis, J.G., Bagley, C.J., Elder, P.A., Bachmann, A.W. and Torpy, D.J. (2005) Plasma free cortisol fraction reflects levels of functioning corticosteroid-binding globulin. *Clinica Chimica Acta* 359(1–2), 189–194. DOI: 10.1016/j.cccn.2005.03.044.

Lo, T.-B.I.N. (1962) The isolation and characterization of methionine sulfoxide analogues of α- and β-melanocyte-stimulating hormones from bovine and equine pituitary glands. *The Journal of Biochemistry* 52(6), 409–422. DOI: 10.1093/oxfordjournals.jbchem.a127637.

Mair, T.S., Sherlock, C.E. and Boden, L.A. (2014) Serum cortisol concentrations in horses with colic. *The Veterinary Journal* 201(3), 370–377. DOI: 10.1016/j.tvjl.2014.06.005.

Marik, P.E. (2007) Mechanisms and clinical consequences of critical illness associated adrenal insufficiency. *Current Opinion in Critical Care* 13(4), 363–369. DOI: 10.1097/MCC.0b013e32818a6d74.

Marik, P.E. (2009) Critical illness-related corticosteroid insufficiency. *Chest* 135(1), 181–193. DOI: 10.1378/chest.08-1149.

Marik, P.E. and Zaloga, G.P. (2002) Adrenal insufficiency in the critically ill: a new look at an old problem. *Chest* 122, 1784–1796.

Marik, P.E. and Zaloga, G.P. (2003) Adrenal insufficiency during septic shock. *Critical Care Medicine* 31(1), 141–145. DOI: 10.1097/00003246-200301000-00022.

Marik, P.E., Kiminyo, K. and Zaloga, G.P. (2002) Adrenal insufficiency in critically ill patients with human immunodeficiency virus. *Critical Care Medicine* 30(6), 1267–1273. DOI: 10.1097/00003246-200206000-00018.

Marklund, L., Moller, M.J., Sandberg, K. and Andersson, L. (1996) A missense mutation in the gene for melanocyte-stimulating hormone receptor (MCIR) is associated with the chestnut coat color in horses. *Mammalian Genome* 7(12), 895–899. DOI: 10.1007/s003359900264.

Marshall, J.B., Kapcala, L.P., Manning, L.D. and McCullough, A.J. (1984) Effect of corticotropin-like intermediate lobe peptide on pancreatic exocrine function in isolated rat pancreatic lobules. *Journal of Clinical Investigation* 74(5), 1886–1889. DOI: 10.1172/JCI111608.

Martin, L.G., Behrend, E.N., Mealey, K.L., Carpenter, D.M. and Hickey, K.C. (2007) Effect of low doses of cosyntropin on serum cortisol concentrations in clinically normal dogs. *American Journal of Veterinary Research* 68(5), 555–560. DOI: 10.2460/ajvr.68.5.555.

Mastro, L.M., Adams, A.A. and Urschel, K.L. (2015) Pituitary pars intermedia dysfunction does not necessarily impair insulin sensitivity in old horses. *Domestic Animal Endocrinology* 50, 14–25. DOI: 10.1016/j.domaniend.2014.07.003.

McFarlane, D. (2011) Equine pituitary pars intermedia dysfunction. *Veterinary Clinics of North America: Equine Practice* 27(1), 93–113. DOI: 10.1016/j.cveq.2010.12.007.

McFarlane, D. and Holbrook, T.C. (2008) Cytokine dysregulation in aged horses and horses with pituitary pars intermedia dysfunction. *Journal of Veterinary Internal Medicine* 22(2), 436–442. DOI: 10.1111/j.1939-1676.2008.0076.x.

McFarlane, D., Donaldson, M.T., McDonnell, S.M. and Cribb, A.E. (2004) Effects of season and sample handling on measurement of plasma alpha-melanocyte-stimulating hormone concentrations in horses and ponies. *American Journal of Veterinary Research* 65(11), 1463–1468. DOI: 10.2460/ajvr.2004.65.1463.

McFarlane, D., Dybdal, N., Donaldson, M.T., Miller, L. and Cribb, A.E. (2005a) Nitration and increased alpha-synuclein expression associated with dopaminergic neurodegeneration in equine pituitary pars intermedia dysfunction. *Journal of Neuroendocrinology* 17(2), 73–80. DOI: 10.1111/j.1365-2826.2005.01277.x.

McFarlane, D., Miller, L.M., Craig, L.E., Dybdal, N.O., Habecker, P.L. *et al.* (2005b) Agreement in histologic assessments of the pituitary pars intermedia in aged horses. *American Journal of Veterinary Research* 66(12), 2055–2059. DOI: 10.2460/ajvr.2005.66.2055.

McFarlane, D., Beech, J. and Cribb, A. (2006) Alpha-melanocyte stimulating hormone release in response to thyrotropin releasing hormone in healthy horses, horses with pituitary pars intermedia dysfunction and equine pars intermedia explants. *Domestic Animal Endocrinology* 30(4), 276–288. DOI: 10.1016/j.domaniend.2005.07.005.

McFarlane, D., Hale, G.M., Johnson, E.M. and Maxwell, L.K. (2010) Fecal egg counts after anthelmintic administration to aged horses and horses with pituitary pars intermedia dysfunction. *Journal of the American Veterinary Medical Association* 236(3), 330–334. DOI: 10.2460/javma.236.3.330.

McFarlane, D., Paradis, M.R., Zimmel, D., Sykes, B., Brorsen, B.W. *et al.* (2011) The effect of geographic location, breed, and pituitary dysfunction on seasonal adrenocorticotropin and α-melanocyte-stimulating hormone plasma concentrations in horses. *Journal of Veterinary Internal Medicine* 25(4), 872–881. DOI: 10.1111/j.1939-1676.2011.0745.x.

McGowan, C.M., Frost, R., Pfeiffer, D.U. and Neiger, R. (2004) Serum insulin concentrations in horses with equine Cushing's syndrome: response to a cortisol inhibitor and prognostic value. *Equine Veterinary Journal* 36(3), 295–298. DOI: 10.2746/0425164044877288.

McGowan, T.W., Pinchbeck, G., Phillips, C.J.C., Perkins, N., Hodgson, D.R. *et al.* (2010) A survey of aged horses in Queensland, Australia. Part 1: management and preventive health care. *Australian Veterinary Journal* 88(11), 420–427. DOI: 10.1111/j.1751-0813.2010.00637.x.

McFarlane, D., Hill, K. and Anton, J. (2015) Neutrophil function in healthy aged horses and horses with pituitary dysfunction. *Veterinary Immunology and Immunopathology* 165(3–4), 99–106. DOI: 10.1016/j.vetimm.2015.04.006.

McGowan, C. (2018) Recommendations from the Australian and New Zealand equine endocrine group and the interpretation of plasma endogenous ACTH concentrations for the diagnosis of pituitary pars intermedia dysfunction (PPID). *Australian Veterinary Journal* 96(9), 317–318. DOI: 10.1111/avj.12743.

McGowan, C.M. and Neiger, R. (2003) Efficacy of trilostane for the treatment of equine Cushing's syndrome. *Equine Veterinary Journal* 35(4), 414–418. DOI: 10.2746/042516403776014271.

McGowan, T.W., Pinchbeck, G.P. and McGowan, C.M. (2013a) Evaluation of basal plasma α-melanocyte-stimulating hormone and adrenocorticotrophic hormone concentrations for the diagnosis of pituitary pars intermedia dysfunction from a population of aged horses. *Equine Veterinary Journal* 45(1), 66–73. DOI: 10.1111/j.2042-3306.2012.00575.x.

McGowan, T.W., Pinchbeck, G.P. and McGowan, C.M. (2013b) Prevalence, risk factors and clinical signs predictive for equine pituitary pars intermedia dysfunction in aged horses. *Equine Veterinary Journal* 45(1), 74–79. DOI: 10.1111/j.2042-3306.2012.00578.x.

Menzies-Gow, N. (2018) Diagnosing and treating laminitis in horses. *Veterinary Record* 183(16), 505–506. DOI: 10.1136/vr.k4485.

Meyer, H.P. and Rothuizen, J. (1993) Determination of the percentage of free cortisol in plasma in the dog by ultrafiltration/dialysis. *Domestic Animal Endocrinology* 10(1), 45–53. DOI: 10.1016/0739-7240(93)90007-X.

Miller, M.A., Pardo, I.D., Jackson, L.P., Moore, G.E. and Sojka, J.E. (2008) Correlation of pituitary histomorphometry with adrenocorticotrophic hormone response to domperidone administration in the diagnosis of equine pituitary pars intermedia dysfunction.

Veterinary Pathology 45(1), 26–38. DOI: 10.1354/vp.45-1-26.

Miller, C., Utter, M.L. and Beech, J. (2013) Evaluation of the effects of age and pituitary pars intermedia dysfunction on corneal sensitivity in horses. *American Journal of Veterinary Research* 74(7), 1030–1035. DOI: 10.2460/ajvr.74.7.1030.

Miller, M.A., Moore, G.E., Bertin, F.R. and Kritchevsky, J.E. (2016) What's new in old horses? postmortem diagnoses in mature and aged Equids. *Veterinary Pathology* 53(2), 390–398. DOI: 10.1177/0300985815608674.

Millington, W.R., Dybdal, N.O., Dawson, R., Manzini, C. and Mueller, G.P. (1988) Equine Cushing's disease: differential regulation of beta-endorphin processing in tumors of the intermediate pituitary. *Endocrinology* 123(3), 1598–1604. DOI: 10.1210/endo-123-3-1598.

Mohammad, Z., Afessa, B. and Finkielman, J.D. (2006) The incidence of relative adrenal insufficiency in patients with septic shock after the administration of etomidate. *Critical Care* 10(4), R105. DOI: 10.1186/cc4979.

Mosier, M.J., Lasinski, A.M. and Gamelli, R.L. (2015) Suspected adrenal insufficiency in critically ill burned patients: etomidate-induced or critical illness-related corticosteroid insufficiency?-A review of the literature. *Journal of burn care & research : official publication of the American Burn Association* 36(2), 272–278. DOI: 10.1097/BCR.0000000000000099.

Muñoz, M.C., Doreste, F., Ferrer, O., González, J. and Montoya, J.A. (1996) Pergolide treatment for Cushing's syndrome in a horse. *Veterinary Record* 139(2), 41–43. DOI: 10.1136/vr.139.2.41.

Nagata, S., Takeda, F., Kurosawa, M., Mima, K., Hiraga, A. *et al.* (1999) Plasma adrenocorticotropin, cortisol and catecholamines response to various exercises. *Equine Veterinary Journal* (30), 570–574. DOI: 10.1111/j.2042-3306.1999.tb05286.x.

Nahon, J.-L. (2006) The melanocortins and melanin-concentrating hormone in the central regulation of feeding behavior and energy homeostasis. *Comptes Rendus Biologies* 329(8), 623–638,discussion 653–655. DOI: 10.1016/j.crvi.2006.03.021.

Oddoze, C., Lombard, E. and Portugal, H. (2012) Stability study of 81 analytes in human whole blood, in serum and in plasma. *Clinical Biochemistry* 45(6), 464–469. DOI: 10.1016/j.clinbiochem.2012.01.012.

Orth, D.N., Holscher, M.A., Wilson, M.G., Nicholson, W.E., Plue, R.E. *et al.* (1982) Equine Cushing's disease: plasma immunoreactive proopiolipomelanocortin peptide and cortisol levels basally and in response to diagnostic tests. *Endocrinology* 110(4), 1430–1441. DOI: 10.1210/endo-110-4-1430.

Pease, A.P., Schott, H.C., Howey, E.B. and Patterson, J.S. (2011) Computed tomographic findings in the pituitary gland and brain of horses with pituitary pars intermedia dysfunction. *Journal of Veterinary Internal Medicine* 25(5), 1144–1151. DOI: 10.1111/j.1939-1676.2011.00784.x.

Perkins, G.A., Lamb, S., Erb, H.N., Schanbacher, B., Nydam, D.V. *et al.* (2002) Plasma adrenocorticotropin (ACTH) concentrations and clinical response in horses treated for equine Cushing s disease with cyproheptadine or pergolide. *Equine Veterinary Journal* 34(7), 679–685. DOI: 10.2746/042516402776250333.

Place, N.J., McGowan, C.M., Lamb, S.V., Schanbacher, B.J., McGowan, T. *et al.* (2010) Seasonal variation in serum concentrations of selected metabolic hormones in horses. *Journal of Veterinary Internal Medicine* 24(3), 650–654. DOI: 10.1111/j.1939-1676.2010.0500.x.

Prutton, J.S.W., Kass, P.H., Watson, J.L. and Pusterla, N. (2015) Pre-analytical stability of adrenocorticotrophic hormone from healthy horses in whole blood, plasma and frozen plasma samples. *The Veterinary Journal* 204(1), 123–124. DOI: 10.1016/j.tvjl.2015.02.010.

Rendle, D.I., Heller, J., Hughes, K.J., Innocent, G.T. and Durham, A.E. (2009) Stability of common biochemistry analytes in equine blood stored at room temperature. *Equine Veterinary Journal* 41(5), 428–432. DOI: 10.2746/042516409X370928.

Rendle, D.I., Litchfield, E., Heller, J. and Hughes, K.J. (2014) Investigation of rhythms of secretion and repeatability of plasma adrenocorticotropic hormone concentrations in healthy horses and horses with pituitary pars intermedia dysfunction. *Equine Veterinary Journal* 46(1), 113–117. DOI: 10.1111/evj.12114.

Rendle, D.I., Litchfield, E., Gough, S., Cowling, A. and Hughes, K.J. (2015) The effects of sample handling and N-phenylmaleimide on concentration of adrenocorticotrophic hormone in equine plasma. *Equine Veterinary Journal* 47(5), 587–591. DOI: 10.1111/evj.12319.

Rendle, D.I., Doran, G., Ireland, J. and Edwards, S. (2019) Pharmacokinetics and pharmacodynamics of pergolide mesylate after oral administration in horses with pituitary pars intermedia dysfunction. *Domestic Animal Endocrinology* 68, 135–141. DOI: 10.1016/j.domaniend.2019.01.008.

Rohrbach, B.W., Stafford, J.R., Clermont, R.S.W., Reed, S.M., Schott, H.C. *et al.* (2012) Diagnostic frequency, response to therapy, and long-term prognosis among horses and ponies with pituitary PAR intermedia dysfunction, 1993–2004. *Journal of Veterinary Internal Medicine* 26(4), 1027–1034. DOI: 10.1111/j.1939-1676.2012.00932.x.

Saiardi, A. and Borrelli, E. (1998) Absence of dopaminergic control on melanotrophs leads to Cushing's-like syndrome in mice. *Molecular Endocrinology* 12(8), 1133–1139. DOI: 10.1210/mend.12.8.0144.

Saland, L.C. (2001) The mammalian pituitary intermediate lobe: an update on innervation and regulation. *Brain Research Bulletin* 54(6), 587–593. DOI: 10.1016/S0361-9230(01)00471-3.

Schott, H.C. (2002) Pituitary pars intermedia dysfunction: equine Cushing's disease. *Veterinary Clinics of North America: Equine Practice* 18(2), 237–270. DOI: 10.1016/S0749-0739(02)00018-4.

Schreiber, C.M., Stewart, A.J., Kwessi, E., Behrend, E.N., Wright, J.C. *et al.* (2012) Seasonal variation in results of diagnostic tests for pituitary pars intermedia dysfunction in older, clinically normal geldings. *Journal of the American Veterinary Medical Association* 241(2), 241–248. DOI: 10.2460/javma.241.2.241.

Secombe, C.J., Tan, R.H.H., Perera, D.I., Byrne, D.P., Watts, S.P. *et al.* (2017) The effect of geographic location on circannual adrenocorticotropic hormone plasma concentrations in horses in Australia. *Journal of Veterinary Internal Medicine* 31(5), 1533–1540. DOI: 10.1111/jvim.14782.

Sgorbini, M., Panzani, D., Maccheroni, M. and Corazza, M. (2004) Equine cushing-like syndrome: diagnosis and therapy in two cases. *Veterinary Research Communications* 28(Suppl 1), 377–380. DOI: 10.1023/B:VERC.0000045368.38959.8b.

Shank, B.R. and Ofner, C.M. (2009) Stability of pergolide mesylate oral liquid at room temperature. *International Journal of Pharmaceutical Compounding* 13(3), 254–258.

Shank, B.R. and Ofner, C.M. (2010) Multitemperature stability and degradation characteristics of pergolide mesylate oral liquid. *Journal of Pharmacy Practice* 23(6), 570–574. DOI: 10.1177/0897190010375851.

Shepard, M.K., Lee, W.L. and Eggleston, R.B. (2015) Perianesthetic development of diaphragmatic hernia in a horse with equine pituitary pars intermedia dysfunction (PpiD). *The Canadian Veterinary Journal* 56(1), 48–52.

Silver, M., Ousey, J.C., Dudan, F.E., Fowden, A.L., Knox, J. *et al.* (1984) Studies on equine prematurity 2: post natal adrenocortical activity in relation to plasma adrenocorticotrophic hormone and catecholamine levels in term and premature foals. *Equine Veterinary Journal* 16(4), 278–286. DOI: 10.1111/j.2042-3306.1984.tb01927.x.

Singh-Asa, P., Jenkin, G. and Thorburn, G.D. (1982) Effects of hydroxysteroid dehydrogenase inhibitors on in-vitro and in-vivo steroidogenesis in the ovine adrenal gland. *Journal of Endocrinology* 92(2), 205–212. DOI: 10.1677/joe.0.0920205.

Soni, A., Pepper, G.M., Wyrwinski, P.M., Ramirez, N.E., Simon, R. *et al.* (1995) Adrenal insufficiency occurring during septic shock: incidence, outcome, and relationship to peripheral cytokine levels. *The American Journal of Medicine* 98(3), 266–271. DOI: 10.1016/S0002-9343(99)80373-8.

Spelta, C.W. and Axon, J.E. (2012) Case series of equine pituitary pars intermedia dysfunction in a tropical climate. *Australian Veterinary Journal* 90(11), 451–456. DOI: 10.1111/j.1751-0813.2012.00997.x.

Spurzem, J.R. (2007) On the diagnosis of adrenal insufficiency in severe sepsis and septic shock. *American Journal of Respiratory and Critical Care Medicine* 175(10), 1095. DOI: 10.1164/ajrccm.175.10.1095.

Stewart, A.J., Wright, J.C., Behrend, E.N., Martin, L.G., Kemppainen, R.J. *et al.* (2013) Validation of a low-dose adrenocorticotropic hormone stimulation test in healthy neonatal foals. *Journal of the American Veterinary Medical Association* 243(3), 399–405. DOI: 10.2460/javma.243.3.399.

Stewart, A.J., Hackett, E., Bertin, F.-R. and Towns, T.J. (2019a) Cortisol and adrenocorticotropic hormone concentrations in horses with systemic inflammatory response syndrome. *Journal of Veterinary Internal Medicine* 33(5), 2257–2266. DOI: 10.1111/jvim.15620.

Stewart, A.J., Yuen, K.A., Hinrichsen, S., Horn, R. and Bertin, F.R. (2019b) Effect of sample handling on ACTH concentrations following thyrotropin-releasing hormone stimulation in horses. *Journal of Veterinary Internal Medicine* 33, 2436–2436.

Talbot, J.A., Kane, J.W. and White, A. (2003) Analytical and clinical aspects of adrenocorticotrophin determination. *Annals of Clinical Biochemistry* 40(Pt 5), 453–471. DOI: 10.1258/000456303322326371.

Tjörnstrand, A., Gunnarsson, K., Evert, M., Holmberg, E., Ragnarsson, O. *et al.* (2014) The incidence rate of pituitary adenomas in Western Sweden for the period 2001–2011. *European Journal of Endocrinology* 171(4), 519–526. DOI: 10.1530/EJE-14-0144.

van der Kolk, J.H., Kalsbeek, H.C., van Garderen, E., Wensing, T. and Breukink, H.J. (1993) Equine pituitary neoplasia: a clinical report of 21 cases (1990–1992). *The Veterinary Record* 133(24), 594–597.

van der Kolk, J.H., Kalsbeek, H.C., Wensing, T. and Breukink, H.J. (1994) Urinary concentration of corticoids in normal horses and horses with hyperadrenocorticism. *Research in Veterinary Science* 56(1), 126–128. DOI: 10.1016/0034-5288(94)90210-0.

van der Kolk, J.H., Wensing, T., Kalsbeek, H.C. and Breukink, H.J. (1995) Laboratory diagnosis of equine pituitary pars intermedia adenoma. *Domestic Animal Endocrinology* 12(1), 35–39. DOI: 10.1016/0739-7240(94)00006-M.

van der Kolk, J.H., Nachreiner, R.F., Schott, H.C., Refsal, K.R. and Zanella, A.J. (2001) Salivary and plasma concentration of cortisol in normal horses and horses with Cushing's disease. *Equine Veterinary Journal* 33(2), 211–213. DOI: 10.1111/j.2042-3306.2001.tb00604.x.

Vila-Pérez, D. and Jordan-García, I. (2015) Relative adrenal insufficiency in pediatric septic shock. *Journal of Pediatric Intensive Care* 4(3), 129–137. DOI: 10.1055/s-0035-1559821.

Wilson, M.G., Nicholson, W.E., Holscher, M.A., Sherrell, B.J., Mount, C.D. *et al.* (1982) Proopiolipomelanocortin peptides in normal pituitary, pituitary tumor, and plasma of normal and Cushing's horses. *Endocrinology* 110(3), 941–954. DOI: 10.1210/endo-110-3-941.

Wong, D.M., Vo, D.T., Alcott, C.J., Peterson, A.D., Sponseller, B.A. *et al.* (2009) Baseline plasma cortisol and ACTH concentrations and response to low-dose ACTH stimulation testing in ill foals. *Journal of the American Veterinary Medical Association* 234(1), 126–132. DOI: 10.2460/javma.234.1.126.

Wylie, C.E., Collins, S.N., Verheyen, K.L.P. and Newton, J.R. (2013) Risk factors for equine laminitis: a case-control study conducted in veterinary-registered horses and ponies in Great Britain between 2009 and 2011. *The Veterinary Journal* 198(1), 57–69. DOI: 10.1016/j.tvjl.2013.08.028.

Zeugswetter, F.K., Zwack, D., Luckschander-Zeller, N. and Schwendenwein, I. (2017) The acute effects of a protein-rich meal on the urinary corticoid:creatinine ratio in healthy dogs. *Journal of Animal Physiology and Animal Nutrition* 101(1), 75–80. DOI: 10.1111/jpn.12510.

5 Diseases of the Endocrine Pancreas and Equine Metabolic Syndrome

Blood glucose is tightly regulated by a complex balance of hyperglycaemic and hypoglycaemic hormones (Ralston, 2002). The regulator of blood glucose concentration that has received the most attention is insulin as, although a few cases of diabetes mellitus with hyperglycaemia have been reported, the most clinically relevant disorder of the carbohydrate metabolism is characterized by insulin dysregulation (ID) (Durham, 2016; Durham *et al.*, 2019).

Regulation of Glucose Metabolism in Horses

Under resting conditions, the equine blood glucose concentration stays between 4 and 6.5 mmol/l (Nadal *et al.*, 1997; Williams *et al.*, 2001). Overall, this concentration is only mildly changed when horses are fasted, exercised or given a variety of feeds (Lawrence *et al.*, 1995; Nadal *et al.*, 1997). More severely acute changes can be observed after intense exercise, systemic disease, stress or ingestion of a high sugar diet, but euglycaemia is rapidly re-established once the event has abated.

A decrease in blood glucose concentration triggers the secretion of glucagon, as well as other hormones with a lesser role such as cortisol and catecholamines (Fields, 1998). Glucagon is a 29-amino-acid peptide secreted by the alpha cells of the islets of Langerhans, the endocrine pancreas functional unit. The secretion of glucagon is constant and free running overall, but it can be enhanced when blood glucose and insulin concentrations are low (Zhang *et al.*, 2016). Glucagon is the product of the cleavage of proglucagon by the proprotein convertase 2 (Orskov *et al.*, 1987). Released in the main circulation, glucagon promotes neoglucogenesis and glycogenolysis by binding to a G protein-coupled receptor and activating a series of enzymatic reactions that lead to the release of glucose-1-phosphate from glycogen-rich cells (Yu *et al.*, 2019). As a catabolic hormone, glucagon also promotes lipolysis leading to the release of fatty acids, increasing the pool of energy generators (Habegger *et al.*, 2010).

An increase in blood glucose concentration triggers the secretion of insulin. Insulin is a 51-amino-acid peptide secreted by the beta cells of the islets of Langerhans (Steiner and Oyer, 1967). It is the product of the successive cleavages of preproinsulin into proinsulin, followed by proinsulin into insulin and C-peptide by three endopeptidases. Hyperglycaemia, detected by insulin-independent glucose transporters 1 and 2 (GLUT1 and GLUT2), is the main trigger for insulin secretion in horses; however, insulin secretion is also triggered by a rise in circulating amino acid concentration, a rise in insulin secretagogues (incretins, for intestinal secretion of insulin) such as glucagon-like peptide-1 (GLP-1) or glucose-dependent insulinotropic peptide (GIP or gastric inhibitory peptide) and a decrease in glucagon concentration (Holz *et al.*, 1993; Bamford *et al.*, 2015; Chameroy *et al.*, 2016; de Laat *et al.*, 2016c). Insulin secretion is biphasic with an early peak about 10 min after hyperglycaemia and a later yet more sustained peak about 2 h after the hyperglycaemic event, possibly caused by the action of incretins (Lorenzo *et al.*, 2010). Insulin promotes cellular glucose uptake by binding to the alpha subunit of its tyrosine kinase receptor. The enzymatic cascade resulting from this binding leads to the exposure of a preformed glucose transporter 4 (GLUT4) on the cell membrane (McManus *et al.*, 2005). In addition, as an anabolic hormone, insulin promotes glycogenesis, DNA replication and protein synthesis and inhibits lipolysis. The main cellular targets of insulin are myocytes, adipocytes and hepatocytes. After binding to its receptor, insulin is cleared either by endocytosis of the ligand–receptor complex or, if released in the main circulation, by the liver or by the kidney (Duckworth *et al.*, 1998). The liver clears the major part of secreted insulin during a first-pass transit while the kidney clears the part released in the systemic circulation. In humans, insulin half-life is estimated to be about

5 min. With a longer half-life of 30 min, C-peptide has been used over insulin as a marker of beta cell function in type-1 diabetes mellitus (Yosten and Kolar, 2015). No clear role for C-peptide has been described in horses, but in humans it would appear that C-peptide is an anti-inflammatory agent promoting endothelial function, vasodilation and decreasing leukocyte adhesion.

In healthy horses, insulin and glucagon are the main regulators of blood glucose concentration. They regulate each other and are also regulated by other hormones whose relevance in horses is not yet fully characterized. Somatostatin is a 14- or 28-amino-acid peptide secreted by the delta cells of the islets of Langerhans as well as the hypothalamus and the proximal duodenum. It is mainly a hormone of the gastrointestinal tract with roles in gastric emptying, but it is also a suppressor of both insulin and glucagon secretion (Tóth *et al.*, 2010b; van der Meulen *et al.*, 2015). Cortisol is another suppressor of insulin secretion, antagonizing its action during stress and inflammation, resulting in hyperglycaemia (Fields, 1998; Bertin *et al.*, 2018; Stewart *et al.*, 2019). On the other hand, free cortisol concentrations have been shown to increase in hyperinsulinaemic horses (Hart *et al.*, 2016). Thyroid hormones, involved in endocrine organ development, would also regulate beta cell differentiation and proliferation. Catecholamines also regulate insulin and glucagon secretion with stimulation of beta-2 adrenergic receptors, increasing insulin secretion but decreasing glucagon secretion, and stimulation of alpha-1 and alpha-2 adrenergic receptors, suppressing insulin secretion but stimulating glucagon secretion (Skoglund *et al.*, 1987; Hirose *et al.*, 1993; Ringer *et al.*, 2013; Grimsrud *et al.*, 2015; de Laat *et al.*, 2016c; Kritchevsky *et al.*, 2020). Systemically, growth hormone antagonizes insulin in glucose and lipid metabolism by reducing the activity of the insulin receptor (Takano *et al.*, 2001). Locally, however, growth hormone promotes beta cell function and insulin secretion (Huang and Chang, 2014).

Insulin Dysregulation

Alterations in insulin secretion and function have been the focus of extensive research in equine medicine, as ID is a core component of equine metabolic syndrome (EMS) and is closely linked to the development of laminitis (Frank *et al.*, 2010b; de Laat *et al.*, 2010; Durham *et al.*, 2019). The term ID refers to the presence of insulin resistance (peripheral or hepatic tissue), the presence of hyperinsulinaemia (spontaneous or evoked) or the presence of both (Frank and Tadros, 2014). The term EMS refers to a collection of clinical signs and laboratory findings associated with ID and resulting in a predisposition toward laminitis. Beyond EMS, ID has also been described in other diseases, such as pituitary pars intermedia dysfunction (PPID) or systemic inflammatory response syndrome, or during physiological challenges such as stress or pregnancy (Fowden *et al.*, 1984; Mills *et al.*, 1997; McGowan *et al.*, 2004; Tóth *et al.*, 2008; Bertin *et al.*, 2018).

Insulin resistance

Insulin resistance and ID have been used interchangeably by some authors; however, with a better understanding of the mechanisms of ID, insulin resistance is now defined as a subset of ID characterized by an inability to increase circulating glucose uptake and utilization due to the absent or decreased response of insulin-sensitive tissues to endogenous or exogenous insulin (Lebovitz, 2001). As stated above, insulin stimulation results in the exposure of GLUT4 for insulin-sensitive cells to allow glucose uptake; therefore, insulin resistance can result from an anomaly at any stage of the process, from an inadequate interaction between insulin and its receptor, to an altered post-receptor signalling pathway or an exposure of a dysfunctional GLUT4 receptor which would be more common in horses (Lebovitz, 2001; Waller *et al.*, 2011a, b).

In other species, insulin resistance results in hyperglycaemia and excessive protein glycosylation; however, resting glucose concentrations in horses are usually within reference intervals or close to the upper limits of the reference interval and advanced glycosylation end products are not detected (Frank *et al.*, 2006; de Laat *et al.*, 2012a). Insulin resistance can be compensated by hyperinsulinaemia; however, in insulin-resistant horses, hyperinsulinaemia, either basal or post-prandial, is not always detected (Dunbar *et al.*, 2016; Bertin and de Laat, 2017).

The main organs and tissues involved in insulin resistance are the liver, skeletal muscles and the adipose tissue, with different degrees of insulin sensitivity (Isganaitis and Lustig, 2005). In the absence of response to insulin, cells fail to absorb glucose and mobilize fat with lipoprotein secretion (Sparks *et al.*, 2012). In the liver, insulin resistance results in the development of hypertriglyceridaemia and very low density lipoprotein (LDL) secretion (Frank *et al.*, 2006; Carter *et al.*, 2009c). Adipose tissue is more sensitive to insulin than other tissues, allowing the accumulation of fatty acids in adipocytes while other tissues are not responding to insulin. This fat accumulation eventually leads to systemic or regional obesity (Shoelson *et al.*, 2007).

As adipocytes accumulate fatty acids, inflammation develops by the secretion of adipokines and by perfusion impairment. Adipokines are hormones secreted by adipose tissue, with leptin and adiponectin being better described in horses. Leptin is a pro-inflammatory hormone and its secretion increases with body adipose mass, with higher concentrations in obese insulin-resistant horses than in lean horses (Buff *et al.*, 2006a; Frank *et al.*, 2006; Carter *et al.*, 2009c; Caltabilota *et al.*, 2010; Morgan *et al.*, 2014). Leptin secretion induces satiety, reduces hepatic fatty acid synthesis and exacerbates endothelial activation and free radical generation (Meier and Gressner, 2004; Singhal, 2005; Korda *et al.*, 2008). Adiponectin, on the other hand, is an anti-inflammatory cytokine and its concentration is negatively correlated with equine body mass index (Kearns *et al.*, 2006). This hormone has many effects including fatty acid oxidation, improvement of glucose tolerance and endothelial protection (Teoh *et al.*, 2008; Shehzad *et al.*, 2012). Both adipokines have paramount effects on the vascular endothelium, to reduce or exacerbate obesity-induced inflammation and perfusion. (Sharma and McNeill, 2005; Singhal, 2005; Korda *et al.*, 2008).

Hypoxia caused by endothelial dysfunction reduces adipocyte mitochondrial function and sustains inflammation with the release of macrophage chemo-attractants and recruitment of inflammatory cells (Cinti *et al.*, 2005; Trayhurn *et al.*, 2008). In obese insulin-resistant horses, positive correlations between systemic and regional adiposity and expression of interleukin 1, interleukin 6 and tumour necrosis factor α have been described (Vick *et al.*, 2007; Suagee *et al.*, 2011a). This sustained inflammation initiates a vicious circle, as production of proinflammatory cytokines has been shown to reduce insulin sensitivity, both in healthy horses receiving lipopolysaccharide perfusions and in spontaneously sick horses (Tóth *et al.*, 2008; Tadros *et al.*, 2013; Bertin *et al.*, 2018). This vicious circle worsens once adipocytes have reached their storage capacity, as erratic lipid deposition ensues with infiltration of the liver, skeletal muscles or the pancreas, further decreasing insulin sensitivity (Yu and Ginsberg, 2005; van Herpen and Schrauwen-Hinderling, 2008).

Hyperinsulinaemia

Hyperinsulinaemia was initially thought to be the consequence of peripheral tissue insulin resistance; however, the presence of hyperinsulinaemia without peripheral tissue insulin resistance suggests that it occurs independently of peripheral tissue insulin resistance (de Laat *et al.*, 2016c). Therefore, hyperinsulinaemia is the consequence of an increased secretion of insulin or the consequence of a decreased hepatic clearance. Although decreased hepatic clearance has been demonstrated in some horses, the inappropriately high insulin secretion appears more consistent with recent studies, making excessive pancreatic stimulation the most likely mechanism of hyperinsulinaemia (Tóth *et al.*, 2010b; de Laat *et al.*, 2016c).

Post-prandial hyperinsulinaemia is triggered by two main mechanisms. The first one is a diet-induced hyperglycaemia that directly acts as a strong beta cell stimulant and is responsible for 76% of the insulin secreted (de Laat *et al.*, 2016c). The second mechanism is mediated by incretins that increase diet-induced hyperinsulinaemia. Incretins are peptides released by the small intestine after non-structural carbohydrate (NSC) and amino acid ingestion and stimulate the release of insulin (Baggio and Drucker, 2007; de Laat *et al.*, 2016c). GLP-1 is secreted by duodenal and jejunal L-cells after ingestion of carbohydrate and increases glucose-stimulated insulin secretion by pancreatic beta cells (Holz *et al.*, 1993). Plasma GLP-1 strongly correlates with equine insulin secretion and is responsible for 23% of the insulin secreted (Bamford *et al.*, 2015; Chameroy *et al.*, 2016; de Laat *et al.*, 2016c). Although basal GLP-1 plasma concentrations do not differ between control and insulin-dysregulated horses, following an oral glucose test, GLP-1 plasma concentrations significantly increase in insulin-dysregulated horses (Bamford *et al.*, 2015; Chameroy *et al.*, 2016; de Laat *et al.*, 2016c). GIP is secreted by the K-cells of the duodenum and jejunum after the ingestion of carbohydrates. Although secreted in larger amounts than GLP-1, GIP is only responsible for about 2% of the insulin secreted and no difference in plasma GIP has been observed following an oral glucose test, between control and insulin-dysregulated ponies (de Laat *et al.*, 2016c). The glucagon-like peptide-2 (GLP-2) is another peptide secreted by the small intestinal L-cells. Unlike the GLP-1, GLP-2 does not directly stimulate pancreatic beta cells but increases small intestinal absorption in a paracrine fashion (Drucker *et al.*, 1996). In insulin-dysregulated ponies, basal GLP-2 has been shown to be higher than in control ponies (de Laat *et al.*, 2018). This increased concentration in GLP-2 suggests that ponies with ID have an increased glucose bioavailability. The magnitude of the hyperinsulinaemic peak differs with diet and more specifically with the NSC composition of this diet, as well as with genetic predisposition: some breeds appear to respond more than others to a given oral glucose challenge (Treiber *et al.*, 2005a; Bamford *et al.*, 2014, 2015).

Fasting hyperinsulinaemia is also described and results more from an excessive and prolonged stimulation of pancreatic beta cells rather than a primary beta cell hyperplasia (Newkirk *et al.*, 2018). In insulin-dysregulated ponies, the increased bioavailability of glucose prolongs the stimulation of pancreatic beta cells and results in sustained insulin secretion. Presence of fasting hyperinsulinaemia would therefore indicate a more severe stage of ID.

Insulin dysregulation and associated diseases

Insulin dysregulation and equine metabolic syndrome

EMS was first introduced in 2002 to describe a collection of clinical signs and laboratory findings linking obesity, insulin resistance and laminitis, becoming a better-characterized collection of risk factors for laminitis in 2010 (Johnson, 2002; Frank *et al.*, 2010b). As the understanding of the disorder improves, the definition and appreciation of the syndrome and the clinical picture it describes change. The central and most important element of EMS is ID as demonstrated by hyperinsulinaemia (basal or post-NSC challenge) and/or peripheral tissue insulin resistance (Durham *et al.*, 2019). The other core elements of EMS are obesity, demonstrated by regional or generalized fat accumulation, and a predisposition toward laminitis (Durham *et al.*, 2019). Additional elements of EMS include hypertriglyceridaemia, increased blood pressure, abnormal plasma concentrations of adipokines, altered reproductive cycle in mares and increased systemic markers of inflammation (Frank *et al.*, 2010b; Durham *et al.*, 2019). For some authors, ID and EMS are used interchangeably; however, ID has been described in other contexts making the overlap between the two entities incomplete (Fig. 5.1).

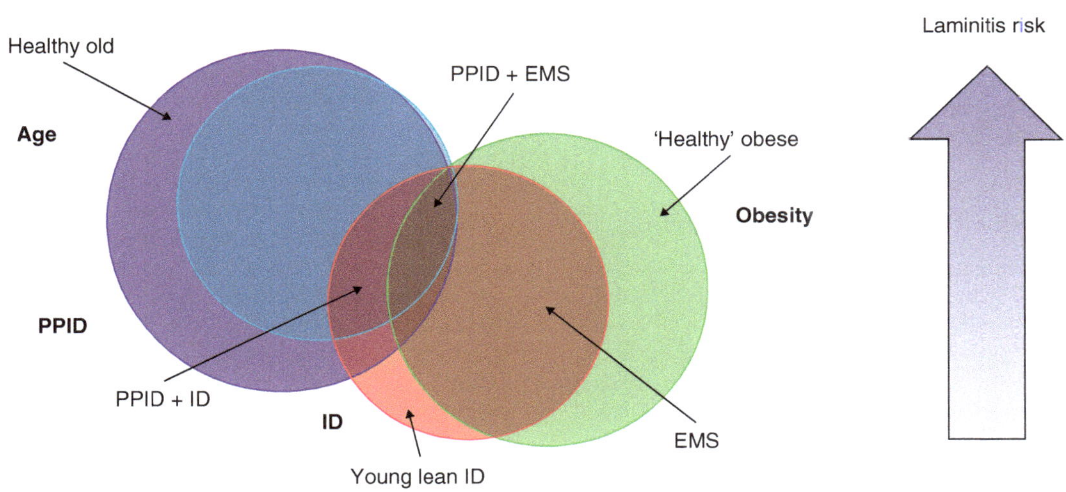

Fig. 5.1. Insulin dysregulation (ID) and associated diseases (pituitary pars intermedia dysfunction, PPID; equine metabolic syndrome, EMS). Modified from the Global Equine Endocrinology Group, 2018 (available at: https://sites.tufts.edu/equineendogroup/, accessed 5 May 2020).

Insulin dysregulation and obesity

Obesity used to be considered as the cause of ID; however, recent studies have described a lean phenotype of insulin-dysregulated horses and have shown that obesity per se was not necessarily associated with ID (Fig. 5.1) (Bamford *et al.*, 2016b; Martin-Gimenez *et al.*, 2016). Obesity results in changes in adipokine (cytokine produced by adipocytes) secretion that impacts glycaemic control, inflammation modulation and cardiovascular function (Radin *et al.*, 2009; Selim *et al.*, 2015). Adiponectin is an adipokine that has some anti-inflammatory effects and a role in glycaemic control (Antuna-Puente *et al.*, 2008). Adiponectin concentration and body mass index are negatively correlated in horses, meaning that obese horses will secrete less adiponectin than lean horses (Kearns *et al.*, 2006). Adiponectin secretion is also highly regulated by NSC ingestion, as feeding horses a diet high in NSC decreases plasma adiponectin (Bamford *et al.*, 2016b). Leptin is another adipokine which signals the fat status of an individual to maintain body condition by decreasing appetite and increasing energy expenditure (Kearns *et al.*, 2006; Van Weyenberg *et al.*, 2013). In some obese horses, hyperleptinaemia has been described, with a possible obesity-associated leptin resistance suspected of worsening pre-existing obesity (Kearns *et al.*, 2006; Van Weyenberg *et al.*, 2013). A correlation between leptin and insulin concentrations is also described but the causality of association is unclear (Morgan *et al.*, 2014). Studies of the consequences of obesity on inflammation modulation have been inconsistent, demonstrating a clear effect of generalized vs localized adiposity and visceral vs subcutaneous fat deposits (Fig. 5.2) (Vick *et al.*, 2007; Burns *et al.*, 2010; Suagee *et al.*, 2011a, 2013).

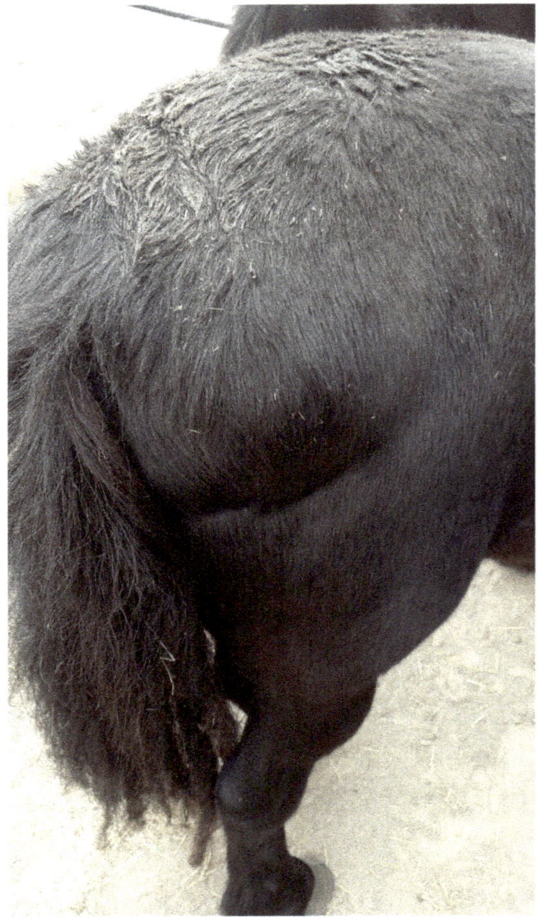

Fig. 5.2. Example of subcutaneous fat deposits in a 10-year-old Shetland mare (Author's own photograph).

Insulin dysregulation and laminitis

Hyperinsulinaemia causes laminitis as demonstrated by the induction of laminitis in healthy Standardbreds and healthy ponies by a 48-h infusion of insulin (Asplin *et al.*, 2007; de Laat *et al.*, 2010). The lesions associated with insulin-induced laminitis are stretching of the lamellar epithelial cells, with cytoskeletal disruption, proliferation and apoptosis, and lengthening and narrowing of the secondary epidermal lamellae (Asplin *et al.*, 2010; de Laat *et al.*, 2011b, 2013; Karikoski *et al.*, 2014). The specific mechanism by which hyperinsulinaemia induces laminitis is currently poorly described as no insulin receptor has been identified in lamellar epithelial cells and many hypotheses, such as hypoperfusion, energy failure, blood flow-induced hyperthermia, glucotoxicity and matrix metalloprotease up regulation, have been disproven (Asplin *et al.*, 2011; de Laat *et al.*, 2011a, de Laat *et al.*, 2012a, b; Stokes *et al.*, 2020a, Stokes *et al.*, 2020b). The currently investigated hypotheses involve the insulin-like growth factor 1 (IGF-1) receptor and the downstream pathways. This receptor shares some similarities with the insulin receptor, is present on lamellar epithelial cells and the downstream pathways have been shown to be activated after insulin infusion or oral administration of NSC (Burns *et al.*, 2013; Lane *et al.*, 2017).

Insulin dysregulation and pituitary pars intermedia dysfunction

Before ID was clearly identified as the core endocrine disorder associated with EMS, the clinical entity was described as peripheral Cushing's syndrome creating some confusion between PPID, ID and EMS (Johnson, 2002). At that time, it was assumed that one disease would lead to another and that both ID and PPID had a common origin. A better understanding of both conditions has considerably challenged this concept and PPID and ID are now considered as different pathological entities, even though they can be found simultaneously in the same animal (Fig. 5.1). The prevalence of ID in horses with PPID ranges from 30% to 75%, depending on the proportion of ponies included in the study and the definition of ID at the time of the study, demonstrating that there is a very incomplete overlap between the two conditions (van der Kolk *et al.*, 1995; McGowan *et al.*, 2013b; Frank and Tadros, 2014; Horn *et al.*, 2019). Many mechanisms could link PPID and ID; however, none has been clearly demonstrated. Hypercortisolaemia and administration of exogenous glucocorticoids increase insulin concentration and decrease insulin sensitivity in horses, suggesting a possible link between the two conditions (Tiley *et al.*, 2007, 2008; Tóth *et al.*, 2010a). However, although this mechanism is common in dogs, less than 20% of horses with PPID have adrenal hyperplasia that could result in increased glucocorticoid secretion, making this hypothesis unlikely (Peterson *et al.*, 1984; Schott, 2002). The increased plasma concentration of proopiomelanocortins (POMC) such as corticotropin-like intermediate peptide (CLIP) and alpha-melanocyte-stimulating hormone (α-MSH) could also be associated with the development of ID in some horses with PPID (Orth *et al.*, 1982; Wilson *et al.*, 1982; Beech *et al.*, 2011; McGowan *et al.*, 2013). CLIP is a direct activator of pancreatic beta cells and acts therefore as an insulin secretagogue while α-MSH regulates energy metabolism and is a leptin antagonist (Frank and Tadros, 2014). Although more research is warranted to unravel the links between ID and PPID, the consensus is that the two diseases are separate entities but that presence of one can worsen the clinical manifestations of the other. Therefore, investigation of both conditions is recommended in most patients.

Epidemiology of insulin dysregulation

The epidemiology of ID and EMS is difficult to describe, as the definition of the terms has changed over time with various inclusion criteria (obesity, actual ID or a combination).

The prevalence of ID varies between 18% and 27% depending on the geographic location (Australia vs USA) and the population of interest (ponies vs horses) (Morgan *et al.*, 2014; Durham *et al.*, 2019). Breed differences in insulin regulation have been described with British native ponies and Andalusian horses being more insulin dysregulated than Standardbreds or Thoroughbreds (Bamford *et al.*, 2014, 2015). Although ID is not considered as a disorder of old age like PPID, insulin sensitivity is found to decrease with age (Hart *et al.*, 2016; Jacob *et al.*, 2018).

The prevalence of equine obesity ranges from 8% to 50% depending on the countries, the breeds included, the use of the horses and the grader (owner or veterinarian); in more recent, veterinarian-based reports, the prevalence of equine obesity varies between 30% and 40% worldwide (Christie *et al.*, 2004; Wyse *et al.*, 2008; Stephenson *et al.*, 2011; Thatcher *et al.*, 2012; Giles *et al.*, 2014; Robin *et al.*, 2015; Jensen *et al.*, 2016; Potter *et al.*, 2016; Kosolofski *et al.*, 2017). Some breeds have a tendency to develop obesity; for example, British native breeds such as Welsh ponies, Rocky Mountain Horses, Tennessee Walking Horses and Warmbloods are more likely to become obese than Standardbreds and Thoroughbreds (Thatcher *et al.*, 2012; Giles *et al.*, 2015; Potter *et al.*, 2016).

The seasonality of ID is controversial as there have been conflicting results. A diagnosis of ID is heavily confounded with diet, both its composition and its availability (Place *et al.*, 2010; Dugdale *et al.*, 2011; Borer-Weir *et al.*, 2013; Selim *et al.*, 2015; Hart *et al.*, 2016). Seasonal factors such as pregnancy can also impact a diagnosis of ID as mares become physiologically insulin dysregulated during gestation (George *et al.*, 2011).

Clinical presentation of insulin dysregulation

The appearance of an insulin-dysregulated horse has been the focus of extensive research with the elaboration of a body condition scoring system (Henneke *et al.*, 1983; Dugdale *et al.*, 2012; Martinson *et al.*, 2014). Obesity used to be considered as a clinical sign of ID; however, as a lean

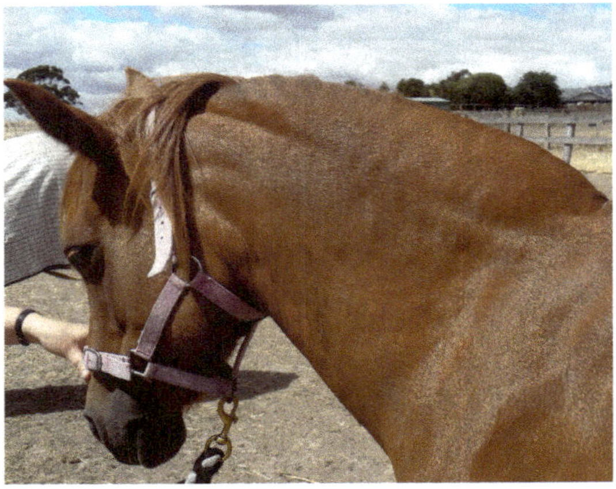

Fig. 5.3. Cresty neck score of 3/5 in an 8-year-old Australian Riding pony with chronic laminitis (courtesy of Dr Nicholas J. Bamford).

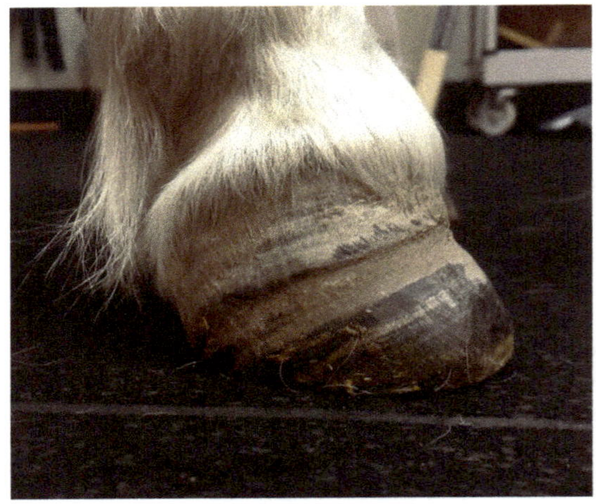

Fig. 5.4. Hoof of a 12-year-old Miniature pony diagnosed with equine metabolic syndrome (EMS). Note the hoof ring, indicative of chronic laminitis (courtesy of Dr Allison J. Stewart).

phenotype of insulin-dysregulated horses has been described and obesity has been shown to be a dispensable element for ID, caution is warranted (Bamford *et al.*, 2016b; Martin-Gimenez *et al.*, 2016; Durham *et al.*, 2019). The body condition scoring system and the cresty neck scoring system have been developed to better describe and quantify the degree of obesity in horses and ponies (Fig. 5.3, see Chapter 1 for definitions of those scoring systems) (Henneke *et al.*, 1983; Carter *et al.*, 2009a; Giles *et al.*, 2015; Martin-Gimenez *et al.*, 2016). Overall, an increased body condition score and an increased cresty neck score correlate with the presence of ID and of laminitis (Frank *et al.*, 2006; Treiber *et al.*, 2006; Vick *et al.*, 2007; Carter *et al.*, 2009a; Suagee *et al.*, 2013; Giles *et al.*, 2015; Selim *et al.*, 2015; Martin-Gimenez *et al.*, 2016). For example, a body condition score >7/9 has a sensitivity of 100% and a specificity of 29–44% to predict laminitis, and a cresty neck score >4 has a sensitivity of 50–83% and a specificity of 78–80% to predict laminitis (Carter *et al.*, 2009c). The variable and low sensitivity and specificity of using morphometric markers to diagnose ID confirms that some obese horses are not insulin dysregulated and that some lean horses can be extremely insulin dysregulated (Bamford *et al.*, 2016b). It is important to remember that more than generalized adiposity, presence of fat deposits in specific locations is more consistent with ID.

Horses with ID tend to have pre-existing changes in their hoof wall, such as abnormal growth rings, appearing even before the first recognized episode of clinical laminitis (Fig. 5.4) (Karikoski *et al.*, 2011).

Unlike sepsis-associated laminitis, the clinical presentation of insulin-associated laminitis seems more insidious (Morgan *et al.*, 2003; Kawasako *et al.*, 2009; McGowan, 2010; Karikoski *et al.*, 2015). Classically, the severity of foot lameness is categorized by the 'Obel scoring system', a system developed for sepsis-associated laminitis and extended to all types of laminitis (Table 5.1) (van Eps and Pollitt, 2006; Meier *et al.*, 2018b; Stokes *et al.*, 2019).

Considering the clinical differences between sepsis-associated laminitis and insulin-associated laminitis, the Obel scoring system often fails to detect mild cases of insulin-associated laminitis and limits the observation of clinical improvement or deterioration of laminitic horses (Meier *et al.*, 2018b). The 'Meier scoring system', or 'modified Obel scoring system', has been developed specifically for cases of insulin-associated laminitis (Meier *et al.*, 2019a). This scoring system is based on the sum of the scores obtained during three stages of examination (standing horse, moving horse and digital pulses, Table 5.2).

Regardless of the scoring system used, it is important to remember that these are clinical scores assessing foot pain and that there can be no correlation between a clinical score and histologic or radiographic changes. A five-point grading system

Table 5.1. Obel scoring system for laminitis severity (Obel, 1948).

Laminitis score	Grade description
Normal, Obel score 0	Horse appears sound
Obel score 1	At rest, the horse shifts its weight between the forelimbs; the horse is sound at the walk, but the gait is stilted at the trot, in a straight line and on turning
Obel score 2	The gait is stilted at the walk and the horse turns with great difficulty; one forelimb can be lifted
Obel score 3	The horse is reluctant to walk, and one forelimb can only be lifted with great difficulty
Obel score 4	The horse will only move if forced to

has been developed to assess the severity of the histopathological changes in experimentally induced laminitis (Table 5.3) (Pollitt, 1996; van Eps *et al.*, 2014).

In vivo, radiographs are a common method to assess laminitis and provide clinically relevant information about disease severity and progression (Fig. 5.5).

The most commonly interpreted view in the case of laminitis is the latero–medial projection in which three measurements and three angles are routinely measured (Cripps and Eustace, 1999; Hampson *et al.*, 2013; Sherlock and Parks, 2013). The first measurement is the coronary–extensor distance which is the distance between the top of the dorsal wall and the proximal limit of the extensor process. In normal feet, the distance should be between −2 and 15 mm and a longer distance would be suggestive of sinking of the third phalanx. The second measurement is the hoof width or wall thickness; this measurement should be between 14 and 22 mm and constant in a given foot. The last measurement is the sole depth, reflecting the distance between the most distal aspect of the third phalanx and the sole. This distance should be greater than 11 to 15 mm; a shorter distance would be consistent with sinking of the third phalanx (Fig. 5.6).

The first angle to be measured is the dorsal hoof wall angle which is the angle subtended by the dorsal hoof wall with the ground. This angle should be between 48° and 54°. The second angle is the parietal surface angle which is the angle subtended by the dorsal cortex of the third phalanx with the ground. This angle should be within 2° of the dorsal hoof wall angle; a greater angle indicates rotation of the third phalanx. The last angle to be measured is the solar margin angle which is the angle created between the distal surface of the solar margin of the third phalanx and the ground. This angle should be less than 8°; a greater angle would be consistent with rotation of the third phalanx (Fig. 5.7).

Diagnosis of insulin dysregulation

With a better understanding of ID, more diagnostic tests have been developed and refined. The ideal test would detect horses in the early stages of ID and address both insulin resistance and hyperinsulinaemia; however, as such a test has not been described, a combination of diagnostic testing is warranted.

Diagnosis of insulin resistance

The techniques used to assess insulin sensitivity in horses and ponies are mostly adapted from human medicine and are a direct or indirect assessment of the availability of insulin-sensitive tissues to respond to endogenous or exogenous insulin with increase cellular uptake of circulating glucose.

FASTING BLOOD GLUCOSE CONCENTRATION. Hyperglycaemia is an indirect measure of peripheral tissue insulin resistance. Although blood glucose concentration might be at the upper end of the reference range in horses with ID, there are many other possible causes of hyperglycaemia; therefore, fasting blood glucose is a poorly sensitive and poorly specific diagnostic test for peripheral tissue insulin resistance (Kronfeld *et al.*, 2005; Frank, 2011).

EUGLYCAEMIC HYPERINSULINAEMIC CLAMP. The euglycaemic hyperinsulinaemic clamp has been considered the 'gold standard' to diagnose peripheral tissue insulin resistance (Kronfeld *et al.*, 2005; Pratt *et al.*, 2005; Geor *et al.*, 2010; Frank and Tadros, 2014). After an insulin priming dose (45 mIU/kg), the horse receives a continuous infusion of insulin (3–6 mIU/kg/min) and blood glucose is maintained at a constant value (5 ± 1 mmol/l) by adjusting the glucose infusion rate (Kronfeld *et al.*, 2005; Pratt *et al.*, 2005; Asplin *et al.*, 2007). At steady state, the glucose infusion rate provides the insulin-induced

Table 5.2. Meier or modified Obel scoring system for insulin-associated laminitis severity (Meier *et al.*, 2019a).

Order of examination	Criteria	Description	Score
Stage 1			
Examine horse standing	Weight shifting	No weight shifting	0
		Weight shifting, including shifting weight between all feet; lying down and/or placing forelimbs in front of body	2
Gently lift each foot up and put back down straightaway	Forelimb lift	Prompt and willingly maintained (each forelimb)	0
		Reluctant and maintained with difficulty (each forelimb)	1
		Unable to lift foot/resists attempts to lift foot (each forelimb)	2
Stage 2			
Conduct on hard surface; walk horse approx. 30 m, side on to examiner	Gait at walk	Normal gait	0
		Mild short, stilted gait; still moves willingly	1
		Moderate short, stilted gait; reluctant/difficulty walking	2
		Severe difficulty walking or unable to walk	6
Turn on short lead, clockwise and anticlockwise	Gait at circle	Normal circling	0
		Mild head rise, difficulty when turning, still moves willingly	1
		Moderate, sharp head rise, reluctance/difficulty turning	2
		Severe difficulty turning, slow and clearly in pain	3
Stage 3			
All feet must be square on ground (unless unable to stand)	Forelimb digital pulse	Normal; able to palpate, normal magnitude but not bounding (each forelimb)	0
		Increased magnitude or bounding digital pulse (each forelimb)	2

glucose disposal rate. A low value indicates tissue insulin resistance whereas a high value indicates effective insulin-induced glucose disposal and insulin sensitivity (Pratt *et al.*, 2005). The interpretation of this test may be difficult in a diagnostic context, in the absence of specific reference intervals or diagnostic cut-off values. For example, a value lower than 7 µmol/kg/min would indicate tissue insulin resistance in the general equine population; however, in Warmbloods, a value lower than 14 µmol/kg/min would indicate tissue insulin resistance (Kronfeld *et al.*, 2005). Despite its practical issues, the euglycaemic hyperinsulinaemic clamp is considered as repeatable and is often used as a reference test (Pratt *et al.*, 2005; Pratt-Phillips *et al.*, 2015). This test carries a small risk of inducing laminitis if performed over more than 24 h with high rates of insulin infusion (de Laat *et al.*, 2010).

Insulin sensitivity tests. The insulin sensitivity test directly assesses the ability of insulin-sensitive tissues to increase glucose uptake after exogenous insulin administration. The complete test assesses insulin sensitivity by measuring blood glucose after intravenous injection of insulin (20–125 mIU/kg) over 5 h (Caltabilota *et al.*, 2010). The shorter test (or 2-step test) assesses insulin sensitivity by measuring blood glucose 30 min after intravenous injection of 100 mIU/kg of exogenous insulin (Bertin and Sojka-Kritchevsky, 2013). The tests carry a small risk of inducing hypoglycaemia but signs of this condition rarely require treatment (Eiler *et al.*, 2005). If needed, an intravenous injection of 30 ml/100 kg of 50% dextrose alleviates signs of hypoglycaemia (Durham, 2016). The 2-step test is widely used in clinical practice (Horn and Bertin, 2019).

Table 5.3. Five-point grading system for severity of laminitis histopathology assessed with haematoxylin and eosin staining (Pollitt, 1996; van Eps *et al.*, 2014).

Histopathology grade	Description
Grade 0	Normal structure, no evidence of laminitis.
Grade 1	At low magnification the keratinized axes of the primary and secondary epidermal lamellae appear normal. The width of the secondary epidermal lamella appears decreased and the secondary epidermal lamellae become elongated. Nuclei become round instead of oval and more centrally located in the basal cell cytoplasm. The nuclei are abnormally close to the basement membrane. The outline between adjacent secondary epidermal lamella is indistinct and the structures become confluent. The clear symmetry of the basement membrane is lost. These early changes are difficult to appreciate.
Grade 2	At low magnification the primary epidermal lamellae appear relatively normal; however, the primary epidermal lamellae tips have a stretched and wavy appearance. The absence of connective tissue between secondary epidermal lamellae is widespread and the rounding of the secondary epidermal lamella basal cell nuclei is more obvious. Neutrophils are present, particularly around vessels adjacent to the primary epidermal lamella tips. At high magnification, many of the basal cell nuclei, particularly those adjacent to the secondary dermal lamellae in which connective tissue is absent, are small and darkly stained. Nearly all the basal cell nuclei are round instead of oval and are situated close to the basement membrane rather than in the normal apical position. The basal cell cytoplasm is pale, cloudy and vacuolated. Many of the secondary epidermal lamellae have tapered tips that stream off into the primary dermal lamellae in the direction of the distal phalanx. Cellular vacuolation, small round nuclei and lamellar attenuation are most pronounced near the tips of secondary epidermal lamellae. The regular symmetrical arrangement of the lamellar anatomy disappears. The basal cells at the tips of primary epidermal lamellae are the least abnormal. Many have oval, normal staining nuclei, situated in the normal position close to the apex of the cell and there are mitotic figures suggesting a proliferative response.
Grade 3	The keratinized axial cores of the primary epidermal lamellae are still intact, but instead of the primary epidermal lamella tips having an overall rounded shape, the tips are tapered and shrunken. The axial cores of the secondary epidermal lamellae are barely recognizable as distinct architectural entities. Most of the epidermal cells form an amorphous mass between alternating primary epidermal and dermal lamellae. The few secondary epidermal lamellae that are recognizable are devoid of connective tissue attachments. At high magnification, the tapered primary epidermal lamella tips consist of wavy empty tubes containing pink material and the occasional epidermal basal cell nucleus. Some of the epidermal cell nuclei are pyknotic. Further from the original primary epidermal lamella tip, the anatomy is recognizable as the remnants of secondary epidermal lamellae. The cytoplasm of the secondary epidermal lamellae basal cells is light pink, cloudy and vacuolated. There is extreme elongation and stretching of the secondary epidermal lamellae. Many of the nuclei are spindle shaped and elongated in the direction of the lamellae. There is no recognizable connective tissue between secondary epidermal lamellae, most of the epidermis appears as an amorphous mass of elongated nuclei and basal cell cytoplasm interspersed between the remnants of the keratinized axes of secondary epidermal lamellae. Although there are many pyknotic nuclei in the epidermal structures, many seem intact and relatively unaffected by surrounding disarray. Blood vessels adjacent to the tips of the primary epidermal lamellae are surrounded by leucocytes but the inflammatory response is minimal. Blood vessels in the sublamellar dermis appear normal. A few lamellar capillaries contain proteinaceous, amorphous, pink staining material but this is not generalized.
Grade 4	Complete physical separation of lamellar epidermis from dermis, with no association between epidermal and dermal tissues.

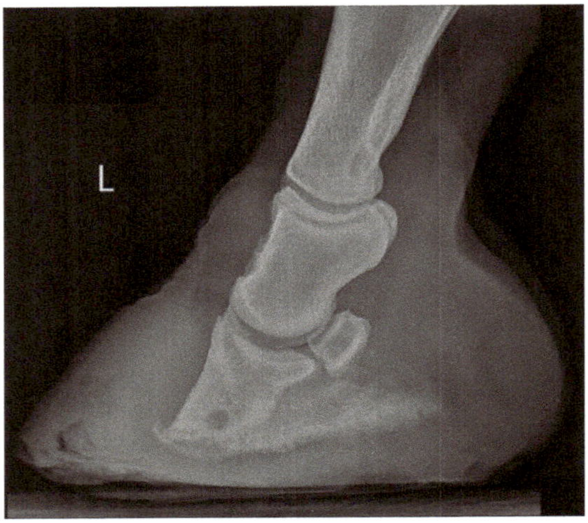

Fig. 5.5. Severe chronic laminitis in a 28-year-old Arab stallion with insulin dysregulation (ID) (Author's own photograph).

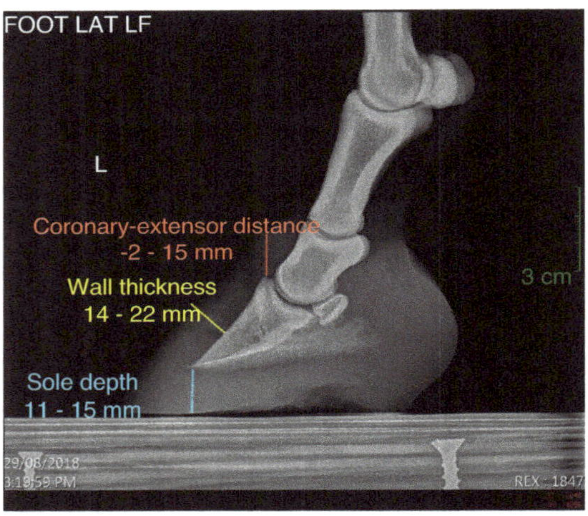

Fig. 5.6. Mild laminitis in a 9-year-old Welsh pony with insulin dysregulation (ID). Note the measurements used to assess the presence of laminitis: coronary–extensor distance in red, hoof width or wall thickness in yellow and sole depth in blue (Author's own photograph).

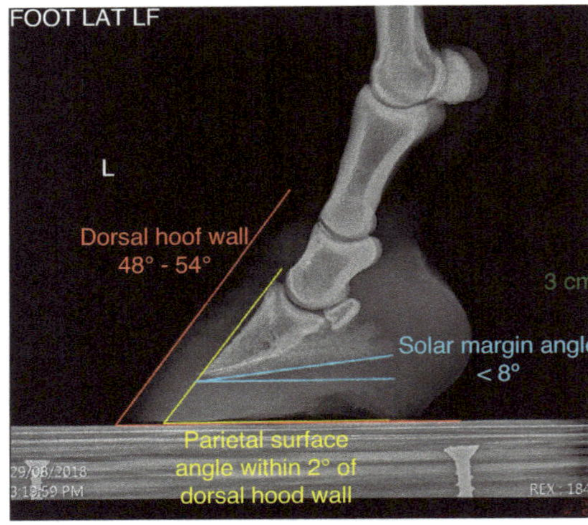

Fig. 5.7. Mild laminitis in a 9-year-old Welsh pony with insulin dysregulation (ID). Note the angles used to assess the presence of laminitis: dorsal hoof wall angle in red, parietal surface angle in yellow and solar margin angle in blue (Author's own photograph).

Frequently sampled intravenous glucose tolerance test. Two versions of the test have been described: one based solely on an intravenous glucose injection (original version of the test) and the other based on an intravenous glucose injection followed by an intravenous insulin injection (modified version of the test). In the original version of the test, 500 mg/kg of dextrose is injected and up to 36 blood samples are collected over 6 h to measure both glucose and insulin (Pratt *et al.*, 2005). This test has been shown to have poor repeatability, with a within-horse coefficient of variability between 24% and 30%; therefore, some changes have been made to limit glucose urinary spilling and variability, resulting in the injection of smaller doses of dextrose (100–300 mg/kg) (Hoffman *et al.*, 2003b; Pratt *et al.*, 2005; Tóth *et al.*, 2009; Bertin *et al.*, 2013; Pratt-Phillips *et al.*, 2015; Dunbar *et al.*, 2016). A minimal model analysis is used to calculate the insulin sensitivity index (Si, reflecting insulin-dependent glucose clearance), the glucose effectiveness (Sg, reflecting insulin-independent glucose clearance), the acute insulin response to glucose (AIRg, reflecting the glucose-induced insulin secretion or beta cell responsiveness) and the glucose half-life (T1/2 g, reflecting overall glucose clearance) (Pratt *et al.*, 2005). The modified version of the test differs from the original version by the intravenous injection of 20–30 mIU/kg of exogenous insulin 20 min after dextrose injection (Hoffman *et al.*, 2003a; Bailey *et al.*, 2007). This modified version allows the calculation of insulin sensitivity (SI, reflecting the efficiency of insulin to accelerate glucose uptake). Peripheral tissue insulin resistance is diagnosed when SI is low (<1 l/min/mIU) whereas a horse is classified as insulin sensitive with a high SI (>1.5 l/min/mIU) (Burns *et al.*, 2010). The modified test is now widely used in research settings (Carter *et al.*, 2009b; Burns *et al.*, 2010; Carter *et al.*, 2010; Frank *et al.*, 2010b; Chameroy *et al.*, 2011; Bamford *et al.*, 2014; Pratt-Phillips *et al.*, 2015; Dunbar *et al.*, 2016).

Combined glucose insulin tolerance test. The combined glucose insulin tolerance test was developed as a simplified combination of the two tests described above and is based on the almost simultaneous intravenous injection of 150 mg/kg of dextrose and 100 mIU/kg of insulin (Eiler *et al.*, 2005). Over 150 min, up to 14 blood samples are collected to measure both glucose and insulin. This simultaneous injection of glucose and insulin results in a biphasic curve with a positive phase (relative hyperglycaemia) and a negative phase (relative hypoglycaemia). The interpretation of the test is either based on the duration of the positive phase (peripheral tissue insulin resistance if the relative hyperglycaemia lasts more than 45 min) or on the insulin concentration after 45 min (peripheral tissue insulin resistance if >100 μIU/ml), or both (Eiler *et al.*, 2005; Argo *et al.*, 2012; Dunbar *et al.*, 2016).

Proxies and surrogate tests. Although these tests seem to be widely used in human medicine, they only have limited value in equine practice (Uwaifo *et al.*, 2002; Gungor *et al.*, 2004). The glucose/insulin ratio is a good estimate of peripheral tissue insulin sensitivity and the insulin/glucose ratio would correlate with insulin secretion (Kronfeld *et al.*, 2005). The homeostasis model assessment of insulin sensitivity (HOMA-IS: 22.5/(glucose × insulin)) and the quantitative insulin sensitivity check index (QUICKI: 1/(log(glucose) + log(insulin)) correlate well with the results of the euglycaemic hyperinsulinaemic clamp (Kronfeld *et al.*, 2005). The reciprocal inverse square of basal insulin (RISQI: insulin − 0.5) and the modified insulin to glucose ratio (MIRG: (800 − 0.3(insulin − 50)2)/(glucose − 30)) correlate well with the SI and AIRg results of the modified frequently sampled intravenous glucose tolerance test (Treiber *et al.*, 2005b). As only very few studies have evaluated the relevance and the validity of these tests in diseased horses, their use is not recommended in clinical practice (Frank, 2011).

Diagnosis of hyperinsulinaemia

The diagnosis of equine hyperinsulinaemia is a developing field and now represents the mainstay for the diagnosis of ID.

Basal serum insulin concentration. Hyperinsulinaemia in a laminitic horse is supportive of ID diagnosis and may not warrant the use of other forms of testing (Frank *et al.*, 2010b; Morgan *et al.*, 2014; Hart *et al.*, 2016). On the other hand, a serum insulin concentration within the reference intervals is non-diagnostic, as horses diagnosed with ID by other tests can present without basal hyperinsulinaemia (Frank *et al.*, 2010b; Dunbar *et al.*, 2016). The threshold for hyperinsulinaemia can be controversial and it is paramount to obtain diagnostic cut-off values from the diagnostic laboratories as different assays will yield different results (Tinworth *et al.*, 2011; Borer-Weir *et al.*, 2012; Banse and McFarlane, 2014; Banse *et al.*, 2014; Warnken *et al.*, 2016). It is considered that in a fasted horse, basal serum insulin concentration should be <20 μIU/ml and in a non-fasted horse, basal insulin concentration should be <60 μIU/ml; however, lower values have been reported (Bertin and de Laat, 2017; Menzies-Gow *et al.*, 2017). Basal serum insulin could have some prognostic value: a basal serum insulin >188 μIU/ml has been shown to have a sensitivity and a specificity >90% to predict laminitis and non-survival (Asplin *et al.*, 2007). Some physiological variability in basal insulin concentration has been described with seasonal and diurnal effects; however, such changes are rather mild and would not alter diagnostic cut-offs (Frank *et al.*, 2010a; Bamford *et al.*, 2015).

Oral sugar and oral glucose tests. The oral sugar test assesses the glucose-induced insulin response to oral administration of NSC and accounts for the enteroinsular axis function (Hoffman *et al.*, 2003b; Borer *et al.*, 2012; de Laat *et al.*, 2016c). A diagnosis of hyperinsulinaemia is based on a serum insulin >60 μIU/ml, 60 or 90 min after oral administration of 0.15 ml/kg of maize syrup to horses fasted overnight (Schuver *et al.*, 2014). The need to fast and the duration of fasting is debatable but it appears that a fast of 3 h is recommended (Bertin *et al.*, 2016). There have been some reports of the poor repeatability of the test; however, this test is now widely used in clinical practice and in research

(Dunbar *et al.*, 2016; Knowles *et al.*, 2016; Smith *et al.*, 2016).

The oral glucose test is based on the same principle as the oral sugar test, using a different source of NSC (Jose-Cunilleras et al., 2002). A diagnosis of hyperinsulinaemia with this test is made on a serum insulin >80 μIU/ml, 120 min after oral administration of 0.75–1 g/kg of dextrose (de Laat and Sillence, 2017). The method of administration of dextrose varies: powdered dextrose mixed with chaff and spontaneously eaten by the horse or a nasogastric intubation of dextrose dissolved in water in a 20% solution (Pratt-Phillips et al., 2015; Smith et al., 2016). This test is widely used in clinical practice and research (Fitzgerald et al., 2019). The oral glucose test could have better repeatability than the oral sugar test and has been shown to correlate well with the results of the euglycaemic hyperinsulinaemic clamp, the modified frequently sampled intravenous glucose tolerance test in healthy horses and with the risk of laminitis in insulin-dysregulated ponies (Pratt-Phillips et al., 2015; Smith et al., 2016; de Laat and Sillence, 2017; Meier et al., 2018b).

Additional testing

Some horses develop peripheral tissue insulin resistance without hyperinsulinaemia (decreased peripheral tissue uptake); others develop hyperinsulinaemia in the absence of peripheral tissue insulin resistance (inappropriate intestinal absorption effect); and some develop both hyperinsulinaemia and peripheral tissue insulin resistance (de Laat *et al.*, 2016c). Therefore, as current tests only investigate one arm of the disease, they might lack sensitivity and fail to diagnose patients that would benefit from earlier therapeutic measures. It is therefore recommended that the diagnosis of ID is done in a stepwise manner, starting with baseline values of insulin and glucose and finishing with a combination of tests that diagnose both peripheral tissue insulin resistance as well as enteroinsular axis dysfunction.

Incretins. The role of incretins in the pathophysiology of ID is becoming clearer; however, a specific role for incretins as a diagnostic tool is not well established and the determination of incretin concentrations is currently restricted to research.

Connecting peptide. Proinsulin is cleaved into C-peptide and insulin. As C-peptide is not degraded as quickly as insulin through hepatic first passage, its half-life is six times longer than that of insulin (Marques *et al.*, 2004). Therefore, C-peptide can be used as a marker of pancreatic secretion and dysfunction in horses (Tóth *et al.*, 2010b; de Laat *et al.*, 2016d).

Adiponectin. The correlation between adiponectin concentrations and insulin concentrations is not clear, with conflicting results; however, beyond ID and obesity, a plasma high molecular weight adiponectin concentration <2.5 μg/ml has a sensitivity and a specificity of 80% to predict the occurrence of pasture-associated laminitis within 3 years (Gordon and McKeever, 2005, Gordon and McKeever, 2006; Bamford *et al.*, 2016b; Menzies-Gow *et al.*, 2017).

Leptin. Leptin is associated with decreased insulin sensitivity, increased body condition score and laminitis; however, its role as a diagnostic target is not clear (Frank *et al.*, 2006; Kearns *et al.*, 2006; Carter *et al.*, 2009c; Caltabilota *et al.*, 2010; Morgan *et al.*, 2014). Nevertheless, a leptin concentration of >7.3 ng/ml has been shown to have a sensitivity of 63–83% to predict endocrinopathic laminitis (Carter *et al.*, 2009c).

Triglycerides. Rather than being a direct marker of ID, triglyceride concentration is associated with obesity and is a poor predictor of ID and laminitis (Treiber *et al.*, 2006; Pleasant *et al.*, 2013; Frank and Tadros, 2014; Morgan *et al.*, 2014; Bamford *et al.*, 2016a; de Laat *et al.*, 2016b; Menzies-Gow *et al.*, 2017).

Management of insulin dysregulation

The management of ID is currently based on four elements of decreasing importance: diet, hoof care, exercise and pharmacologic aids.

Dietary management

Reduction in digestible energy intake overall and reduction in NSC intake specifically is the mainstay of the management of horses with ID and EMS (Geor and Harris, 2009).

A general rule to allow progressive weight reduction in obese horses is to decrease their dry matter intake to 1.25–1.5% of their body weight in hay, depending on the amount of weight to lose, to provide between 65% and 95% of the horses' maintenance requirements (Argo *et al.*, 2012, 2015; Bruynsteen *et al.*, 2015). This degree of restriction has been shown to result in both weight loss and improved insulin regulation (Freestone *et al.*, 1992; Buff *et al.*, 2006b; Van Weyenberg *et al.*, 2008; Dugdale *et al.*, 2010; Ungru *et al.*, 2012; Argo *et al.*, 2015; Morgan *et al.*, 2016). To avoid excessive restriction, it should be noted that hay is only about 90% dry matter so the actual amount of hay to be provided to a horse is around 1.5–1.7% of its body weight (Argo *et al.*, 2012, 2015; Bruynsteen *et al.*, 2015). With this degree of restriction, a decrease in body condition score (toward 'moderate') and a weight loss of up to 1% of body weight per week can be expected (Dugdale *et al.*, 2010; Bamford *et al.*, 2019). The response to diet restriction, however, varies tremendously between horses, as some can take significantly longer than others to lose weight and appear as weight-loss resistant (Dugdale *et al.*, 2010; Argo *et al.*, 2012). In these cases, further restriction to 1% of their body weight of hay as dry matter (about 1.1% of hay) can be considered. Close monitoring of these animals is warranted as excessive restrictions and rapid weight loss is associated with a negative energy balance, resulting in excessive lipolysis and hypertriglyceridaemia or hyperlipaemia (Freestone *et al.*, 1991; Dunkel *et al.*, 2014; Bruynsteen *et al.*, 2015; Brøkner *et al.*, 2016). As weight loss is never an emergency, further dietary restrictions should be undertaken over the course of 2 weeks with frequent weight and serum triglyceride concentration monitoring. Long periods of fasting are not recommended as fasting increases peripheral tissue insulin resistance and further complications such as behavioural issues can also arise (Freestone *et al.*, 1991; Bertin *et al.*, 2016). Therefore, feeding strategies to keep an animal busy have yielded better long-term results. Feeding in a hay net prolongs hay intake time by 60% and dynamic feeding systems provide a combination of exercise and prolonged hay intake time, decreasing the ingestion of bedding material (Glunk *et al.*, 2015; de Laat *et al.*, 2016a). Other strategies to decrease dry matter intake include restricted grazing and the use of a grazing muzzle (Frank *et al.*, 2010b). Restricted grazing has been shown to have a limited effect on actual dry matter intake as horses and ponies can ingest large amounts of grass, up to 90% of their requirements, in a period of time as short as 3 h (Glunk *et al.*, 2015). Grazing muzzles, on the other hand, have been shown to reduce dry matter intake by up to 25% (Durham *et al.*, 2019). The use of grazing muzzles is not as straightforward as expected. To work, the muzzles have to be correctly fitted and the grass has to be cut to the right length so the horse will not remove it too easily and can actually graze; grass cut too short or too long will not go through the muzzle.

In addition to the quantity of dry matter ingested, hay quality and composition are key elements to consider when managing an insulin-dysregulated horse. This critical step is, however, only rarely taken by owners and veterinary practitioners and the nutrient composition of the forage fed to horses is usually unknown (Harris *et al.*, 2017). A hay containing less than 10% of NSC is recommended in horses with ID to limit their insulin response (Borgia *et al.*, 2011). Hays from legume plants tend to be richer in NSC; hays with a usually low NSC content include lucerne or Timothy hay; while oat and barley yield hays with a usually higher NSC content. Most hays like Rhodes hay and grass hay will have variable NSC content and hay analysis is strongly encouraged. Addition of straw in the diet can also be used to manage ID horses. Being poorly digestible with high fibre and low NSC content, straw represents a low-calorie option. Furthermore, mixing hay with straw decreases the palatability of the hay resulting in a longer ingestion time and an overall lower dry matter intake. One strategy to reduce the NSC intake of insulin-dysregulated horses consists in soaking hay: properly soaked hay reduces its water-soluble carbohydrate content and reduces the glycaemic and insulinaemic responses to the hay (Carslake *et al.*, 2018). The reduction in water-soluble carbohydrate content increases with water temperature and duration of soaking, with a decrease of up to 49% after 16 h at 16°C with agitation (Longland *et al.*, 2014; Moore-Colyer *et al.*, 2014; Argo *et al.*, 2015). In warmer climates, a shorter soaking time of only 1 to 2 h is recommended as bacterial and mould growth can become problematic unless the hay is steamed before being given to horses (Moore-Colyer *et al.*, 2014). As water-soluble carbohydrates are not the only nutrient lost in water, protein, mineral and vitamin supplementation with a ration balancer is recommended to cover requirements (Mack *et al.*, 2014; Argo *et al.*, 2015). Dietary supplements to provide a specific element such as chromium, magnesium or short-chain fructo-oligosaccharides have shown some potentially beneficial effects on insulin regulation; however, further research is necessary (Chameroy *et al.*, 2011; Respondek *et al.*, 2011; McGowan *et al.*, 2013).

Once a new diet is implemented, follow-up to ensure its adequacy is warranted. Frequent monitoring of body weight and assessment of the insulin response after ingestion of the new diet are the best tools to demonstrate success or failure of the management plan (Morgan *et al.*, 2016). Pasture access should be eliminated for insulin-dysregulated horses in the early stages of management; however, following control of their body weight and improvement of their insulin regulation, those horses can eventually be put back on pasture (Van Weyenberg *et al.*, 2008; Morgan *et al.*, 2016).

Hoof care

As most horses with ID suffer or have suffered from laminitis, proper hoof care is paramount in all cases. A close relationship between the owner, the farrier and the veterinarian is often required to obtain good results. When the lamella has separated, the return to a normal mechanical function is a very slow process that can take up to 12 months (O'Grady, 2010). During an acute episode, absolute stall rest is recommended to reduce stress on the inflamed lamella; however, limited movement, in a deeply bedded stall and depending on the degree of pain, can be beneficial to allow proper hoof perfusion (Stokes *et al.*, 2020a). Although insulin-associated laminitis is a chronic process, continuous digital hypothermia during acute crises limits lamellar failure in experimentally induced insulin-associated laminitis (Stokes *et al.*, 2019). Long-term management of chronic laminitis is based on three principles: prevention of further hoof distortion, pain management and promotion of hoof growth (O'Grady, 2010). To limit further hoof distortion, the hoof needs to be trimmed to realign the distal surface of the solar margin of the third phalanx and the ground (reduction of the solar margin angle) and to reposition the hoof breakover point (realignment of the dorsal hoof wall angle and the parietal surface angle). As mentioned above, this is a slow process and it requires several trimming sessions guided by frequent radiographic monitoring. Depending on the severity of the lesions, sole depth and pain, initial trimming sessions are usually 4 weeks apart with longer intervals as the hoof grows appropriately (Hampson *et al.*, 2011). Beyond the careful use of non-steroidal anti-inflammatory drugs, pain management is achieved by limiting the stress on the hoof wall and taking advantage of a ground surface capable of weight bearing, like the sole or the frog. Sole padding, shoeing and deep bedding are the main options used in these cases. A large array of shoes has been recommended for chronic laminitis treatment; however, it appears that they all have their advantages and pitfalls. Reverse shoes, egg-bar shoes, heart-bar shoes or wooden shoes have the merit of supporting the heel, but a heel elevation is not recommended in all cases (O'Grady, 2010). Therefore, rather than a one-shoe-fits-all approach, a case-by-case and stage-by-stage approach is warranted. Promotion of hoof growth requires foot movement, and this step is often limited by the degree of pain. As the horse improves with improved insulin regulation and progressive hoof trimming, movement can increase, and the hoof can grow better. After 6 to 12 months of proper therapeutic farriery and adequate dietary management, insulin-dysregulated horses can be ridden again.

Exercise

Associated with a proper diet and after management of the laminitic crisis, exercise promotes weight loss and insulin sensitivity. At low intensity (5 min of trot daily for 2 weeks), exercise decreases obesity-associated inflammation; however, higher levels of exercise (45 min of fast trotting to achieve 70% of the maximum heart rate or 150–180 beats per minute daily for 1 week) would be required to achieve a significant improvement in insulin regulation (McCutcheon *et al.*, 2002; Stewart-Hunt *et al.*, 2006; Carter *et al.*, 2010; Menzies-Gow *et al.*, 2014; Bonelli *et al.*, 2017). Exercise on its own only brings short-term improvement and several studies have had disappointing results. However, when exercise is combined with an improved diet and associated with weight loss, it can improve insulin regulation for a longer period of time, even at low intensity (Freestone *et al.*, 1992; Duren *et al.*, 1999; Geor *et al.*, 2000; Powell *et al.*, 2002; Carter *et al.*, 2010; de Laat *et al.*, 2016a; Bamford *et al.*, 2019). Therefore, a routine of moderate exercise is recommended for insulin-dysregulated horses. This routine has to take into account the risk of laminitis; frequent monitoring to detect early signs of laminitis is warranted.

Pharmacologic options

Dietary management, hoof care and exercise routine are the main treatments for ID. In some cases, drugs can improve case management and accelerate results but should never be used without the interventions described above.

Metformin. In human medicine, this adenosine monophosphate-activated protein kinase (AMPK) agonist is usually prescribed to improve peripheral tissue insulin sensitivity, mainly in myocytes (Hardie, 2011). Although the drug is commonly prescribed in horses with ID, metformin is poorly absorbed in the equine gastrointestinal tract and does not appear to improve peripheral tissue insulin sensitivity (Hustace *et al.*, 2009; Tinworth *et al.*, 2010, 2012). Instead, the suggested mechanism of action of metformin in horses would be a local effect on enterocytes of the proximal small intestine. Through this mechanism, metformin alters enteric glucose absorption and subsequent insulin secretion (Rendle *et al.*, 2013). Therefore, although the drug has no effect on peripheral tissue insulin resistance, it appears to have a beneficial effect in horses with post-prandial hyperinsulinaemia (Tinworth *et al.*, 2012; Rendle *et al.*, 2013). Doses range from 15 mg/kg to 30 mg/kg administered orally every 8 to 12 h, depending on the feeding schedule of the horse (Durham *et al.*, 2008). Considering its local effect, metformin should be administered 30 to 60 min before feeding the horse for a maximum effect (Rendle *et al.*, 2013).

Pioglitazone. This thiazolidinedione is an anti-type-2 diabetes drug prescribed in humans. There are a few reports of its use in horses, but results are generally disappointing with low plasma concentrations and a limited effect on insulin regulation (Suagee *et al.*, 2011b; Wearn *et al.*, 2011, Wearn *et al.*, 2012). Its use is therefore not recommended.

Levothyroxine. This synthetic thyroid hormone was initially used when the combination of obesity and laminitis was thought to result from a thyroid dysfunction. With the identification of ID as the core element of EMS, the rationale for thyroid hormone supplementation is weak; however, in horses with weight-loss resistance, prolonged treatment with levothyroxine, in addition to an adequate diet for an insulin-dysregulated horse, allows a more rapid weight management (Frank *et al.*, 2005, 2008b). This effect would be mediated by the overall increase in metabolic rate fostering weight loss. Treatment is administered orally at 0.05 to 0.2 mg/kg daily for up to 48 weeks, or until the targeted weight loss has been achieved (Frank *et al.*, 2005). Even at high doses and for long courses, this treatment is well tolerated by horses (Frank *et al.*, 2008a; Bertin *et al.*, 2019). Discontinuation of treatment should be progressive over 1 month, with the dose halved for 2 weeks and halved again for another 2 weeks.

Sodium–glucose cotransport -2 inhibitors. This class of drugs promotes urinary glucose excretion from the renal proximal tubule. Early studies have been very promising in the possible management of insulin-dysregulated horses with drugs such as canagliflozin and velagliflozin (Frank, 2018; Meier *et al.*, 2018a). The use of these drugs has been shown to be safe and associated with a decreased risk of laminitis in insulin-dysregulated ponies (Meier *et al.*, 2018a, 2019b) Although the results are promising, the drugs are expensive and further research on this class is required before recommendations can be made.

Pergolide. In horses with PPID, pergolide is the drug of choice to manage the disease (Horn *et al.*, 2019). There is, however, very limited evidence to support its use in horses with ID, as other dopamine agonists have failed to provide any beneficial effect (Durham *et al.*, 2019).

Monitoring and prognosis for insulin dysregulation and equine metabolic syndrome

As for all endocrine disorders, management of ID and EMS is a long process and frequent monitoring of the horse, as well as establishment of a veterinarian–owner–farrier partnership, are key for success. Setting realistic weight loss and exercise objectives is important to keep the owner on board with treatment. When results are disappointing, levothyroxine can be added to the treatment. Re-examination of insulin-dysregulated horses should also focus on retesting insulin concentrations, ideally after ingestion of their improved diet to detect any insulin peak and potentially adapt the diet or add metformin if necessary. With time and diligent observance of recommendations, the prognosis for ID in horses and ponies is good.

Diabetes Mellitus

The characteristic of diabetes mellitus is the presence of sustained, and often severe, hyperglycaemia measured on several occasions (Durham *et al.*, 2009; Navas de Solis and Foreman, 2010). This persistent hyperglycaemia can be associated with glycosuria and polyuria/polydipsia, with cases reported to consume up to 360 ml/kg/day of water (Giri *et al.*, 2011). Unlike other species, diabetes in horses is rare but both type-1 and type-2 diabetes have been reported.

Type-1 diabetes mellitus

Insulin-dependent or type-1 diabetes mellitus results from a direct lesion of the endocrine pancreas, resulting in a decrease in beta cell function and a decreased or absent insulin secretion. Only a handful of cases have been reported indicating that the condition is rare. Three causes of type-1 diabetes mellitus have been reported: lymphocytic infiltration of the pancreas leading to loss of beta cells; infectious pancreatitis also leading to loss of beta cells; and systemic inflammation leading to decreased beta cell function (Jeffrey, 1968; Navas de Solis and Foreman, 2010; Giri *et al.*, 2011; Newman, 2015; Bertin *et al.*, 2018). The first two mechanisms seem to result in permanent damages while the third mechanism seems only to cause transient and reversible type-1 diabetes mellitus.

Horses with type-1 diabetes mellitus are usually presented for investigation of weight loss, low body condition score and depression. There is usually a discrepancy between the ravenous appetite of the animals and their body condition scores. Haematology is usually unremarkable although a mild anaemia can be reported. Serum chemistry reveals marked hyperglycaemia (16–23 mmol/l), marked hyponatraemia, high anion gap and hypertriglyceridaemia of variable magnitude (6.5–34.1 mmol/l) associated with increased activities of liver enzymes (gamma-glutamyl transferase and aspartate aminotransferase) (Navas de Solis and Foreman, 2010; Giri *et al.*, 2011).

Diagnosis of type-1 diabetes mellitus

Diagnosis is achieved by demonstration of profound hyperglycaemia on multiple occasions, persistent glycosuria and low serum insulin concentration. The concept of hypoinsulinaemia is rarely used as no lower limits of insulin reference intervals have been reported; however, in suspected cases, insulin concentrations are reported to be undetectable or well below the mean value of age-matched controls despite hyperglycaemia (Forhead *et al.*, 2004; Holdstock *et al.*, 2004; Navas de Solis and Foreman, 2010; Giri *et al.*, 2011). Determination of fructosamine concentration and glycosylated haemoglobin (Hb A1c) concentration is also recommended in cases suspected of diabetes mellitus as the concentration of these compounds is less impacted by daily variations in glucose concentration (Scroggie *et al.*, 2003). In healthy controls, fructosamine concentrations are reported to range from 195.5 to 402 µmol/l while Hb A1c is reported to range from 2.5% to 5.0% (Giri *et al.*, 2011; Knowles *et al.*, 2012, 2014).

Treatment of type-1 diabetes mellitus

Treatment of type-1 diabetes mellitus relies on the provision of exogenous insulin to maintain blood glucose concentrations below 11 mmol/l (Giri *et al.*, 2011). Different forms of insulin have been used: intramuscular, intravenous or subcutaneous injections of regular insulin at 0.1–0.5 IU/kg twice a day; constant-rate intravenous infusion of regular insulin at 0.01–0.1 IU/kg/h; subcutaneous injections of intermediate-acting insulin at 0.4 IU/kg once a day; intramuscular injections of ultralente insulin at 0.3–0.4 IU/kg once a day; subcutaneous injections of protamine zinc insulin at 0.15–1.0 IU/kg once to twice a day; and subcutaneous injections of insulin glargine at 0.2–0.4 IU/kg once a day (Jeffrey, 1968; Navas de Solis and Foreman, 2010; Giri *et al.*, 2011). In other species, protamine zinc insulin and insulin glargine have been shown to provide better glycaemic control than regular or ultralente insulin; however, equine data are lacking (Marshall *et al.*, 2008). The dose and type of insulin used, as well as the duration of insulin therapy, varies with individual response to treatment and is limited by owners' financial commitment as long-acting insulins are expensive (Giri *et al.*, 2011). Treatment monitoring is performed by frequent measures of blood glucose concentrations; however, similar to diagnosis, determination of fructosamine concentration and Hb A1c concentration is recommended as it limits the risk of overinterpretation of hyper- and hypoglycaemic events (Seino *et al.*, 2010; Giri *et al.*, 2011). Mild to moderate hypoglycaemic episodes are reported in cases treated with exogenous insulin, mainly after exercise; however, these seem self limiting and successful management is reported with spontaneous resolution after 1 month of treatment or horses returning to their expected use after 3–12 months (Jeffrey, 1968; Navas de Solis and Foreman, 2010; Giri *et al.*, 2011).

Additional treatment used in type-1 diabetes mellitus includes metformin to decrease intestinal glucose absorption, decrease hepatic glucose production and improve peripheral tissue insulin sensitivity; however, given the limited intestinal absorption of metformin in horses, this drug might only have an effect on intestinal glucose absorption (Hustace *et al.*, 2009). Providing food with low glycaemic index and high fibre as well as high fat content is recommended in humans with diabetes mellitus; this would also be indicated in horses to improve insulin sensitivity and reduce blood glucose concentration (Giri *et al.*, 2011). Increasing the horse's activity with regular exercise would also be beneficial in these cases to increase insulin sensitivity (Powell *et al.*, 2002; Bamford *et al.*, 2019).

Type-2 diabetes mellitus

Non-insulin-dependent or type-2 diabetes mellitus results from a deficiency in insulin secretion subsequent to peripheral tissue insulin resistance (Staempfli *et al.*, 1988; Durham *et al.*, 2009). As the condition is rare in horses, the staging system developed in human medicine has not been transposed. In humans, stage 1 type-2 diabetes mellitus comprises compensated peripheral tissue insulin resistance with normoglycaemia, normal beta cell function and hyperinsulinaemia; stage 2 type-2 diabetes mellitus comprises uncompensated peripheral tissue insulin resistance with mild to moderate hyperglycaemia, mild beta cell dysfunction and variable serum insulin (high or normal); and stage 3 type-2 diabetes mellitus comprises uncompensated peripheral tissue insulin resistance with marked hyperglycaemia, severe beta cell dysfunction and variable serum insulin (low or normal) (Martin *et al.*, 1992; Kahn, 2001, 2003). Although this condition is rare in horses, with only a few case studies, it appears to be more common than type-1 diabetes mellitus (Oyaert and Muyelle, 1965; Tasker *et al.*, 1966; Johnson *et al.*, 2012). In most reports, the disease is described in cases previously diagnosed with PPID; however, many of these cases were reported before ID, EMS and PPID were properly described (Loeb *et al.*, 1966; Holscher *et al.*, 1978; van der Kolk *et al.*, 1993; Munoz *et al.*, 1996).

Similarly to type-1 diabetes mellitus, horses with type-2 diabetes mellitus are often presented for weight loss despite a good appetite and polydipsia associated or not with documented polyuria (McCoy, 1986; Muylle *et al.*, 1986; Field and Wolf, 1988; Johnson *et al.*, 2005; Durham *et al.*, 2009). In many of these cases, clinical signs of advanced PPID such as hypertrichosis, hyperhidrosis and laminitis are described, as type-2 diabetes mellitus is rarely a primary condition (Baker and Ritchie, 1974; Holscher *et al.*, 1978; Ruoff *et al.*, 1986; Fey *et al.*, 1998; Dunkel *et al.*, 2014). Among seven cases incidentally diagnosed with hyperlipaemia, six were eventually diagnosed with type-2 diabetes mellitus, five of which had been previously diagnosed with PPID. In another case report, the disease was thought to be subsequent to a granulosa cell tumour (GCT) and the mare presented for infertility (McCoy, 1986; Dunkel *et al.*, 2014). Serum chemistry of horses with type-2 diabetes mellitus yields severe hyperglycaemia (12.6–24.5 mmol/l), hypertriglyceridaemia and often increased liver enzyme activity (alkaline phosphatase and gamma-glutamyl transferase) (Ruoff *et al.*, 1986; Johnson *et al.*, 2005; Durham *et al.*, 2009). Serum insulin concentrations are variable with some reports of hypoinsulinaemia and some reports of hyperinsulinaemia which are, retrospectively, possibly consistent with EMS (Ruoff *et al.*, 1986; Staempfli *et al.*, 1988; Johnson *et al.*, 2005).

Diagnosis of type-2 diabetes mellitus

Unlike type-1 diabetes mellitus, a diagnosis of type-2 diabetes mellitus requires the demonstration of both improper insulin production and peripheral tissue insulin resistance. A complete investigation of insulin and glucose dynamics, such as the modified frequently sampled intravenous glucose tolerance test, with minimal model analysis to demonstrate peripheral tissue insulin resistance (low insulin sensitivity) and poor beta cell function (low acute insulin response to glucose), would be considered a 'gold standard' for a diagnosis of type-2 diabetes mellitus; however, simpler tests such as a low response to an insulin tolerance test or a glucose tolerance test have also been used (King *et al.*, 1962; Loeb *et al.*, 1966; Baker and Ritchie, 1974; Field and Wolf, 1988; Kahn *et al.*, 2001; Johnson *et al.*, 2005; Durham *et al.*, 2009).

More recent reports have also determined serum fructosamine concentrations and serum C-peptide concentrations to diagnose type-2 diabetes mellitus (Johnson *et al.*, 2005; Durham *et al.*, 2009). Reference values for fructosamine concentrations consistent with persistent hyperglycaemia are presented above, while C-peptide concentrations lower than 0.64 ± 0.17 pmol/ml would indicate poor beta cell function (Johnson *et al.*, 2005). It is important to note that, in these studies, presence of peripheral tissue insulin resistance had been previously established using one of the tests mentioned above.

Treatment of type-2 diabetes mellitus

Management of type-2 diabetes mellitus relies on the treatment of the underlying condition, improvement of insulin secretion, improvement of peripheral tissue insulin sensitivity and reduction in intestinal glucose absorption. In cases in which PPID is present, management of the condition with pergolide mesylate has improved the clinical signs and laboratory abnormalities (Munoz *et al.*, 1996; Fey *et al.*, 1998; Dunkel *et al.*, 2014). In other horses, in addition to the dietary and exercise management described above, daily administration of metformin orally (1–15 mg/kg) to decrease intestinal glucose absorption and twice daily administration of glibenclamide orally (glyburide, 0.1–0.3 mg/kg) to stimulate insulin secretion, have provided encouraging results with clinical improvement as well as serum insulin and blood glucose concentrations within reference intervals after a few months of treatment (Johnson *et al.*, 2005; Durham *et al.*, 2009). Pioglitazone, a thiazolidinedione anti-diabetic drug used in humans, has been investigated in horses to increase insulin sensitivity and reduce blood glucose concentration; however, although pharmacokinetic studies have been promising, little effect has been demonstrated clinically (Suagee *et al.*, 2011b; Wearn *et al.*, 2011, Wearn *et al.*, 2012). Treatment with exogenous insulin administration has had very limited success in several reports, likely because of peripheral insulin resistance (King *et al.*, 1962; Loeb *et al.*, 1966; Baker and Ritchie, 1974; Field and Wolf, 1988). In one case, however, daily administration of exogenous lente insulin subcutaneously (1500 IU) resulted in clinical improvement for up to 7 weeks until the horse developed antibodies against both porcine and bovine insulin (Staempfli *et al.*, 1988).

References

Antuna-Puente, B., Feve, B., Fellahi, S. and Bastard, J.-P. (2008) Adipokines: the missing link between insulin resistance and obesity. *Diabetes & Metabolism* 34(1), 2–11. DOI: 10.1016/j.diabet.2007.09.004.

Argo, C.M., Curtis, G.C., Grove-White, D., Dugdale, A.H.A., Barfoot, C.F. *et al.* (2012) Weight loss resistance: a further consideration for the nutritional management of obese Equidae. *The Veterinary Journal* 194(2), 179–188. DOI: 10.1016/j.tvjl.2012.09.020.

Argo, C.M., Dugdale, A.H.A. and McGowan, C.M. (2015) Considerations for the use of restricted, soaked grass hay diets to promote weight loss in the management of equine metabolic syndrome and obesity. *The Veterinary Journal* 206(2), 170–177. DOI: 10.1016/j.tvjl.2015.07.027.

Asplin, K.E., Sillence, M.N., Pollitt, C.C. and McGowan, C.M. (2007) Induction of laminitis by prolonged hyperinsulinaemia in clinically normal ponies. *The Veterinary Journal* 174(3), 530–535. DOI: 10.1016/j.tvjl.2007.07.003.

Asplin, K.E., Patterson-Kane, J.C., Sillence, M.N., Pollitt, C.C. and McGowan, C.M. (2010) Histopathology of insulin-induced laminitis in ponies. *Equine Veterinary Journal* 42(8), 700–706. DOI: 10.1111/j.2042-3306.2010.00111.x.

Asplin, K.E., Curlewis, J.D., McGowan, C.M., Pollitt, C.C. and Sillence, M.N. (2011) Glucose transport in the equine hoof. *Equine Veterinary Journal* 43(2), 196–201. DOI: 10.1111/j.2042-3306.2010.00127.x.

Baggio, L.L. and Drucker, D.J. (2007) Biology of incretins: GLP-1 and GIP. *Gastroenterology* 132(6), 2131–2157. DOI: 10.1053/j.gastro.2007.03.054.

Bailey, S.R., Menzies-Gow, N.J., Harris, P.A., Habershon-Butcher, J.L., Crawford, C. *et al.* (2007) Effect of dietary fructans and dexamethasone administration on the insulin response of ponies predisposed to laminitis. *Journal of the American Veterinary Medical Association* 231(9), 1365–1373. DOI: 10.2460/javma.231.9.1365.

Baker, J.R. and Ritchie, H.E. (1974) Diabetes mellitus in the horse: a case report and review of the literature. *Equine Veterinary Journal* 6(1), 7–11. DOI: 10.1111/j.2042-3306.1974.tb03919.x.

Bamford, N.J., Potter, S.J., Harris, P.A. and Bailey, S.R. (2014) Breed differences in insulin sensitivity and insulinemic responses to oral glucose in horses and ponies of moderate body condition score. *Domestic Animal Endocrinology* 47, 101–107. DOI: 10.1016/j.domaniend.2013.11.001.

Bamford, N.J., Baskerville, C.L., Harris, P.A. and Bailey, S.R. (2015) Postprandial glucose, insulin, and glucagon-like peptide-1 responses of different equine breeds adapted to meals containing micronized maize. *Journal of Animal Science* 93(7), 3377–3383. DOI: 10.2527/jas.2014-8736.

Bamford, N.J., Potter, S.J., Baskerville, C.L., Harris, P.A. and Bailey, S.R. (2016a) Effect of increased adiposity on insulin sensitivity and adipokine concentrations in different equine breeds adapted to cereal-rich or fat-rich meals. *The Veterinary Journal* 214, 14–20. DOI: 10.1016/j.tvjl.2016.02.002.

Bamford, N.J., Potter, S.J., Harris, P.A. and Bailey, S.R. (2016b) Effect of increased adiposity on insulin sensitivity and adipokine concentrations in horses and ponies fed a high fat diet, with or without a once daily high glycaemic meal. *Equine Veterinary Journal* 48(3), 368–373. DOI: 10.1111/evj.12434.

Bamford, N.J., Potter, S.J., Baskerville, C.L., Harris, P.A. and Bailey, S.R. (2019) Influence of dietary restriction and low-intensity exercise on weight loss and insulin sensitivity in obese equids. *Journal of Veterinary Internal Medicine* 33(1), 280–286. DOI: 10.1111/jvim.15374.

Banse, H.E., McCann, J., Yang, F., Wagg, C. and McFarlane, D. (2014) Comparison of two methods for measurement of equine insulin. *Journal of Veterinary Diagnostic Investigation* 26(4), 527–530. DOI: 10.1177/1040638714536560.

Beech, J., McFarlane, D., Lindborg, S., Sojka, J.E. and Boston, R.C. (2011) α-melanocyte--stimulating hormone and adrenocorticotropin concentrations in response to thyrotropin-releasing hormone and comparison with adrenocorticotropin concentration after domperidone administration in healthy horses and horses with pituitary pars intermedia dysfunction. *Journal of the American Veterinary Medical Association* 238(10), 1305–1315. DOI: 10.2460/javma.238.10.1305.

Banse, H.E. and McFarlane, D. (2014) Comparison of three methods for evaluation of equine insulin regulation in horses of varied body condition score. *Journal of Equine Veterinary Science* 34(6), 742–748. DOI: 10.1016/j.jevs.2014.01.001.

Bertin, F.R. and de Laat, M.A. (2017) The diagnosis of equine insulin dysregulation. *Equine Veterinary Journal* 49(5), 570–576. DOI: 10.1111/evj.12703.

Bertin, F.R. and Sojka-Kritchevsky, J.E. (2013) Comparison of a 2-step insulin-response test to conventional insulin-sensitivity testing in horses. *Domestic Animal Endocrinology* 44(1), 19–25. DOI: 10.1016/j.domaniend.2012.07.003.

Bertin, F.R., Pader, K.S., Lescun, T.B. and Sojka-Kritchevsky, J.E. (2013) Short-term effect of ovariectomy on measures of insulin sensitivity and response to dexamethasone administration in horses. *American Journal of Veterinary Research* 74(12), 1506–1513. DOI: 10.2460/ajvr.74.12.1506.

Bertin, F.R., Taylor, S.D., Bianco, A.W. and Sojka-Kritchevsky, J.E. (2016) The effect of fasting duration on baseline blood glucose concentration, blood insulin concentration, glucose/insulin ratio, oral sugar test, and insulin response test results in horses. *Journal of Veterinary Internal Medicine* 30(5), 1726–1731. DOI: 10.1111/jvim.14529.

Bertin, F.-R., Ruffin-Taylor, D. and Stewart, A.J. (2018) Insulin dysregulation in horses with systemic inflammatory response syndrome. *Journal of Veterinary Internal Medicine* 32(4), 1420–1427. DOI: 10.1111/jvim.15138.

Bertin, F.R., Eichstadt Forsythe, L. and Kritchevsky, J.E. (2019) Effects of high doses of levothyroxine sodium on serum concentrations of triiodothyronine and thyroxine in horses. *American Journal of Veterinary Research* 80(6), 565–571. DOI: 10.2460/ajvr.80.6.565.

Bonelli, F., Sgorbini, M., Meucci, V., Sighieri, C. and Baragli, P. (2017) How swimming affects plasma insulin and glucose concentration in thoroughbreds: a pilot study. *The Veterinary Journal* 226, 1–3. DOI: 10.1016/j.tvjl.2017.06.006.

Borer-Weir, K.E., Bailey, S.R., Menzies-Gow, N.J., Harris, P.A. and Elliott, J. (2012) Evaluation of a commercially available radioimmunoassay and species-specific ELISAs for measurement of high concentrations of insulin in equine serum. *American Journal of Veterinary Research* 73(10), 1596–1602. DOI: 10.2460/ajvr.73.10.1596.

Borer-Weir, K.E., Menzies-Gow, N.J., Bailey, S.R., Harris, P.A. and Elliott, J. (2013) Seasonal and annual influence on insulin and cortisol results from overnight dexamethasone suppression tests in normal ponies and ponies predisposed to laminitis. *Equine Veterinary Journal* 45(6), 688–693. DOI: 10.1111/evj.12053.

Borer, K.E., Bailey, S.R., Menzies-Gow, N.J., Harris, P.A. and Elliott, J. (2012) Effect of feeding glucose, fructose, and inulin on blood glucose and insulin concentrations in normal ponies and those predisposed to laminitis. *Journal of Animal Science* 90(9), 3003–3011. DOI: 10.2527/jas.2011-4236.

Borgia, L., Valberg, S., McCue, M., Watts, K. and Pagan, J. (2011) Glycaemic and insulinaemic responses to feeding hay with different non-structural carbohydrate content in control and polysaccharide storage myopathy-affected horses. *Journal of Animal Physiology and Animal Nutrition* 95(6), 798–807. DOI: 10.1111/j.1439-0396.2010.01116.x.

Bruynsteen, L., Moons, C.P.H., Janssens, G.P.J., Harris, P.A., Vandevelde, K. *et al.* (2015) Level of energy restriction alters body condition score and morphometric profile in obese Shetland ponies. *The Veterinary Journal* 206(1), 61–66. DOI: 10.1016/j.tvjl.2015.06.006.

Brøkner, C., Austbø, D., Næsset, J.A., Blache, D., Bach Knudsen, K.E. *et al*. (2016) Metabolic response to dietary fibre composition in horses. *Animal* 10(7), 1155–1163. DOI: 10.1017/S1751731115003006.

Buff, P.R., Johnson, P.J., Wiedmeyer, C.E., Ganjam, V.K., Messer Iv, N.T. *et al*. (2006a) Modulation of leptin, insulin, and growth hormone in obese pony mares under chronic nutritional restriction and supplementation with ractopamine hydrochloride. *Veterinary Therapeutics: Research in Applied Veterinary Medicine* 7, 64–72.

Buff, P.R., Spader, B.R., Morrison, C.D. and Keisler, D.H. (2006b) Endocrine responses in mares undergoing abrupt changes in nutritional management. *Journal of Animal Science* 84(10), 2700–2707. DOI: 10.2527/jas.2005-741.

Burns, T.A., Geor, R.J., Mudge, M.C., McCutcheon, L.J., Hinchcliff, K.W. *et al*. (2010) Proinflammatory cytokine and chemokine gene expression profiles in subcutaneous and visceral adipose tissue depots of insulin-resistant and insulin-sensitive light breed horses. *Journal of Veterinary Internal Medicine* 24(4), 932–939. DOI: 10.1111/j.1939-1676.2010.0551.x.

Burns, T.A., Watts, M.R., Weber, P.S., McCutcheon, L.J., Geor, R.J. *et al*. (2013) Distribution of insulin receptor and insulin-like growth factor-1 receptor in the digital laminae of mixed-breed ponies: an immunohistochemical study. *Equine Veterinary Journal* 45(3), 326–332. DOI: 10.1111/j.2042-3306.2012.00631.x.

Caltabilota, T.J., Earl, L.R., Thompson, D.L., Clavier, S.E. and Mitcham, P.B. (2010) Hyperleptinemia in mares and geldings: assessment of insulin sensitivity from glucose responses to insulin injection. *Journal of Animal Science* 88(9), 2940–2949. DOI: 10.2527/jas.2010-2879.

Carslake, H.B., Argo, C.M., Pinchbeck, G.L., Dugdale, A.H.A. and McGowan, C.M. (2018) Insulinaemic and glycaemic responses to three forages in ponies. *The Veterinary Journal* 235, 83–89. DOI: 10.1016/j.tvjl.2018.03.008.

Carter, R.A., Geor, R.J., Burton Staniar, W., Cubitt, T.A. and Harris, P.A. (2009a) Apparent adiposity assessed by standardised scoring systems and morphometric measurements in horses and ponies. *The Veterinary Journal* 179(2), 204–210. DOI: 10.1016/j.tvjl.2008.02.029.

Carter, R.A., McCutcheon, L.J., George, L.A., Smith, T.L., Frank, N. *et al*. (2009b) Effects of diet-induced weight gain on insulin sensitivity and plasma hormone and lipid concentrations in horses. *American Journal of Veterinary Research* 70(10), 1250–1258. DOI: 10.2460/ajvr.70.10.1250.

Carter, R.A., Treiber, K.H., Geor, R.J., Douglass, L. and Harris, P.A. (2009c) Prediction of incipient pasture-associated laminitis from hyperinsulinaemia, hyperleptinaemia and generalised and localised obesity in a cohort of ponies. *Equine Veterinary Journal* 41(2), 171–178. DOI: 10.2746/042516408X342975.

Carter, R.A., McCutcheon, L.J., Valle, E., Meilahn, E.N. and Geor, R.J. (2010) Effects of exercise training on adiposity, insulin sensitivity, and plasma hormone and lipid concentrations in overweight or obese, insulin-resistant horses. *American Journal of Veterinary Research* 71(3), 314–321. DOI: 10.2460/ajvr.71.3.314.

Chameroy, K.A., Frank, N., Elliott, S.B. and Boston, R.C. (2011) Effects of a supplement containing chromium and magnesium on morphometric measurements, resting glucose, insulin concentrations and insulin sensitivity in laminitic obese horses. *Equine Veterinary Journal* 43(4), 494–499. DOI: 10.1111/j.2042-3306.2010.00302.x.

Chameroy, K.A., Frank, N., Elliott, S.B. and Boston, R.C. (2016) Comparison of plasma active glucagon-like peptide 1 concentrations in normal horses and those with equine metabolic syndrome and in horses placed on a high-grain diet. *Journal of Equine Veterinary Science* 40, 16–25. DOI: 10.1016/j.jevs.2016.01.009.

Christie, J.L., Hewson, C.J., Riley, C.B., McNiven, M.A., Dohoo, I.R. *et al*. (2004) Demographics, management, and welfare of nonracing horses in Prince Edward island. *The Canadian Veterinary Journal* 45(12), 1004–1011.

Cinti, S., Mitchell, G., Barbatelli, G., Murano, I., Ceresi, E. *et al*. (2005) Adipocyte death defines macrophage localization and function in adipose tissue of obese mice and humans. *Journal of Lipid Research* 46(11), 2347–2355. DOI: 10.1194/jlr.M500294-JLR200.

Cripps, P.J. and Eustace, R.A. (1999) Radiological measurements from the feet of normal horses with relevance to laminitis. *Equine Veterinary Journal* 31(5), 427–432. DOI: 10.1111/j.2042-3306.1999.tb03844.x.

de Laat, M.A. and Sillence, M.N. (2017) The repeatability of an oral glucose test in ponies. *Equine Veterinary Journal* 49(2), 238–243. DOI: 10.1111/evj.12579.

de Laat, M.A., McGowan, C.M., Sillence, M.N. and Pollitt, C.C. (2010) Equine laminitis: induced by 48 h hyperinsulinaemia in standardbred horses. *Equine Veterinary Journal* 42(2), 129–135. DOI: 10.2746/042516409X475779.

de Laat, M.A., Kyaw-Tanner, M.T., Nourian, A.R., McGowan, C.M., Sillence, M.N. *et al*. (2011a) The developmental and acute phases of insulin-induced laminitis involve minimal metalloproteinase activity. *Veterinary Immunology and Immunopathology* 140(3–4), 275–281. DOI: 10.1016/j.vetimm.2011.01.013.

de Laat, M.A., van Eps, A.W., McGowan, C.M., Sillence, M.N. and Pollitt, C.C. (2011b) Equine laminitis: comparative histopathology 48 hours after experimental induction with insulin or alimentary oligofructose in standardbred horses. *Journal of Comparative Pathology* 145(4), 399–409. DOI: 10.1016/j.jcpa.2011.02.001.

de Laat, M.A., Kyaw-Tanner, M.T., Sillence, M.N., McGowan, C.M. and Pollitt, C.C. (2012a) Advanced glycation endproducts in horses with insulin-induced laminitis. *Veterinary Immunology and Immunopathology* 145(1–2), 395–401. DOI: 10.1016/j.vetimm.2011.12.016.

de Laat, M.A., Pollitt, C.C., Walsh, D.M., McGowan, C.M. and Sillence, M.N. (2012b) Persistent digital hyperthermia over a 48h period does not induce laminitis in horses. *The Veterinary Journal* 192(3), 435–440. DOI: 10.1016/j.tvjl.2011.09.016.

de Laat, M.A., Patterson-Kane, J.C., Pollitt, C.C., Sillence, M.N. and McGowan, C.M. (2013) Histological and morphometric lesions in the pre-clinical, developmental phase of insulin-induced laminitis in standardbred horses. *The Veterinary Journal* 195(3), 305–312. DOI: 10.1016/j.tvjl.2012.07.003.

de Laat, M.A., Hampson, B.A., Sillence, M.N. and Pollitt, C.C. (2016a) Sustained, low-intensity exercise achieved by a dynamic feeding system decreases body fat in ponies. *Journal of Veterinary Internal Medicine* 30(5), 1732–1738. DOI: 10.1111/jvim.14577.

de Laat, M.A., Hampson, B.A., Sillence, M.N. and Pollitt, C.C. (2016b) Sustained, low-intensity exercise achieved by a dynamic feeding system decreases body fat in ponies. *Journal of Veterinary Internal Medicine* 30(5), 1732–1738. DOI: 10.1111/jvim.14577.

de Laat, M.A., McGree, J.M. and Sillence, M.N. (2016c) Equine hyperinsulinemia: investigation of the enteroinsular axis during insulin dysregulation. *American Journal of Physiology-Endocrinology and Metabolism* 310(1), E61–E72. DOI: 10.1152/ajpendo.00362.2015.

de Laat, M.A., van Haeften, J.J. and Sillence, M.N. (2016d) The effect of oral and intravenous dextrose on C-peptide secretion in ponies1. *Journal of Animal Science* 94(2), 574–580. DOI: 10.2527/jas.2015-9817.

de Laat, M.A., Fitzgerald, D.M., Sillence, M.N. and Spence, R.J. (2018) Glucagon-Like peptide-2: a potential role in equine insulin dysregulation. *Equine Veterinary Journal* 50(6), 842–847. DOI: 10.1111/evj.12825.

Drucker, D.J., Erlich, P., Asa, S.L. and Brubaker, P.L. (1996) Induction of intestinal epithelial proliferation by glucagon-like peptide 2. *Proceedings of the National Academy of Sciences* 93(15), 7911–7916. DOI: 10.1073/pnas.93.15.7911.

Duckworth, W.C., Bennett, R.G. and Hamel, F.G. (1998) Insulin degradation: progress and potential. *Endocrine Reviews* 19(5), 608–624. DOI: 10.1210/edrv.19.5.0349.

Dugdale, A.H.A., Curtis, G.C., Cripps, P., Harris, P.A. and Argo, C.M. (2010) Effect of dietary restriction on body condition, composition and welfare of overweight and obese pony mares. *Equine Veterinary Journal* 42(7), 600–610. DOI: 10.1111/j.2042-3306.2010.00110.x.

Dugdale, A.H.A., Curtis, G.C., Cripps, P.J., Harris, P.A. and Argo, C.M. (2011) Effects of season and body condition on appetite, body mass and body composition in AD libitum fed pony mares. *The Veterinary Journal* 190(3), 329–337. DOI: 10.1016/j.tvjl.2010.11.009.

Dugdale, A.H.A., Grove-White, D., Curtis, G.C., Harris, P.A. and Argo, C.M. (2012) Body condition scoring as a predictor of body fat in horses and ponies. *The Veterinary Journal* 194(2), 173–178. DOI: 10.1016/j.tvjl.2012.03.024.

Dunbar, L.K., Mielnicki, K.A., Dembek, K.A., Toribio, R.E. and Burns, T.A. (2016) Evaluation of four diagnostic tests for insulin dysregulation in adult light-breed horses. *Journal of Veterinary Internal Medicine* 30(3), 885–891. DOI: 10.1111/jvim.13934.

Dunkel, B., Wilford, S.A., Parkinson, N.J., Ward, C., Smith, P. *et al.* (2014) Severe hypertriglyceridaemia in horses and ponies with endocrine disorders. *Equine Veterinary Journal* 46(1), 118–122. DOI: 10.1111/evj.12089.

Duren, S.E., Pagan, J.D., Harris, P.A.T.A. and Crandell, K.G. (1999) Time of feeding and fat supplementation affect plasma concentrations of insulin and metabolites during exercise. *Equine Veterinary Journal* 31(S30), 479–484. DOI: 10.1111/j.2042-3306.1999.tb05269.x.

Durham, A.E., Rendle, D.I. and Newton, J.R. (2008) The effect of metformin on measurements of insulin sensitivity and β cell response in 18 horses and ponies with insulin resistance. *Equine Veterinary Journal* 40(5), 493–500. DOI: 10.2746/042516408X273648.

Durham, A.E., Hughes, K.J., Cottle, H.J., Rendle, D.I. and Boston, R.C. (2009) Type 2 diabetes mellitus with pancreatic β cell dysfunction in 3 horses confirmed with minimal model analysis. *Equine Veterinary Journal* 41(9), 924–929. DOI: 10.2746/042516409X452152.

Durham, A.E. (2016) Endocrine disease in aged horses. *Veterinary Clinics of North America: Equine Practice* 32(2), 301–315.

Durham, A.E., Frank, N., McGowan, C.M., Menzies-Gow, N.J., Roelfsema, E. *et al.* (2019) ECEIM consensus statement on equine metabolic syndrome. *Journal of Veterinary Internal Medicine* 33(2), 335–349. DOI: 10.1111/jvim.15423.

Eiler, H., Frank, N., Andrews, F.M., Oliver, J.W. and Fecteau, K.A. (2005) Physiologic assessment of blood glucose homeostasis via combined intravenous glucose and insulin testing in horses. *American Journal of Veterinary Research* 66(9), 1598–1604. DOI: 10.2460/ajvr.2005.66.1598.

Fey, K., Jonigkeit, E. and Moritz, A. (1998) [Equine Cushing syndrome (ECS). Case report, review of its diagnosis and therapy and substantial differences from Cushing syndrome in dogs]. *Tierarztl Prax Ausg G Grosstiere Nutztiere* 26, 41–47.

Field, J.R. and Wolf, C. (1988) Cushing's syndrome in a horse. *Equine Veterinary Journal* 20(4), 301–304. DOI: 10.1111/j.2042-3306.1988.tb01530.x.

Fields, M. (1998) Nutritional factors adversely influencing the glucose/insulin system. *Journal of the*

American College of Nutrition 17(4), 317–321. DOI: 10.1080/07315724.1998.10718768.

Fitzgerald, D.M., Pollitt, C.C., Walsh, D.M., Sillence, M.N. and de Laat, M.A. (2019) The effect of different grazing conditions on the insulin and incretin response to the oral glucose test in ponies. *BMC Veterinary Research* 15(1), 345. DOI: 10.1186/s12917-019-2088-1.

Forhead, A.J., Ousey, J.C., Allen, W.R. and Fowden, A.L. (2004) Postnatal insulin secretion and sensitivity after manipulation of fetal growth by embryo transfer in the horse. *Journal of Endocrinology* 181(3), 459–467. DOI: 10.1677/joe.0.1810459.

Fowden, A.L., Comline, R.S. and Silver, M. (1984) Insulin secretion and carbohydrate metabolism during pregnancy in the mare. *Equine Veterinary Journal* 16(4), 239–246. DOI: 10.1111/j.2042-3306.1984.tb01919.x.

Frank, N. (2011) Equine metabolic syndrome. *Veterinary Clinics of North America: Equine Practice* 27(1), 73–92.

Frank, N. (2018) Safety and efficacy of canagliflozin and octreotide for managing insulin dysregulation in horses. *Journal of Veterinary Internal Medicine* 32, 2129–2129.

Frank, N. and Tadros, E.M. (2014) Insulin dysregulation. *Equine Veterinary Journal* 46(1), 103–112. DOI: 10.1111/evj.12169.

Frank, N., Sommardahl, C.S., Eiler, H., Webb, L.L., Denhart, J.W. *et al.* (2005) Effects of oral administration of levothyroxine sodium on concentrations of plasma lipids, concentration and composition of very-low-density lipoproteins, and glucose dynamics in healthy adult mares. *American Journal of Veterinary Research* 66(6), 1032–1038. DOI: 10.2460/ajvr.2005.66.1032.

Frank, N., Elliott, S.B., Brandt, L.E. and Keisler, D.H. (2006) Physical characteristics, blood hormone concentrations, and plasma lipid concentrations in obese horses with insulin resistance. *Journal of the American Veterinary Medical Association* 228(9), 1383–1390. DOI: 10.2460/javma.228.9.1383.

Frank, N., Buchanan, B.R. and Elliott, S.B. (2008a) Effects of long-term oral administration of levothyroxine sodium on serum thyroid hormone concentrations, clinicopathologic variables, and echocardiographic measurements in healthy adult horses. *American Journal of Veterinary Research* 69(1), 68–75. DOI: 10.2460/ajvr.69.1.68.

Frank, N., Elliott, S.B. and Boston, R.C. (2008b) Effects of long-term oral administration of levothyroxine sodium on glucose dynamics in healthy adult horses. *American Journal of Veterinary Research* 69(1), 76–81. DOI: 10.2460/ajvr.69.1.76.

Frank, N., Elliott, S.B., Chameroy, K.A., Tóth, F., Chumbler, N.S. *et al.* (2010a) Association of season and pasture grazing with blood hormone and metabolite concentrations in horses with presumed pituitary pars intermedia dysfunction. *Journal of Veterinary Internal Medicine* 24(5), 1167–1175. DOI: 10.1111/j.1939-1676.2010.0547.x.

Frank, N., Geor, R.J., Bailey, S.R., Durham, A.E., Johnson, P.J. *et al.* (2010b) Equine metabolic syndrome. *Journal of Veterinary Internal Medicine* 24(3), 467–475. DOI: 10.1111/j.1939-1676.2010.0503.x.

Freestone, J.F., Wolfsheimer, K.J., Ford, R.B., Church, G. and Bessin, R. (1991) Triglyceride, insulin, and cortisol responses of ponies to fasting and dexamethasone administration. *Journal of Veterinary Internal Medicine* 5(1), 15–22. DOI: 10.1111/j.1939-1676.1991.tb00925.x.

Freestone, J.F., Beadle, R., Shoemaker, K., Bessin, R.T., Wolfsheimer, K.J. *et al.* (1992) Improved insulin sensitivity in hyperinsulinaemic ponies through physical conditioning and controlled feed intake. *Equine Veterinary Journal* 24(3), 187–190. DOI: 10.1111/j.2042-3306.1992.tb02812.x.

Geor, R.J. and Harris, P. (2009) Dietary management of obesity and insulin resistance: countering risk for laminitis. *The Veterinary Clinics of North America. Equine Practice* 25(1), 51–65. DOI: 10.1016/j.cveq.2009.02.001.

Geor, R.J., Hinchcliff, K.W. and Sams, R.A. (2000) Glucose infusion attenuates endogenous glucose production and enhances glucose use of horses during exercise. *Journal of Applied Physiology* 88(5), 1765–1776. DOI: 10.1152/jappl.2000.88.5.1765.

Geor, R.J., Stewart-Hunt, L. and McCutcheon, L.J. (2010) Effects of prior exercise on insulin-mediated and noninsulin-mediated glucose uptake in horses during a hyperglycaemic clamp. *Equine Veterinary Journal* 42, 129–134. DOI: 10.1111/j.2042-3306.2010.00218.x.

George, L.A., Staniar, W.B., Cubitt, T.A., Treiber, K.H., Harris, P.A. *et al.* (2011) Evaluation of the effects of pregnancy on insulin sensitivity, insulin secretion, and glucose dynamics in thoroughbred mares. *American Journal of Veterinary Research* 72(5), 666–674. DOI: 10.2460/ajvr.72.5.666.

Giles, S.L., Rands, S.A., Nicol, C.J. and Harris, P.A. (2014) Obesity prevalence and associated risk factors in outdoor living domestic horses and ponies. *PeerJ* 2(1), e299. DOI: 10.7717/peerj.299.

Giles, S.L., Nicol, C.J., Rands, S.A. and Harris, P.A. (2015) Assessing the seasonal prevalence and risk factors for nuchal crest adiposity in domestic horses and ponies using the cresty neck score. *BMC Veterinary Research* 11(1), 13. DOI: 10.1186/s12917-015-0327-7.

Giri, J.K., Magdesian, K.G. and Gaffney, P.M. (2011) Insulin-dependent diabetes mellitus associated with presumed autoimmune polyendocrine syndrome in a mare. *The Canadian Veterinary Journal* 52(5), 506–512.

Glunk, E.C., Hathaway, M.R., Grev, A.M., Lamprecht, E.D., Maher, M.C. *et al.* (2015) The effect of a limit-fed diet and slow-feed hay nets on morphometric measurements and postprandial metabolite and hormone patterns in adult horses. *Journal of Animal Science* 93(8), 4144–4152. DOI: 10.2527/jas.2015-9150.

Gordon, M.E. and McKeever, K.H. (2005) Diurnal variation of ghrelin, leptin, and adiponectin in standardbred mares. *Journal of Animal Science* 83(10), 2365–2371. DOI: 10.2527/2005.83102365x.

Gordon, M.E. and McKeever, K.H. (2006) Oral and intravenous carbohydrate challenges decrease active ghrelin concentrations and alter hormones related to control of energy metabolism in horses. *Journal of Animal Science* 84(7), 1682–1690. DOI: 10.2527/jas.2005-484.

Grimsrud, K.N., Ait-Oudhia, S., Durbin-Johnson, B.P., Rocke, D.M., Mama, K.R. *et al.* (2015) Pharmacokinetic and pharmacodynamic analysis comparing diverse effects of detomidine, medetomidine, and dexmedetomidine in the horse: a population analysis. *Journal of Veterinary Pharmacology and Therapeutics* 38(1), 24–34. DOI: 10.1111/jvp.12139.

Gungor, N., Saad, R., Janosky, J. and Arslanian, S. (2004) Validation of surrogate estimates of insulin sensitivity and insulin secretion in children and adolescents. *The Journal of Pediatrics* 144(1), 47–55. DOI: 10.1016/j.jpeds.2003.09.045.

Habegger, K.M., Heppner, K.M., Geary, N., Bartness, T.J., DiMarchi, R. *et al.* (2010) The metabolic actions of glucagon revisited. *Nature Reviews Endocrinology* 6(12), 689–697. DOI: 10.1038/nrendo.2010.187.

Hampson, B.A., Connelley, A.D., de Laat, M.A., Mills, P.C. and Pollitt, C.C. (2011) Sole depth and weight-bearing characteristics of the palmar surface of the feet of feral horses and domestic thoroughbreds. *American Journal of Veterinary Research* 72(6), 727–735. DOI: 10.2460/ajvr.72.6.727.

Hampson, B.A., de Laat, M.A., Mills, P.C., Walsh, D.M. and Pollitt, C.C. (2013) The feral horse foot. Part B: radiographic, gross visual and histopathological parameters of foot health in 100 Australian feral horses. *Australian Veterinary Journal* 91(1–2), 23–30. DOI: 10.1111/avj.12017.

Hardie, D.G. (2011) Energy sensing by the AMP-activated protein kinase and its effects on muscle metabolism. *Proceedings of the Nutrition Society* 70(1), 92–99. DOI: 10.1017/S0029665110003915.

Harris, P.A., Ellis, A.D., Fradinho, M.J., Jansson, A., Julliand, V. *et al.* (2017) Review: feeding conserved forage to horses: recent advances and recommendations. *Animal* 11(6), 958–967. DOI: 10.1017/S1751731116002469.

Hart, K.A., Wochele, D.M., Norton, N.A., McFarlane, D., Wooldridge, A.A. *et al.* (2016) Effect of age, season, body condition, and endocrine status on serum free cortisol fraction and insulin concentration in horses. *Journal of Veterinary Internal Medicine* 30(2), 653–663. DOI: 10.1111/jvim.13839.

Henneke, D.R., Potter, G.D., Kreider, J.L. and Yeates, B.F. (1983) Relationship between condition score, physical measurements and body fat percentage in mares. *Equine Veterinary Journal* 15(4), 371–372.10.1111/j.2042-3306.1983.tb01826.x DOI: 10.1111/j.2042-3306.1983.tb01826.x.

Hirose, H., Maruyama, H., Ito, K., Kido, K., Koyama, K. *et al.* (1993) Effects of alpha 2- and beta-adrenergic agonism on glucagon secretion from perfused pancreata of normal and streptozocin-induced diabetic rats. *Metabolism* 42(8), 1072–1076. DOI: 10.1016/0026-0495(93)90025-J.

Hoffman, R.M., Boston, R.C., Stefanovski, D., Kronfeld, D.S. and Harris, P.A. (2003a) Obesity and diet affect glucose dynamics and insulin sensitivity in thoroughbred geldings. *Journal of Animal Science* 81(9), 2333–2342. DOI: 10.2527/2003.8192333x.

Hoffman, R.M., Kronfeld, D.S., Cooper, W.L. and Harris, P.A. (2003b) Glucose clearance in grazing mares is affected by diet, pregnancy, and lactation. *Journal of Animal Science* 81(7), 1764–1771. DOI: 10.2527/2003.8171764x.

Holdstock, N.B., Allen, V.L., Bloomfield, M.R., Hales, C.N. and Fowden, A.L. (2004) Development of insulin and proinsulin secretion in newborn pony foals. *Journal of Endocrinology* 181(3), 469–476. DOI: 10.1677/joe.0.1810469.

Holscher, M.A., Linnabary, R.L., Netsky, M.G. and Owen, H.D. (1978) Adenoma of the pars intermedia and hirsutism in a pony. *Veterinary Medicine, Small Animal Clinician : VM, SAC* 73(9), 1197–1200.

Holz, G.G., Kiihtreiber, W.M. and Habener, J.F. (1993) Pancreatic beta-cells are rendered glucose-competent by the insulinotropic hormone glucagon-like peptide-1(7-37). *Nature* 361(6410), 362–365. DOI: 10.1038/361362a0.

Horn, R. and Bertin, F.-R. (2019) Evaluation of combined testing to simultaneously diagnose pituitary pars intermedia dysfunction and insulin dysregulation in horses. *Journal of Veterinary Internal Medicine* 33(5), 2249–2256. DOI: 10.1111/jvim.15617.

Horn, R., Bamford, N.J., Afonso, T., Sutherland, M., Buckerfield, J. *et al.* (2019) Factors associated with survival, laminitis and insulin dysregulation in horses diagnosed with equine pituitary pars intermedia dysfunction. *Equine Veterinary Journal* 51(4), 440–445. DOI: 10.1111/evj.13041.

Huang, Y. and Chang, Y. (2014) Regulation of pancreatic islet beta-cell mass by growth factor and hormone signaling. *Progress in Molecular Biology and Translational Science* 121, 321–349. DOI: 10.1016/B978-0-12-800101-1.00010-7.

Hustace, J.L., Firshman, A.M. and Mata, J.E. (2009) Pharmacokinetics and bioavailability of metformin in horses. *American Journal of Veterinary Research* 70(5), 665–668. DOI: 10.2460/ajvr.70.5.665.

Isganaitis, E. and Lustig, R.H. (2005) Fast food, central nervous system insulin resistance, and obesity. *Arteriosclerosis, Thrombosis, and Vascular*

Biology 25(12), 2451–2462. DOI: 10.1161/01.ATV.0000186208.06964.91.

Jacob, S.I., Geor, R.J., Weber, P.S.D., Harris, P.A. and McCue, M.E. (2018) Effect of age and dietary carbohydrate profiles on glucose and insulin dynamics in horses. *Equine Veterinary Journal* 50(2), 249–254. DOI: 10.1111/evj.12745.

Jeffrey, J.R. (1968) Diabetes mellitus secondary to chronic pancreatitis in a pony. *Journal of the American Veterinary Medical Association* 153(9), 1168–1175.

Jensen, R.B., Danielsen, S.H. and Tauson, A.-H. (2016) Body condition score, morphometric measurements and estimation of body weight in mature Icelandic horses in Denmark. *Acta Veterinaria Scandinavica* 58(S1), 59. DOI: 10.1186/s13028-016-0240-5.

Johnson, P.J. (2002) The equine metabolic syndrome peripheral Cushing's syndrome. *The Veterinary clinics of North America. Equine Practice* 18(2), 271–293. DOI: 10.1016/s0749-0739(02)00006-8.

Johnson, P.J., Scotty, N.C., Wiedmeyer, C., Messer, N.T. and Kreeger, J.M. (2005) Diabetes mellitus in a domesticated Spanish Mustang. *Journal of the American Veterinary Medical Association* 226(4), 542–588. DOI: 10.2460/javma.2005.226.584.

Johnson, P.J., Wiedmeyer, C.E., LaCarrubba, A., Ganjam, V.K. and Messer, N.T. (2012) Diabetes, insulin resistance, and metabolic syndrome in horses. *Journal of Diabetes Science and Technology* 6(3), 534–540. DOI: 10.1177/193229681200600307.

Jose-Cunilleras, E., Hinchcliff, K.W., Sams, R.A., Devor, S.T. and Linderman, J.K. (2002) Glycemic index of a meal fed before exercise alters substrate use and glucose flux in exercising horses. *Journal of Applied Physiology* 92(1), 117–128. DOI: 10.1152/jappl.2002.92.1.117.

Kahn, S.E. (2001) Clinical review 135: the importance of beta-cell failure in the development and progression of type 2 diabetes. *The Journal of Clinical Endocrinology and Metabolism* 86(9), 4047–4058. DOI: 10.1210/jcem.86.9.7713.

Kahn, S.E. (2003) The relative contributions of insulin resistance and beta-cell dysfunction to the pathophysiology of type 2 diabetes. *Diabetologia* 46(1), 3–19. DOI: 10.1007/s00125-002-1009-0.

Kahn, S.E., Montgomery, B., Howell, W., Ligueros-Saylan, M., Hsu, C.-H. *et al.* (2001) Importance of early phase insulin secretion to intravenous glucose tolerance in subjects with type 2 diabetes mellitus. *The Journal of Clinical Endocrinology & Metabolism* 86(12), 5824–5829. DOI: 10.1210/jcem.86.12.8105.

Karikoski, N.P., Horn, I., McGowan, T.W. and McGowan, C.M. (2011) The prevalence of endocrinopathic laminitis among horses presented for laminitis at a first-opinion/referral equine hospital. *Domestic Animal Endocrinology* 41(3), 111–117. DOI: 10.1016/j.domaniend.2011.05.004.

Karikoski, N.P., Patterson-Kane, J.C., Asplin, K.E., McGowan, T.W., McNutt, M. *et al.* (2014) Morphological and cellular changes in secondary epidermal laminae of horses with insulin-induced laminitis. *American Journal of Veterinary Research* 75(2), 161–168. DOI: 10.2460/ajvr.75.2.161.

Karikoski, N.P., McGowan, C.M., Singer, E.R., Asplin, K.E., Tulamo, R.-M. *et al.* (2015) Pathology of natural cases of equine endocrinopathic laminitis associated with hyperinsulinemia. *Veterinary Pathology* 52(5), 945–956. DOI: 10.1177/0300985814549212.

Kawasako, K., Higashi, T., Nakaji, Y., Komine, M., Hirayama, K. *et al.* (2009) Histologic evaluation of the diversity of epidermal laminae in hooves of horses without clinical signs of laminitis. *American Journal of Veterinary Research* 70(2), 186–193. DOI: 10.2460/ajvr.70.2.186.

Kearns, C.F., McKeever, K.H., Roegner, V., Brady, S.M. and Malinowski, K. (2006) Adiponectin and leptin are related to fat mass in horses. *The Veterinary Journal* 172(3), 460–465. DOI: 10.1016/j.tvjl.2005.05.002.

King, J.M., Kavanaugh, J.F. and Bentinck-Smith, J. (1962) Diabetes mellitus with pituitary neoplasms in a horse and a dog. *The Cornell Veterinarian* 52, 133–145.

Knowles, E.J., Withers, J.M. and Mair, T.S. (2012) Increased plasma fructosamine concentrations in laminitic horses. *Equine Veterinary Journal* 44(2), 226–229. DOI: 10.1111/j.2042-3306.2011.00419.x.

Knowles, E.J., Menzies-Gow, N.J. and Mair, T.S. (2014) Plasma fructosamine concentrations in horses with pituitary *pars intermedia* dysfunction with and without laminitis. *Equine Veterinary Journal* 46(2), 249–251. DOI: 10.1111/evj.12090.

Knowles, E.J., Harris, P.A., Elliott, J. and Menzies-Gow, N.J. (2016) Use of the oral sugar test in ponies when performed with or without prior fasting. *Equine Veterinary Journal*.

Korda, M., Kubant, R., Patton, S. and Malinski, T. (2008) Leptin-induced endothelial dysfunction in obesity. *American Journal of Physiology-Heart and Circulatory Physiology* 295(4), H1514–H1521. DOI: 10.1152/ajpheart.00479.2008.

Kosolofski, H.R., Gow, S.P. and Robinson, K.A. (2017) Prevalence of obesity in the equine population of Saskatoon and surrounding area. *The Canadian Veterinary Journal* 58(9), 967–970.

Kritchevsky, J.E., Muir, G.S., Leschke, D.H.Z., Hodgson, J.K., Hess, E.K. *et al.* (2020) Blood glucose and insulin concentrations after alpha-2-agonists administration in horses with and without insulin dysregulation. *Journal of Veterinary Internal Medicine* 34(2), 902–908. DOI: 10.1111/jvim.15747.

Kronfeld, D.S., Treiber, K.H. and Geor, R.J. (2005) Comparison of nonspecific indications and quantitative methods for the assessment of insulin resistance in horses and ponies. *Journal of the American*

Veterinary Medical Association 226(5), 712–719. DOI: 10.2460/javma.2005.226.712.

Lane, H.E., Burns, T.A., Hegedus, O.C., Watts, M.R., Weber, P.S. *et al.* (2017) Lamellar events related to insulin-like growth factor-1 receptor signalling in two models relevant to endocrinopathic laminitis. *Equine Veterinary Journal* 49(5), 643–654. DOI: 10.1111/evj.12663.

Lawrence, L.M., Williams, J., Soderholm, L.V., Roberts, A.M. and Hintz, H.F. (1995) Effect of feeding state on the response of horses to repeated bouts of intense exercise. *Equine Veterinary Journal* 27(1), 27–30. DOI: 10.1111/j.2042-3306.1995.tb03028.x.

Lebovitz, H. (2001) Insulin resistance: definition and consequences. *Experimental and Clinical Endocrinology & Diabetes* 109(Suppl 2), S135–S148. DOI: 10.1055/s-2001-18576.

Loeb, W.F., Capen, C.C. and Johnson, L.E. (1966) Adenomas of the pars intermedia associated with hyperglycemia and glycosuria in two horses. *The Cornell Veterinarian* 56(4), 623–639.

Longland, A.C., Barfoot, C. and Harris, P.A. (2014) Effect of period, water temperature and agitation on loss of water-soluble carbohydrates and protein from grass hay: implications for equine feeding management. *Veterinary Record* 174(3), 68. DOI: 10.1136/vr.101820.

Lorenzo, C., Wagenknecht, L.E., Rewers, M.J., Karter, A.J., Bergman, R.N. *et al.* (2010) Disposition index, glucose effectiveness, and conversion to type 2 diabetes: the insulin resistance atherosclerosis study (IRAS). *Diabetes Care* 33(9), 2098–2103. DOI: 10.2337/dc10-0165.

Mack, S.J., Dugdale, A.H., Argo, C.M., Morgan, R.A. and McGowan, C.M. (2014) Impact of water-soaking on the nutrient composition of UK hays. *Veterinary Record* 174(18), 452.1–45452. DOI: 10.1136/vr.102074.

Marques, R.G., Fontaine, M.J. and Rogers, J. (2004) C-peptide: much more than a byproduct of insulin biosynthesis. *Pancreas* 29, 231–238.

Marshall, R.D., Rand, J.S. and Morton, J.M. (2008) Glargine and protamine zinc insulin have a longer duration of action and result in lower mean daily glucose concentrations than lente insulin in healthy cats. *Journal of Veterinary Pharmacology and Therapeutics* 31(3), 205–212. DOI: 10.1111/j.1365-2885.2008.00947.x.

Martin, B.C., Warram, J.H., Krolewski, A.S., Soeldner, J.S., Kahn, C.R. *et al.* (1992) Role of glucose and insulin resistance in development of type 2 diabetes mellitus: results of a 25-year follow-up study. *The Lancet* 340(8825), 925–929. DOI: 10.1016/0140-6736(92)92814-V.

Martinson, K.L., Coleman, R.C., Rendahl, A.K., Fang, Z. and McCue, M.E. (2014) Estimation of body weight and development of a body weight score for adult equids using morphometric measurements. *Journal of Animal Science* 92(5), 2230–2238. DOI: 10.2527/jas.2013-6689.

Martin-Gimenez, T., de Blas, I., Aguilera-Tejero, E., Diez de Castro, E. and Aguirre-Pascasio, C.N. (2016) Endocrine, morphometric, and ultrasonographic characterization of neck adiposity in Andalusian horses. *Domestic Animal Endocrinology* 56, 57–62. DOI: 10.1016/j.domaniend.2016.02.003.

McCoy, D.J. (1986) Diabetes mellitus associated with bilateral granulosa cell tumors in a mare. *Journal of the American Veterinary Medical Association* 188(7), 733–735.

McCutcheon, L.J., Geor, R.J. and Hinchcliff, K.W. (2002) Changes in skeletal muscle GLUT4 content and muscle membrane glucose transport following 6 weeks of exercise training. *Equine Veterinary Journal* 34(S34), 199–204. DOI: 10.1111/j.2042-3306.2002.tb05418.x.

McGowan, C.M. (2010) Endocrinopathic Laminitis. *The Veterinary clinics of North America. Equine practice* 26(2), 233–237.

McGowan, C.M., Frost, R., Pfeiffer D.U. and Neiger, R. (2004) Serum insulin concentrations in horses with equine Cushing's syndrome: response to a cortisol inhibitor and prognostic value. *Equine Veterinary Journal* 36(3), 295–298. DOI: 10.2746/0425164044877288.

McGowan, C.M., Dugdale, A.H., Pinchbeck, G.L. and Argo, C.M. (2013) Dietary restriction in combination with a nutraceutical supplement for the management of equine metabolic syndrome in horses. *The Veterinary Journal* 196(2), 153–159. DOI: 10.1016/j.tvjl.2012.10.007.

McGowan, T.W., Pinchbeck, G.P. and McGowan, C.M. (2013b) Prevalence, risk factors and clinical signs predictive for equine pituitary pars intermedia dysfunction in aged horses. *Equine Veterinary Journal* 45(1), 74–79. DOI: 10.1111/j.2042-3306.2012.00578.x.

McManus, E.J., Sakamoto, K., Armit, L.J., Ronaldson, L., Shpiro, N. *et al.* (2005) Role that phosphorylation of GSK3 plays in insulin and Wnt signalling defined by knockin analysis. *The EMBO Journal* 24(8), 1571–1583. DOI: 10.1038/sj.emboj 7600633.

Meier, A., Reiche, D., de Laat, M., Pollitt, C., Walsh, D. *et al.* (2018a) The sodium-glucose co-transporter 2 inhibitor velagliflozin reduces hyperinsulinemia and prevents laminitis in insulin-dysregulated ponies. *Plos One* 13(9), e0203655. DOI: 10.1371/journal.pone.0203655.

Meier, A.D., de Laat, M.A., Reiche, D.B., Pollitt, C.C., Walsh, D.M. *et al.* (2018b) The oral glucose test predicts laminitis risk in ponies fed a diet high in nonstructural carbohydrates. *Domestic Animal Endocrinology* 63, 1–9. DOI: 10.1016/j.domaniend.2017.10.008.

Meier, A., de Laat, M., Pollitt, C., Walsh, D., McGree, J. *et al.* (2019a) A "modified Obel" method for the severity scoring of (endocrinopathic) equine laminitis. *PeerJ* 7(3), e7084. DOI: 10.7717/peerj.7084.

Meier, A., de Laat, M., Reiche, D., Fitzgerald, D. and Sillence, M. (2019b) The efficacy and safety of velagliflozin over 16 weeks as a treatment for insulin dysregulation in ponies. *BMC Veterinary Research* 15(1), 65. DOI: 10.1186/s12917-019-1811-2.

Meier, U. and Gressner, A.M. (2004) Endocrine regulation of energy metabolism: review of pathobiochemical and clinical chemical aspects of leptin, ghrelin, adiponectin, and resistin. *Clinical Chemistry* 50(9), 1511–1525. DOI: 10.1373/clinchem.2004.032482.

Menzies-Gow, N.J., Wray, H., Bailey, S.R., Harris, P.A. and Elliott, J. (2014) The effect of exercise on plasma concentrations of inflammatory markers in normal and previously laminitic ponies. *Equine Veterinary Journal* 46(3), 317–321. DOI: 10.1111/evj.12132.

Menzies-Gow, N.J., Harris, P.A. and Elliott, J. (2017) Prospective cohort study evaluating risk factors for the development of pasture-associated laminitis in the United Kingdom. *Equine Veterinary Journal* 49(3), 300–306. DOI: 10.1111/evj.12606.

Mills, P.C., Ng, J.C., Kramer, H. and Auer, D.E. (1997) Stress response to chronic inflammation in the horse. *Equine Veterinary Journal* 29(6), 483–486. DOI: 10.1111/j.2042-3306.1997.tb03163.x.

Moore-Colyer, M.J.S., Lumbis, K., Longland, A. and Harris, P. (2014) The effect of five different wetting treatments on the nutrient content and microbial concentration in hay for horses. *PLoS One* 9(11), e114079. DOI: 10.1371/journal.pone.0114079.

Morgan, R.A., McGowan, T.W. and McGowan, C.M. (2014) Prevalence and risk factors for hyperinsulinaemia in ponies in Queensland, Australia. *Australian Veterinary Journal* 92(4), 101–106. DOI: 10.1111/avj.12159.

Morgan, R.A., Keen, J.A. and McGowan, C.M. (2016) Treatment of equine metabolic syndrome: a clinical case series. *Equine Veterinary Journal* 48(4), 422–426. DOI: 10.1111/evj.12445.

Morgan, S.J., Hood, D.M., Wagner, I.P. and Postl, S.P. (2003) Submural histopathologic changes attributable to peracute laminitis in horses. *American Journal of Veterinary Research* 64(7), 829–834. DOI: 10.2460/ajvr.2003.64.829.

Munoz, M.C., Doreste, F., Ferrer, O., Gonzalez, J. and Montoya, J.A. (1996) Pergolide treatment for Cushing's syndrome in a horse. *Veterinary Record* 139(2), 41–43. DOI: 10.1136/vr.139.2.41.

Muylle, E., van den Hende, C., Deprez, P., Nuytten, J. and Oyaert, W. (1986) Non-insulin dependent diabetes mellitus in a horse. *Equine Veterinary Journal* 18(2), 145–146. DOI: 10.1111/j.2042-3306.1986.tb03572.x.

Nadal, M.R., Thompson, D.L. and Kincaid, L.A. (1997) Effect of feeding and feed deprivation on plasma concentrations of prolactin, insulin, growth hormone, and metabolites in horses. *Journal of Animal Science* 75(3), 736–744. DOI: 10.2527/1997.753736x.

Navas de Solis, C. and Foreman, J.H. (2010) Transient diabetes mellitus in a neonatal thoroughbred foal. *Journal of Veterinary Emergency and Critical Care* 20(6), 611–615. DOI: 10.1111/j.1476-4431.2010.00588.x.

Newkirk, K.M., Ehrensing, G., Odoi, A., Boston, R.C. and Frank, N. (2018) Immunohistochemical expression of insulin, glucagon, and somatostatin in pancreatic islets of horses with and without insulin resistance. *American Journal of Veterinary Research* 79(2), 191–198. DOI: 10.2460/ajvr.79.2.191.

Newman, S.J. (2015) Equine pancreatic disease: a review and characterization of the lesions of four cases (2005–2014). *Journal of Veterinary Diagnostic Investigation: Official Publication of the American Association of Veterinary Laboratory Diagnosticians, Inc* 27(1), 92–96. DOI: 10.1177/1040638714560606.

Obel, N. (1948) Studies on the histopathology of acute laminitis. *Almqvist & Wiksells Boktryckeri*, 1–95.

Orskov, C., Holst, J.J., Poulsen, S.S. and Kirkegaard, P. (1987) Pancreatic and intestinal processing of proglucagon in man. *Diabetologia* 30(11), 874–881. DOI: 10.1007/bf00274797.

Orth, D.N., Holscher, M.A., Wilson, M.G., Nicholson, W.E., Plue, R.E. *et al.* (1982) Equine Cushing's disease: plasma immunoreactive proopiolipomelanocortin peptide and cortisol levels basally and in response to diagnostic tests. *Endocrinology* 110(4), 1430–1441. DOI: 10.1210/endo-110-4-1430.

Oyaert, W. and Muyelle, E. (1965) Diabetes mellitus in a horse. *Dtsch Tierarztl Wochenschr* 72, 232–233.

O'Grady, S.E. (2010) Farriery for chronic laminitis. *Veterinary Clinics of North America: Equine Practice* 26(2), 407–423.

Peterson, M.E., Altszuler, N. and Nichols, C.E. (1984) Decreased insulin sensitivity and glucose tolerance in spontaneous canine hyperadrenocorticism. *Research in Veterinary Science* 36(2), 177–182. DOI: 10.1016/S0034-5288(18)31975-1.

Place, N.J., McGowan, C.M., Lamb, S.V., Schanbacher, B.J., McGowan, T. *et al.* (2010) Seasonal variation in serum concentrations of selected metabolic hormones in horses. *Journal of Veterinary Internal Medicine* 24(3), 650–654. DOI: 10.1111/j.1939-1676.2010.0500.x.

Pleasant, R.S., Suagee, J.K., Thatcher, C.D., Elvinger, F. and Geor, R.J. (2013) Adiposity, plasma insulin, leptin, lipids, and oxidative stress in mature light breed horses. *Journal of Veterinary Internal Medicine* 27(3), 576–582. DOI: 10.1111/jvim.12056.

Pollitt, C.C. (1996) Basement membrane pathology: a feature of acute equine laminitis. *Equine Veterinary Journal* 28(1), 38–46. DOI: 10.1111/j.2042-3306.1996.tb01588.x.

Potter, S.J., Bamford, N.J., Harris, P.A. and Bailey, S.R. (2016) Prevalence of obesity and owners' perceptions of body condition in pleasure horses and ponies in south-eastern Australia. *Australian Veterinary Journal* 94(11), 427–432. DOI: 10.1111/avj.12506.

Powell, D.M., Reedy, S.E., Sessions, D.R. and Fitzgerald, B.P. (2002) Effect of short-term exercise training on insulin sensitivity in obese and lean mares. *Equine*

Veterinary Journal 34(S34), 81–84. DOI: 10.1111/j.2042-3306.2002.tb05396.x.

Pratt, S.E., Geor, R.J. and McCutcheon, L.J. (2005) Repeatability of 2 methods for assessment of insulin sensitivity and glucose dynamics in horses. *Journal of Veterinary Internal Medicine* 19(6), 883–888. DOI: 10.1111/j.1939-1676.2005.tb02782.x.

Pratt-Phillips, S.E., Geor, R.J. and McCutcheon, L.J. (2015) Comparison among the euglycemic-hyperinsulinemic clamp, insulin-modified frequently sampled intravenous glucose tolerance test, and oral glucose tolerance test for assessment of insulin sensitivity in healthy Standardbreds. *American Journal of Veterinary Research* 76(1), 84–91. DOI: 10.2460/ajvr.76.1.84.

Radin, M.J., Sharkey, L.C. and Holycross, B.J. (2009) Adipokines: a review of biological and analytical principles and an update in dogs, cats, and horses. *Veterinary Clinical Pathology* 38(2), 136–156. DOI: 10.1111/j.1939-165X.2009.00133.x.

Ralston, S.L. (2002) Insulin and glucose regulation. *Veterinary Clinics of North America: Equine Practice* 18(2), 295–304.

Rendle, D.I., Rutledge, F., Hughes, K.J., Heller, J. and Durham, A.E. (2013) Effects of metformin hydrochloride on blood glucose and insulin responses to oral dextrose in horses. *Equine Veterinary Journal* 45(6), 751–754. DOI: 10.1111/evj.12068.

Respondek, F., Myers, K., Smith, T.L., Wagner, A. and Geor, R.J. (2011) Dietary supplementation with short-chain fructo-oligosaccharides improves insulin sensitivity in obese horses. *Journal of Animal Science* 89(1), 77–83. DOI: 10.2527/jas.2010-3108.

Ringer, S.K., Schwarzwald, C.C., Portier, K., Mauch, J., Ritter, A. *et al.* (2013) Blood glucose, acid–base and electrolyte changes during loading doses of alpha2-adrenergic agonists followed by constant rate infusions in horses. *The Veterinary Journal* 198(3), 684–689. DOI: 10.1016/j.tvjl.2013.09.063.

Robin, C.A., Ireland, J.L., Wylie, C.E., Collins, S.N., Verheyen, K.L.P. *et al.* (2015) Prevalence of and risk factors for equine obesity in Great Britain based on owner-reported body condition scores. *Equine Veterinary Journal* 47(2), 196–201. DOI: 10.1111/evj.12275.

Ruoff, W.W., Baker, D.C., Morgan, S.J. and Abbitt, B. (1986) Type II diabetes mellitus in a horse. *Equine Veterinary Journal* 18(2), 143–144. DOI: 10.1111/j.2042-3306.1986.tb03571.x.

Schott, H.C. (2002) Pituitary pars intermedia dysfunction: equine Cushing's disease. *Veterinary Clinics of North America: Equine Practice* 18(2), 237–270.

Schuver, A., Frank, N., Chameroy, K.A. and Elliott, S.B. (2014) Assessment of insulin and glucose dynamics by using an oral sugar test in horses. *Journal of Equine Veterinary Science* 34(4), 465–470. DOI: 10.1016/j.jevs.2013.09.006.

Scroggie, D.A., Albright, A. and Harris, M.D. (2003) The effect of glucosamine-chondroitin supplementation on glycosylated hemoglobin levels in patients with type 2 diabetes mellitus: a placebo-controlled, double-blinded, randomized clinical trial. *Archives of Internal Medicine* 163(13), 1587–1590. DOI: 10.1001/archinte.163.13.1587.

Seino, Y., Nanjo, K., Tajima, N., Kadowaki, T., Kashiwagi, A. *et al.* (2010) Report of the Committee on the classification and diagnostic criteria of diabetes mellitus. *Diabetology International* 1(1), 2–20. DOI: 10.1007/s13340-010-0006-7.

Selim, S., Elo, K., Jaakkola, S., Karikoski, N., Boston, R. *et al.* (2015) Relationships among body condition, insulin resistance and subcutaneous adipose tissue gene expression during the grazing season in mares. *PLoS One* 10(5), e0125968. DOI: 10.1371/journal.pone.0125968.

Sharma, V. and McNeill, J.H. (2005) The emerging roles of leptin and ghrelin in cardiovascular physiology and pathophysiology. *Current Vascular Pharmacology* 3(2), 169–180. DOI: 10.2174/1570161053586868.

Shehzad, A., Iqbal, W., Shehzad, O. and Lee, Y.S. (2012) Adiponectin: regulation of its production and its role in human diseases. *Hormones* 11(1), 8–20. DOI: 10.1007/BF03401534.

Sherlock, C. and Parks, A. (2013) Radiographic and radiological assessment of laminitis. *Equine Veterinary Education* 25(10), 524–535. DOI: 10.1111/eve.12065.

Shoelson, S.E., Herrero, L. and Naaz, A. (2007) Obesity, inflammation, and insulin resistance. *Gastroenterology* 132(6), 2169–2180. DOI: 10.1053/j.gastro.2007.03.059.

Singhal, A. (2005) Endothelial dysfunction: role in obesity-related disorders and the early origins of CVD. *Proceedings of the Nutrition Society* 64(1), 15–22. DOI: 10.1079/PNS2004404.

Skoglund, G., Lundquist, I. and Ahrén, B. (1987) Alpha 1- and alpha 2-adrenoceptor activation increases plasma glucagon levels in the mouse. *European Journal of Pharmacology* 143(1), 83–88. DOI: 10.1016/0014-2999(87)90737-0.

Smith, S., Harris, P.A. and Menzies-Gow, N.J. (2016) Comparison of the in-feed glucose test and the oral sugar test. *Equine Veterinary Journal* 48(2), 224–227. DOI: 10.1111/evj.12413.

Sparks, J.D., Sparks, C.E. and Adeli, K. (2012) Selective hepatic insulin resistance, VLDL overproduction, and hypertriglyceridemia. *Arteriosclerosis, Thrombosis, and Vascular Biology* 32(9), 2104–2112. DOI: 10.1161/ATVBAHA.111.241463.

Staempfli, H.R., Eigenmann, E.J. and Clarke, L.M. (1988) Insulin treatment and development of anti-insulin antibodies in a horse with diabetes mellitus associated with a functional pituitary adenoma. *The Canadian Veterinary Journal* 29(11), 934–936.

Steiner, D.F. and Oyer, P.E. (1967) The biosynthesis of insulin and a probable precursor of insulin by a human islet cell adenoma. *Proceedings of the National Academy of Sciences* 57(2), 473–480. DOI: 10.1073/pnas.57.2.473.

Stephenson, H.M., Green, M.J. and Freeman, S.L. (2011) Prevalence of obesity in a population of horses in the UK. *Veterinary Record* 168(5), 131. DOI: 10.1136/vr.c6281.

Stewart-Hunt, L., Geor, R.J. and McCutcheon, L.J. (2006) Effects of short-term training on insulin sensitivity and skeletal muscle glucose metabolism in standardbred horses. *Equine Veterinary Journal* (36), 226–232. DOI: 10.1111/j.2042-3306.2006.tb05544.x.

Stewart, A.J., Hackett, E., Bertin, F.-R. and Towns, T.J. (2019) Cortisol and adrenocorticotropic hormone concentrations in horses with systemic inflammatory response syndrome. *Journal of Veterinary Internal Medicine* 33(5), 2257–2266. DOI: 10.1111/jvim.15620.

Stokes, S.M., Belknap, J.K., Engiles, J.B., Stefanovski, D., Bertin, F.R. *et al.* (2019) Continuous digital hypothermia prevents lamellar failure in the euglycaemic hyperinsulinaemic clamp model of equine laminitis. *Equine Veterinary Journal* 51(5), 658–664. DOI: 10.1111/evj.13072.

Stokes, S.M., Bertin, F.R., Stefanovski, D., Belknap, J.K., Medina-Torres, C.E. *et al.* (2020a) Lamellar energy metabolism and perfusion in the euglycaemic hyperinsulinaemic clamp model of equine laminitis. *Equine Veterinary Journal* 52(4), 577–584. DOI: 10.1111/evj.13224.

Stokes, S.M., Bertin, F.-R., Stefanovski, D., Poulsen, L., Belknap, J.K. *et al.* (2020b) The effect of continuous digital hypothermia on lamellar energy metabolism and perfusion during laminitis development in two experimental models. *Equine Veterinary Journal* 52(4), 585–592. DOI: 10.1111/evj.13215.

Suagee, J.K., Corl, B.A., Crisman, M.V., Hulver, M.W., McCutcheon, L.J. *et al.* (2011a) Effects of acute hyperinsulinemia on inflammatory proteins in horses. *Veterinary Immunology and Immunopathology* 142(3–4), 141–146. DOI: 10.1016/j.vetimm.2011.05.001.

Suagee, J.K., Corl, B.A., Wearn, J.G., Crisman, M.V., Hulver, M.W. *et al.* (2011b) Effects of the insulin-sensitizing drug pioglitazone and lipopolysaccharide administration on insulin sensitivity in horses. *Journal of Veterinary Internal Medicine* 25(2), 356–364. DOI: 10.1111/j.1939-1676.2011.0681.x.

Suagee, J.K., Corl, B.A., Crisman, M.V., Pleasant, R.S., Thatcher, C.D. *et al.* (2013) Relationships between body condition score and plasma inflammatory cytokines, insulin, and lipids in a mixed population of light-breed horses. *Journal of Veterinary Internal Medicine* 27(1), 157–163. DOI: 10.1111/jvim.12021.

Tadros, E.M., Frank, N., De Witte, F.G. and Boston, R.C. (2013) Effects of intravenous lipopolysaccharide infusion on glucose and insulin dynamics in horses with equine metabolic syndrome. *American Journal of Veterinary Research* 74(7), 1020–1029. DOI: 10.2460/ajvr.74.7.1020.

Takano, A., Haruta, T., Iwata, M., Usui, I., Uno, T. *et al.* (2001) Growth hormone induces cellular insulin resistance by uncoupling phosphatidylinositol 3-kinase and its downstream signals in 3T3-L1 adipocytes. *Diabetes* 50(8), 1891–1900. DOI: 10.2337/diabetes.50.8.1891.

Tasker, J.B., Whiteman, C.E. and Martin, B.R. (1966) Diabetes mellitus in the horse. *Journal of the American Veterinary Medical Association* 149(4), 393–399.

Teoh, H., Quan, A., Bang, K.W.A., Wang, G., Lovren, F. *et al.* (2008) Adiponectin deficiency promotes endothelial activation and profoundly exacerbates sepsis-related mortality. *American Journal of Physiology-Endocrinology and Metabolism* 295(3), E658–E664. DOI: 10.1152/ajpendo.90384.2008.

Thatcher, C.D., Pleasant, R.S., Geor, R.J. and Elvinger, F. (2012) Prevalence of overconditioning in mature horses in Southwest Virginia during the summer. *Journal of Veterinary Internal Medicine* 26(6), 1413–1418. DOI: 10.1111/j.1939-1676.2012.00995.x.

Tiley, H.A., Geor, R.J. and McCutcheon, L.J. (2007) Effects of dexamethasone on glucose dynamics and insulin sensitivity in healthy horses. *American Journal of Veterinary Research* 68(7), 753–759. DOI: 10.2460/ajvr.68.7.753.

Tiley, H.A., Geor, R.J. and McCutcheon, L.J. (2008) Effects of dexamethasone administration on insulin resistance and components of insulin signaling and glucose metabolism in equine skeletal muscle. *American Journal of Veterinary Research* 69(1), 51–58. DOI: 10.2460/ajvr.69.1.51.

Tinworth, K.D., Edwards, S., Noble, G.K., Harris, P.A., Sillence, M.N. *et al.* (2010) Pharmacokinetics of metformin after enteral administration in insulin-resistant ponies. *American Journal of Veterinary Research* 71(10), 1201–1206. DOI: 10.2460/ajvr.71.10.1201.

Tinworth, K.D., Wynn, P.C., Boston, R.C., Harris, P.A., Sillence, M.N. *et al.* (2011) Evaluation of commercially available assays for the measurement of equine insulin. *Domestic Animal Endocrinology* 41(2), 81–90. DOI: 10.1016/j.domaniend.2011.05.001.

Tinworth, K.D., Boston, R.C., Harris, P.A., Sillence, M.N., Raidal, S.L. *et al.* (2012) The effect of oral metformin on insulin sensitivity in insulin-resistant ponies. *The Veterinary Journal* 191(1), 79–84. DOI: 10.1016/j.tvjl.2011.01.015.

Trayhurn, P., Wang, B. and Wood, I.S. (2008) Hypoxia in adipose tissue: a basis for the dysregulation of tissue function in obesity? *British Journal of Nutrition* 100(2), 227–235. DOI: 10.1017/S0007114508971282.

Treiber, K.H., Boston, R.C., Kronfeld, D.S., Staniar, W.B. and Harris, P.A. (2005a) Insulin resistance and compensation in thoroughbred weanlings adapted to high-glycemic meals. *Journal of Animal Science* 83(10), 2357–2364. DOI: 10.2527/2005.83102357x.

Treiber, K.H., Kronfeld, D.S., Hess, T.M., Boston, R.C. and Harris, P.A. (2005b) Use of proxies and reference quintiles obtained from minimal model analysis for determination of insulin sensitivity and pancreatic beta-cell responsiveness in horses. *American Journal of Veterinary Research* 66(12), 2114–2121. DOI: 10.2460/ajvr.2005.66.2114.

Treiber, K.H., Kronfeld, D.S., Hess, T.M., Byrd, B.M., Splan, R.K. *et al.* (2006) Evaluation of genetic and metabolic predispositions and nutritional risk factors for pasture-associated laminitis in ponies. *Journal of the American Veterinary Medical Association* 228(10), 1538–1545. DOI: 10.2460/javma.228.10.1538.

Tóth, F., Frank, N., Elliott, S.B., Geor, R.J. and Boston, R.C. (2008) Effects of an intravenous endotoxin challenge on glucose and insulin dynamics in horses. *American Journal of Veterinary Research* 69(1), 82–88. DOI: 10.2460/ajvr.69.1.82.

Tóth, F., Frank, N., Elliott, S.B., Perdue, K., Geor, R.J. *et al.* (2009) Optimisation of the frequently sampled intravenous glucose tolerance test to reduce urinary glucose spilling in horses. *Equine Veterinary Journal* 41(9), 844–851. DOI: 10.2746/042516409X439661.

Tóth, F., Frank, N., Geor, R.J. and Boston, R.C. (2010a) Effects of pretreatment with dexamethasone or levothyroxine sodium on endotoxin-induced alterations in glucose and insulin dynamics in horses. *American Journal of Veterinary Research* 71(1), 60–68. DOI: 10.2460/ajvr.71.1.60.

Tóth, F., Frank, N., Martin-Jiménez, T., Elliott, S.B., Geor, R.J. *et al.* (2010b) Measurement of C-peptide concentrations and responses to somatostatin, glucose infusion, and insulin resistance in horses. *Equine Veterinary Journal* 42(2), 149–155. DOI: 10.2746/042516409X478497.

Ungru, J., Blüher, M., Coenen, M., Raila, J., Boston, R. *et al.* (2012) Effects of body weight reduction on blood adipokines and subcutaneous adipose tissue adipokine mRNA expression profiles in obese ponies. *Veterinary Record* 171(21), 528. DOI: 10.1136/vr.100911.

Uwaifo, G.I., Fallon, E.M., Chin, J., Elberg, J., Parikh, S.J. *et al.* (2002) Indices of insulin action, disposal, and secretion derived from fasting samples and clamps in normal glucose-tolerant black and white children. *Diabetes Care* 25(11), 2081–2087. DOI: 10.2337/diacare.25.11.2081.

van der Kolk, J.H., Kalsbeek, H.C., van Garderen, E., Wensing, T. and Breukink, H.J. (1993) Equine pituitary neoplasia: a clinical report of 21 cases (1990–1992). *The Veterinary Record* 133(24), 594–597.

van der Kolk, J.H., Wensing, T., Kalsbeek, H.C. and Breukink, H.J. (1995) Laboratory diagnosis of equine pituitary pars intermedia adenoma. *Domestic Animal Endocrinology* 12(1), 35–39. DOI: 10.1016/0739-7240(94)00006-M.

van der Meulen, T., Donaldson, C.J., Cáceres, E., Hunter, A.E., Cowing-Zitron, C. *et al.* (2015) Urocortin3 mediates somatostatin-dependent negative feedback control of insulin secretion. *Nature Medicine* 21(7), 769–776. DOI: 10.1038/nm.3872.

van Eps, A.W. and Pollitt, C.C. (2006) Equine laminitis induced with oligofructose. *Equine Veterinary Journal* 38(3), 203–208. DOI: 10.2746/042516406776866327.

van Eps, A.W., Pollitt, C.C., Underwood, C., Medina-Torres, C.E., Goodwin, W.A. *et al.* (2014) Continuous digital hypothermia initiated after the onset of lameness prevents lamellar failure in the oligofructose laminitis model. *Equine Veterinary Journal* 46(5), 625–630. DOI: 10.1111/evj.12180.

van Herpen, N.A. and Schrauwen-Hinderling, V.B. (2008) Lipid accumulation in non-adipose tissue and lipotoxicity. *Physiology & Behavior* 94(2), 231–241. DOI: 10.1016/j.physbeh.2007.11.049.

Van Weyenberg, S., Hesta, M., Buyse, J. and Janssens, G.P.J. (2008) The effect of weight loss by energy restriction on metabolic profile and glucose tolerance in ponies. *Journal of Animal Physiology and Animal Nutrition* 92(5), 538–545. DOI: 10.1111/j.1439-0396.2007.00744.x.

Van Weyenberg, S., Buyse, J., Kalmar, I.D., Swennen, Q. and Janssens, G.P.J. (2013) Voluntary feed intake and leptin sensitivity in AD libitum fed obese ponies following a period of restricted feeding: a pilot study. *Journal of Animal Physiology and Animal Nutrition* 97(4), 624–631. DOI: 10.1111/j.1439-0396.2012.01300.x.

Vick, M.M., Adams, A.A., Murphy, B.A., Sessions, D.R., Horohov, D.W. *et al.* (2007) Relationships among inflammatory cytokines, obesity, and insulin sensitivity in the horse. *Journal of Animal Science* 85(5), 1144–1155. DOI: 10.2527/jas.2006-673.

Waller, A.P., Burns, T.A., Mudge, M.C., Belknap, J.K. and Lacombe, V.A. (2011a) Insulin resistance selectively alters cell-surface glucose transporters but not their total protein expression in equine skeletal muscle. *Journal of Veterinary Internal Medicine* 25(2), 315–321. DOI: 10.1111/j.1939-1676.2010.0674.x.

Waller, A.P., Kohler, K., Burns T.A., Mudge, M.C., Belknap, J.K. *et al.* (2011b) Naturally occurring compensated insulin resistance selectively alters glucose transporters in visceral and subcutaneous adipose tissues without change in AS160 activation. *Biochimica et Biophysica Acta (BBA) - Molecular Basis of Disease* 1812(9), 1098–1103. DOI: 10.1016/j.bbadis.2011.02.007.

Warnken, T., Huber, K. and Feige, K. (2016) Comparison of three different methods for the quantification of equine insulin. *BMC Veterinary Research* 12(1), 196. DOI: 10.1186/s12917-016-0828-z.

Wearn, J.M.G., Crisman, M.V., Davis, J.L., Geor, R.J., Hodgson, D.R. *et al.* (2011) Pharmacokinetics of pioglitazone after multiple oral dose administration in horses. *Journal of Veterinary Pharmacology and Therapeutics* 34(3), 252–258. DOI: 10.1111/j.1365-2885.2010.01217.x.

Wearn, J.G., Suagee, J.K., Crisman, M.V., Corl, B.A., Hulver, M.W. *et al.* (2012) Effects of the insulin sensitizing drug, pioglitazone, and lipopolysaccharide administration on markers of systemic inflammation and clinical parameters in horses. *Veterinary Immunology and Immunopathology* 145(1–2), 42–49. DOI: 10.1016/j.vetimm.2011.10.007.

Williams, C.A., Kronfeld, D.S., Staniar, W.B. and Harris, P.A. (2001) Plasma glucose and insulin responses of thoroughbred mares fed a meal high in starch and sugar or fat and fiber. *Journal of Animal Science* 79(8), 2196–2201. DOI: 10.2527/2001.7982196x.

Wilson, M.G., Nicholson, W.E., Holscher, M.A., Sherrell, B.J., Mount, C.D. *et al.* (1982) Proopiolipomelanocortin peptides in normal pituitary, pituitary tumor, and plasma of normal and Cushing's horses. *Endocrinology* 110(3), 941–954. DOI: 10.1210/endo-110-3-941.

Wyse, C.A., McNie, K.A., Tannahill, V.J., Tannahil, V.J., Murray, J.K. *et al.* (2008) Prevalence of obesity in riding horses in Scotland. *Veterinary Record* 162(18), 590–591. DOI: 10.1136/vr.162.18.590.

Yosten, G.L.C. and Kolar, G.R. (2015) The physiology of proinsulin C-peptide: unanswered questions and a proposed model. *Physiology* 30(4), 327–332. DOI: 10.1152/physiol.00008.2015.

Yu, Q., Shuai, H., Ahooghalandari, P., Gylfe, E. and Tengholm, A. (2019) Glucose controls glucagon secretion by directly modulating cAMP in alpha cells. *Diabetologia* 62(7), 1212–1224. DOI: 10.1007/s00125-019-4857-6.

Yu, Y.-H. and Ginsberg, H.N. (2005) Adipocyte signaling and lipid homeostasis: sequelae of insulin-resistant adipose tissue. *Circulation Research* 96(10), 1042–1052. DOI: 10.1161/01.RES.0000165803.47776.38.

Zhang, X.-X., Pan, Y.-H., Huang, Y.-M. and Zhao, H.-L. (2016) Neuroendocrine hormone amylin in diabetes. *World Journal of Diabetes* 7(9), 189–197. DOI: 10.4239/wjd.v7.i9.189.

6 Hyperlipaemia and Lipid Metabolism Disorders

Disorders of lipid metabolism are characterized by the increase in circulating lipids following a negative energy balance caused by stress, anorexia, gastrointestinal disease, gestation or lactation. These disorders are recognized by the opalescence of the serum resulting from excessive fat mobilization and circulation of high triglyceride concentrations. Moderate increases can have mild clinical consequences; however, severe increases can lead to severe systemic complications and death (McKenzie, 2011).

Lipid Metabolism

Lipid absorption

In horses, lipids are absorbed as fatty acids from the gastrointestinal tract. While some short chain fatty acids are bound to albumin and transported in the portal circulation, most fatty acids are transformed into phospholipids and triglycerides by gastrointestinal epithelial cells before being transported in the portal circulation or being incorporated as chylomicrons and transported in the lymphatic circulation. Since horses are hindgut fermenters, they can shift between a traditional monogastric glucose-oriented metabolism to a ruminant fatty acid-oriented metabolism (Argenzio and Hintz, 1972; Naylor *et al.*, 1980). In this case, the most important fatty acids absorbed are acetate, propionate and butyrate (Bergman, 1990).

Lipid transformations

Regardless of their form of transportation, fatty acids are delivered to the liver. There, depending on energy demands and hormonal stimulation, fatty acids can be esterified with glycerol into triglycerides to be exported or oxidized into acetyl coenzyme A (acetyl CoA) to provide energy.

In the form of triglycerides, fatty acids are incorporated with cholesterol, proteins and carbohydrates in hepatocytes to form very-low-density lipoproteins (VLDL, rich in triglycerides) or high-density lipoproteins (HDL, rich in phospholipids and proteins) and are released in the systemic circulation. Circulating VLDL are then used as sources of triglycerides for adipocytes and all lipoprotein–lipase-containing cells, leading to the formation of low-density lipoproteins (LDL) and intermediate-density lipoproteins (IDL) depending on the concentration of triglycerides.

In the cells, in the form of acetyl CoA, fatty acids can enter the Krebs cycle or be transformed into steroids, cholesterol, ketones and other fatty acids such as acetoacetate and beta-hydroxybutyrate (van der Kolk *et al.*, 1995). The formation of ketones, originating from partial oxidation of fatty acids, is quite limited in horses, unlike in other herbivores (Rose and Sampson, 1982).

Regulation of lipid metabolism

The major regulator of lipid metabolism is energy demand: positive energy balance favours lipogenesis whereas negative energy balance favours lipolysis and lipid mobilization.

After a meal, glucose absorption results in glucose-dependent insulinotropic peptide (GIP) by the K-cells of the duodenum and jejunum and in insulin secretion from the beta cells of the islets of Langerhans (de Laat *et al.*, 2016). Insulin increases glucose uptake by insulin-sensitive tissues to maintain blood glucose in a narrow range, and glucose is used either as a source of energy or transformed into glycogen in the muscles or the liver, or stored as fat in adipocytes. As an anabolic hormone, insulin also inhibits the hormone-sensitive lipase (HSL), preventing the breakdown of triglycerides from adipose tissue into glycerol and fatty acids, and stimulates the lipoprotein–lipase activity, increasing the uptake of triglycerides by peripheral tissues (Suagee *et al.*, 2010). GIP is another stimulator of lipoprotein–lipase activity (Schmidt *et al.*, 2001).

When glucose becomes scarce, which is observed with food deprivation, lactation or disease state, insulin secretion decreases and glucagon secretion increases resulting in metabolic stress, a shift toward the use of lipids as a source of energy and overall catabolism (Naylor *et al.*, 1980; Freestone *et al.*, 1991; Frank *et al.*, 2002). As mentioned above, insulin regulates HSL: if insulin secretion decreases, HSL activity increases resulting in the formation of glycerol and fatty acids (Naylor *et al.*, 1980). Glycerol can be metabolized locally or converted into glucose to provide energy; fatty acids can be metabolized locally to provide energy through beta oxidation (Hughes *et al.*, 2004). If lipolysis is excessive, fatty acids are released in the systemic circulation to be taken up by the liver and esterified into triglycerides, to recirculate or be oxidized to provide energy, although this pathway is limited (Naylor *et al.*, 1980; Freestone *et al.*, 1991). This metabolic stress also increases the secretion of glucocorticoids such as cortisol, that antagonizes insulin actions and up regulates HSL activity resulting in further lipolysis, and the secretion of catecholamines such as norepinephrine, that increases fatty acid release from adipocytes (van der Kolk *et al.*, 1995; Breidenbach *et al.*, 1999; Lavery and Glover, 2000; Langin, 2006).

Several other factors such as breed, age or endocrine background, can lead or predispose to impaired lipid metabolism and unregulated lipolysis. In ponies, the regulation of triglyceride release from adipocytes has been shown to be more susceptible to norepinephrine, leading to higher concentrations of circulating fatty acids and triglycerides (Breidenbach *et al.*, 1999). In donkeys, circulating triglyceride concentrations are above horse reference intervals and even more so in obese donkeys, in which a correlation has been documented between body condition score and circulating triglycerides (Díez *et al.*, 2012). In some horses with pituitary pars intermedia dysfunction (PPID), disturbances in insulin and cortisol concentrations have been shown to increase rates of lipolysis and ketogenesis, predisposing these horses to excessive lipid mobilization (van der Kolk *et al.*, 1995). There is conflicting evidence regarding the role of insulin dysregulation (ID) in the regulation of lipid metabolism. In physiologic conditions insulin inhibits HSL, limiting lipolysis; however, a correlation between plasma insulin and triglycerides has been documented suggesting that hyperinsulinaemia could trigger lipolysis. Ponies, and especially obese or fasting ponies, tend to have reduced response to insulin secretion suggesting that the hyperinsulinaemia observed in these animals is a compensation of insulin resistance leading to poor HSL inhibition and increased lipolysis (Oikawa *et al.*, 2006). That being said, horses with normal insulin responses can still develop lipid disorders (Argenzio and Hintz, 1972; Freestone *et al.*, 1991; Forhead *et al.*, 1994; van der Kolk *et al.*, 1995; Forhead and Dobson, 1997).

Hyperlipaemia

Hyperlipaemia is a syndrome characterized by an opalescence of the serum and a circulating triglyceride concentration above 5.5 mmol/l (Gay *et al.*, 1978; McKenzie, 2011). This disease is associated with fatty infiltration of the liver and can be life threatening (Murray, 1985). A milder form of the disease is described with circulating triglyceride concentrations below 5.5 mmol/l and is called *hyperlipidaemia* (Waitt and Cebra, 2009). In this case, fatty infiltration of the liver is rare and opalescence of the serum is inconsistent (Dunkel and McKenzie, 2003). Milder increases of circulating triglycerides above reference intervals (1.1 mmol/l) are called *hypertriglyceridaemia* (McKenzie, 2011).

Epidemiology of hyperlipaemia

Hyperlipaemia mainly occurs in ponies and is more rarely seen in horses with an incidence as high as 5% (Jeffcott and Field, 1985a, b; Watson *et al.*, 1992a). The disease is reported on all continents although the majority of published reports include ponies from British breeds such as Shetlands or Welsh Mountain ponies, which could correspond to a true genetic predisposition (Jeffcott and Field, 1985a, b; Watson *et al.*, 1992a). Donkeys are another group of equids commonly affected by hyperlipaemia and seem especially prone to the disorder (Moore *et al.*, 1994; Durham, 2006; Waitt and Cebra, 2009). The disease is commonly reported in obese animals, in females (representing between 74% and 100% of cases, mainly during late gestation or early lactation), when pastures are unavailable, when feed supplies are short or when a primary condition (such as enterocolitis or colic) reduces the horse dietary intake (Jeffcott and Field, 1985b; Watson *et al.*, 1993; Waitt and Cebra, 2009). The association with parturition could suggest a seasonal predisposition for the disease but no consistent association between season and hyperlipaemia has yet been proven (Watson *et al.*, 1992a). The majority of the cases are adults over 4 years of age and with a peak around 9 years of age but a few case reports exist from younger horses (Jeffcott and Field, 1985b; Gilbert, 1986; Hughes *et al.*, 2002).

Pathogenesis of hyperlipaemia

Hyperlipaemia can be a primary condition but more commonly develops after stressful episodes (Jeffcott and Field, 1985b). About half of the ponies diagnosed with hyperlipaemia were exposed to some kind of stress within the 4 weeks preceding hyperlipaemia. As mentioned above, stress-induced cortisol secretion antagonizes insulin effects, inducing a state of insulin resistance leading to decreased HSL inhibition and uncontrolled lipolysis (Jeffcott and Field, 1985a). This effect is even more pronounced in obese animals in which insulin sensitivity and regulation are already compromised (Hughes *et al.*, 2004; McKenzie, 2011). Typical stressors include transport, gestation, lactation, systemic disease, such as colic or enterocolitis, as well as limited feed availability, all creating a state of negative energy balance either by increased demand or by decreased intake (Watson *et al.*, 1992a, 1993; Hughes *et al.*, 2004; Conwell, 2010). In horses, azotaemia is also a common predisposing factor for hyperlipaemic episodes as it interferes with lipoprotein–lipase activity (Watson *et al.*, 1992a; Hughes *et al.*, 2002).

During episodes of negative energy balance and lipolysis, concentrations of circulating fatty acids, cholesterol, triglyceride and VLDL increase tremendously (Watson *et al.*, 1992a, 1993; Tóth *et al.*, 2018). This increased fatty acid flux stimulates hepatic triglyceride synthesis and VLDL release (Fig. 6.1) (Watson *et al.*, 1992a). In other species, fatty acids are used as sources of energy; the ketone pathway is poorly developed in horses resulting in large amounts of triglycerides being produced and VLDL being released (McKenzie, 2011). Electrophoretic analysis of VLDL fractions have shown that hyperlipaemic ponies have more circulating VLDL and that the fraction of larger VLDL, VLDL1, is greater than in control ponies in which the portion of smaller VLDL, VLDL2, is dominant (Watson *et al.*, 1992a). In addition, the larger VLDL1 are richer in apolipoprotein B48 and E but poorer in lipoprotein

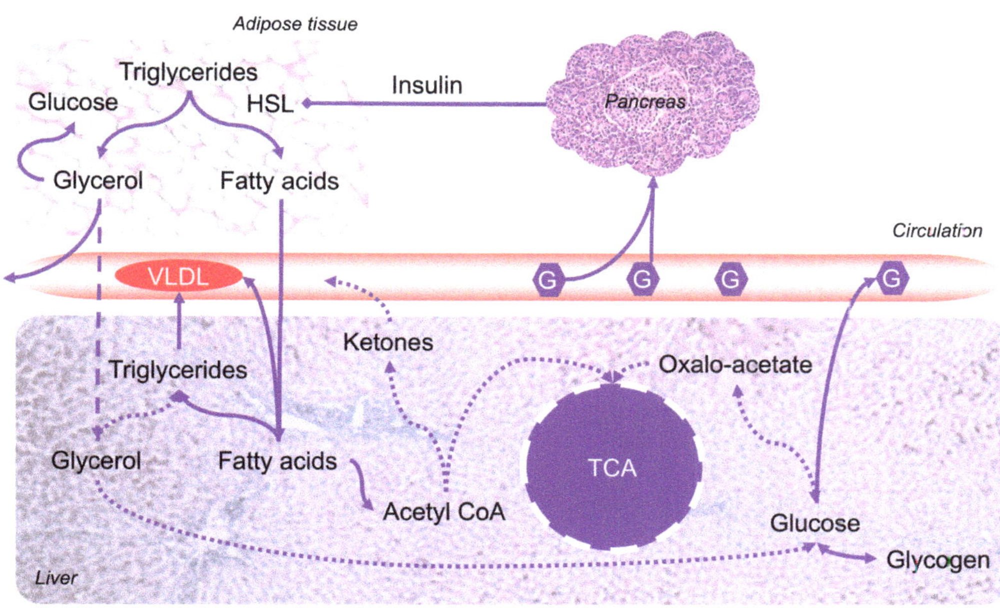

Fig. 6.1. Simplified pathogenesis of hyperlipaemia in horses, showing the tricarboxylic acid cycle (TCA, or Krebs cycle) and the circulation of very-low-density lipoprotein (VLDL), hormone-sensitive lipase (HSL), glucose (G) and acetyl coenzyme A (acetyl CoA) (Author's own).

B100. This lower B100/B48 ratio allows the incorporation of a larger amount of triglyceride and suggests an up-regulation of hepatic triglyceride release through VLDL1. As the release of VLDL increases, the activity of lipoprotein–lipase and hepatic lipase increases resulting in a fatty infiltration of tissues, including the liver (Watson *et al.*, 1993). Therefore, rather than a defective hepatic catabolism of lipid, overproduction of VLDL would cause hyperlipaemia and liver fatty infiltration (Watson *et al.*, 1992a, 1993).

Depending on the magnitude of the increase and the nature of the increased fraction, three types of hyperlipaemia have been described: type 1, characterized by a marked increase in VLDL only; type 2, characterized by a marked increase in chylomicrons and VLDL; and type 3, characterized by moderate increases in chylomicrons and VLDL (Wensing *et al.*, 1975). Although consistent with lipoprotein electrophoresis profiles, this classification is not as commonly used as the classification by concentrations of circulating triglycerides.

Clinical signs of hyperlipaemia

Clinical signs of hyperlipaemia are vague and progressive as the disease is often secondary to another disorder. Clinical signs become more obvious after 3 to 7 days; however, at this stage the disease can already be irreversible (Jeffcott and Field, 1985b; Mogg and Palmer, 1995; Hughes *et al.*, 2004). The first signs can be missed and hyperlipaemia can be an incidental finding (Dunkel *et al.*, 2014). When present, the signs are mild and mainly consist in behavioural changes (Gay *et al.*, 1978; Murray, 1985). As the disease progresses, dysfunctions of the gastrointestinal tract, the liver and the nervous system become more obvious (Gay *et al.*, 1978; Murray, 1985; Mogg and Palmer, 1995; Conwell, 2010). Interestingly, icterus is an inconsistent finding of hyperlipaemia. In the final stages of the disease, the neurologic signs are dominant and the animal progresses to terminal agony (Table 6.1) (Gay *et al.*, 1978; Murray, 1985; Moore *et al.*, 1994).

Diagnosis of hyperlipaemia

A clinical diagnosis of hyperlipaemia is not possible considering the vague clinical signs (Hughes *et al.*, 2004). However, as predisposing factors such as obesity, gestation, lactation or gastrointestinal disease are well recognized, they should be used to improve detection of cases, even if the plasma of the animal does not appear opalescent (Fig. 6.2) (Murray, 1985; Dunkel and McKenzie, 2003).

Table 6.1. Clinical signs of equine hyperlipaemia and their frequency (Gay *et al.*, 1978; Jeffcott and Field, 1985b; Murray, 1985; Moore *et al.*, 1994; Mogg and Palmer, 1995; Hughes *et al.*, 2004; Oikawa *et al.*, 2006; Conwell, 2010; Dunkel *et al.*, 2014).

Disease stage	Clinical signs	Frequency in the reported studies
Early stage	Depression and drowsiness	95%
	Inappetence and anorexia	87%
	Adipsia	64%
	None	43%
	Weight loss	43%
	Ileus	Inconsistent
Intermediate stage	Fever	66%
	Colic	64%
	Ventral and limb oedema	53%
	Diarrhoea	47%
	Muscle fasciculations	46%
	Tachycardia	33%
	Incoordination	Inconsistent
	Icterus	Inconsistent
	Tachypnoea	Inconsistent but marked
Terminal stage	Central nervous system signs: convulsions, nystagmus, mania	33%
	Death	22–80%

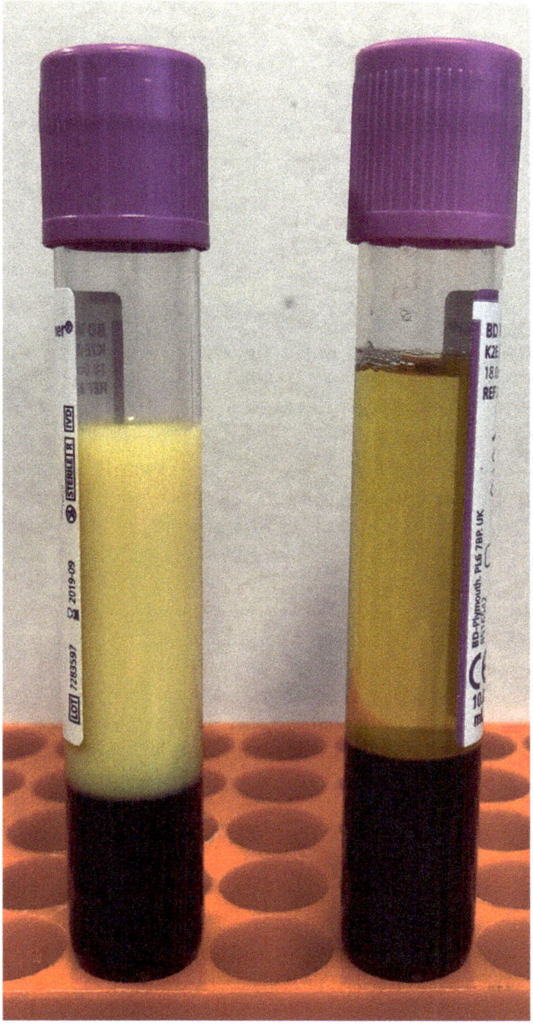

Fig. 6.2. Lipaemic plasma from a mixed breed pony with enterocolitis (left). Note the difference with plasma from a healthy horse (right) (courtesy of Dr Nicholas J. Bamford).

Clinical pathology

A definitive diagnosis of hyperlipaemia is made by the determination of circulating triglycerides. In healthy horses, triglyceride concentration is below 1.1 mmol/l; however, in some physiological conditions, higher triglyceride concentrations could be considered normal. For example, in late pregnancy, concentrations of 2.8 mmol/l have been reported and in donkeys, concentrations of 2.9 mmol/l have been documented (Watson *et al.*, 1990, 1993; Hughes *et al.*, 2004). For triglyceride concentrations between 1.1 mmol/l and 5.5 mmol/l, hyperlipidaemia is rarely of clinical significance although warrants monitoring (Hughes *et al.*, 2004; Dunkel *et al.*, 2014). Above 5.5 mmol/l, hyperlipaemia is associated with clinical signs and hepatic lipidosis (Watson *et al.*, 1992b). In severe cases, the triglyceride concentrations can be 40- to 80-fold of reference intervals (Murray, 1985; Oikawa *et al.*, 2006; Dunkel *et al.*, 2014). The prognostic value of triglyceride concentration is controversial as some studies have failed to identify any association with survival, whereas in one study, all the horses in which triglycerides were above 13.6 mmol/l died and all but one of the horses in which triglycerides were below 13.6 mmol/l survived (Watson *et al.*, 1992a; Mogg and Palmer, 1995; Dunkel *et al.*, 2014). More than the actual value, the trend in triglyceride concentrations in the face of therapy are more informative for survival (Mogg and Palmer, 1995; Oikawa *et al.*, 2006). Monitoring of circulating triglyceride concentrations in patients at risk of hyperlipaemia is therefore indicated. As such, point-of-care handheld analysers have been developed for equine patients and are shown to provide accurate and reliable measurements, given that adequate reference intervals are developed (Naylor and Durward-Akhurst, 2012; Pongratz *et al.*, 2016).

Beyond high circulating triglyceride concentrations, horses with hyperlipaemia often exhibit metabolic acidosis, renal azotaemia and evidence of liver disease with increased aspartate aminotransferase and gamma-glutamyl transpeptidase activities (Murray, 1985; Watson *et al.*, 1992a, b; Moore *et al.*, 1994; Hughes *et al.*, 2002; Dunkel and McKenzie, 2003; Dunkel *et al.*, 2014) When tested, liver function can be compromised as indicated by the prolonged bromsulfthalein excretion half-time reported in some cases (Murray, 1985). As mentioned above, since the ketone pathway is poorly developed in horses, ketonaemia and ketonuria are not reported in equine hyperlipaemia (Hughes *et al.*, 2004).

Anatomical pathology

Liver biopsies can confirm hepatic lipidosis (Dunkel *et al.*, 2014). In such cases, hepatocytes are extremely vacuolated and resemble adipocytes (Murray, 1985). At necropsy, there is a widespread proliferation of lipids on the carcass (Gay *et al.*,

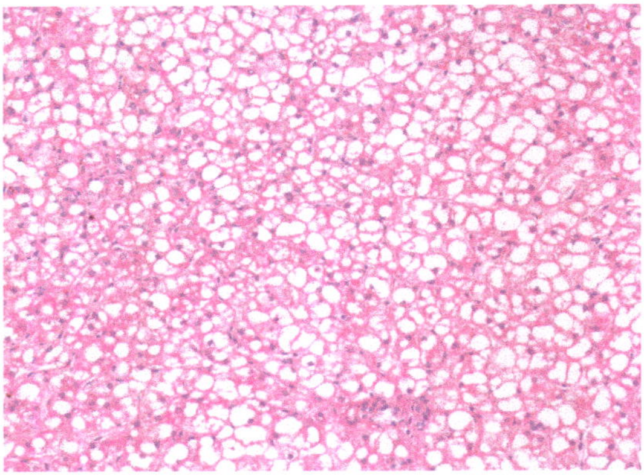

Fig. 6.3. Liver biopsy from a 12-year-old mixed breed pony with hepatic lipidosis. Note that hepatocytes are enlarged by a discrete clear cytoplasmic vacuole that displaces the nucleus at the periphery (courtesy of Dr Chiara Palmieri).

1978). The liver and kidneys are the organs that are usually the most severely affected (Fig. 6.3) (Dunkel *et al.*, 2014). In some cases, the liver has been reported to rupture because of the severe fatty infiltration (Mogg and Palmer, 1995).

Management of hyperlipaemia

The prognosis for patients that have developed hyperlipaemia is quite poor; therefore, successful management requires prompt identification of affected patients, ideally before the concentration of circulating triglycerides becomes too high and before clinical signs develop (Watson *et al.*, 1992b; Dunkel and McKenzie, 2003). As predisposing factors are well documented, frequent monitoring of circulating triglycerides is recommended, mainly for ponies, donkeys and miniature breeds (Mogg and Palmer, 1995; McKenzie, 2011). Treatment of hyperlipaemia is based on addressing two components: the predisposing factor and the negative energy balance.

Addressing predisposing factors

Correction of predisposing factors, such as pregnancy, lactation or being a pony, might not be easy or even possible; however, efforts should be made to identify and treat any underlying disease. In mild cases, correction of the underlying disease, usually of gastrointestinal or endocrine origin, is enough to resolve the episode of hyperlipaemia; however, in the most severe cases, drastic treatment such as termination of gestation must be considered (Gay *et al.*, 1978; Dunkel *et al.*, 2014). In all cases, supporting care including fluid therapy to correct azotaemia, electrolyte and acid–base abnormalities, and close monitoring of circulating triglyceride concentrations are recommended (Murray, 1985; Hughes *et al.*, 2004).

Addressing the negative energy balance

Determination of a hospitalized patient's daily energy requirements is challenging. In a healthy mature horse, the daily energy requirement is estimated to be around 140 kJ/kg/day (33 kcal/kg/day) (Council, 2007). During hospitalization, horses are contained in stalls and have virtually no activity, so their daily energy requirement drops to around 30% (Pagan and Hintz, 1986). On the other hand, standard equine hospital procedures, such as anaesthesia or surgery, increase the daily energy requirement by 10% and this increase could be greater with more invasive procedures or more severe conditions (Cruz *et al.*, 2006). Overall, it is considered that the daily energy requirement of a sick horse is around 92–96 kJ/kg/day (23–23 kcal/kg/day) (McKenzie, 2011). That being said, providing about 60% of the daily energy requirement would be sufficient, as provision of excessive enteral or parenteral nutrition is associated with potentially severe complications (Dunkel and Wilkins, 2004; Durham, 2006).

Enteral nutrition should be the first line of treatment, as long as the gastrointestinal tract is functional. If spontaneous feed intake does not match the daily energy requirement, support should be provided. Frequent oral administration of small quantities of carbohydrate solution, such as 60 ml of maize syrup, molasses or dextrose every 2 h, has been shown to be well tolerated and provides about 21 kJ/kg/day (5 kcal/kg/day) (Watson *et al.*, 1992b; McKenzie, 2011). Although this is far from the recommended daily energy requirement, this amount could be enough to stimulate endogenous insulin secretion and inhibit HSL activity, limiting lipolysis (Watson *et al.*, 1992b; McKenzie, 2011). As many of the horses suffering from hyperlipaemia have some degree of peripheral tissue insulin resistance, monitoring of blood glucose is recommended to detect hyperglycaemia. If more energy is required, repeated nasogastric intubation or placement of an indwelling enteral feeding tube might be required (Golenz *et al.*, 1992; Toth *et al.*, 2014). The advantage of repeated nasogastric intubation stems from the size of the tube used and the more fibrous diet that can therefore be provided. However, repeated nasogastric intubations are stressful and an indwelling tube might be preferred for prolonged treatments. In those cases, the use of commercial enteric formulations delivered every 4 h through enteral feeding tubes has been shown to reverse hyperlipaemia within 48 h (Golenz *et al.*, 1992; Hughes *et al.*, 2004). Careful monitoring of the gastrointestinal function is required in cases in which enteral feeding is elected, as the occurrence of complications such as diarrhoea or gastrointestinal reflux warrant the use of alternative methods (Dunkel and McKenzie, 2003; Durham, 2006).

When the gastrointestinal tract is not functional, parenteral nutrition is indicated (Moore *et al.*, 1994; Durham *et al.*, 2004) If parenteral nutrition is to be provided for a short period of time, infusion of a 5% dextrose solution at 5 ml/kg/h providing about 21 kJ/kg/day (5 kcal/kg/day) is enough to stimulate endogenous insulin secretion, inhibit HSL activity and decrease circulating triglycerides (Murray, 1985; Dunkel and McKenzie, 2003; McKenzie, 2011). If a fluid pump is available, a 50% dextrose solution at 0.5 ml/kg/h can also be used (McKenzie, 2011). Possible complications include hyperglycaemia and electrolytic disorders that need to be monitored and addressed (Murray, 1985; Hughes *et al.*, 2004). In one study, infusion of a 5% dextrose solution was continued for 8 days; however, when parenteral nutrition is considered for more than 24 h, a parenteral nutrition solution containing amino acids in addition to carbohydrates should be used, as the amino acids can provide a source for neoglucogenesis, limiting protein catabolism (Murray, 1985; McKenzie, 2011). Lipid-free solutions are commonly used as there is a concern that lipid-containing solutions might exacerbate hyperlipaemia (Magdesian, 2010). The infusion of parenteral nutrition solution containing both amino acids and carbohydrates can provide 63 kJ/kg/day (15 kcal/kg/day) representing about 70% of the estimated daily energy requirement for a hospitalized sick mature horse (Durham, 2006). Although hyperglycaemia is a common complication of parenteral nutrition solutions, decreases in circulating triglyceride concentrations are rapidly observed after initiation of the treatment. Discontinuation of parenteral nutrition and transition to enteral nutrition are critical steps that can lead to profound hypoglycaemia. Gradual reduction in infusion rate, such as a 25% decrease every 6 h, and monitoring of blood glucose are warranted (McKenzie, 2011).

Additional treatments

Insulin is often used in cases of hyperlipidaemia, either to directly inhibit HSL or to regulate hyperglycaemia (Murray, 1985). Although the rationale behind using insulin in these cases is clear, its clinical value is controversial. Some reports have failed to observe any beneficial effect of insulin injection on survival; however, others have found a beneficial effect, mainly when insulin was used to regulate parenteral nutrition-induced hyperglycaemia (Watson *et al.*, 1992b; Moore *et al.*, 1994; Durham, 2006; Waitt and Cebra, 2009). This discrepancy could come from the selection of cases that received insulin in these studies. More severe cases with pre-existing insulin resistance and no parenteral nutrition are less likely to survive and to respond favourably. If used, insulin can be administered subcutaneously or as a continuous-rate infusion. Subcutaneous injection should be started at 0.15 IU/kg twice a day with 0.05 IU/kg increments if hyperglycaemia persists. Delayed hypoglycaemia is a possible complication of subcutaneous insulin injections and should be monitored. For a continuous-rate infusion, the starting dose should be 0.07 IU/kg/h and blood glucose should also be monitored at least hourly until it has stabilized, to ensure euglycaemia (3.4–8.8 mmol/l). If dose adjustments are required, the insulin rate can be increased progressively, and blood glucose monitored again until it has stabilized. At such a dose, the risk of iatrogenic insulin-induced laminitis is considered minimal (Meier *et al.*, 2018; Stokes *et al.*, 2019). If insulin and glucose are administered simultaneously, only one infusion rate should be modified at a time and blood glucose monitored until it has stabilized (McKenzie, 2011).

Heparin is the second drug used for treatment of hyperlipaemia as it promotes lipoprotein–lipase activity and triglyceride use by peripheral tissues (Watson *et al.*, 1992a). As mentioned above, lipoprotein–lipase activity is increased in cases of hyperlipaemia, so reports on the effect of heparin have been inconsistent. If treatment with heparin is elected, a dose ranging from 40 to 100 IU/kg administered either intravenously or subcutaneously, once or every 8 h, can be used (Watson *et al.*, 1992a; Mogg and Palmer, 1995). Regardless of the route and the dose, heparin treatment should be as short as possible in order to minimize bleeding disorders (McKenzie, 2011).

Prevention

Nutrition of hospitalized patients is often overlooked but close attention to actual dietary intake is warranted, mainly when considering horses with gastrointestinal disorders, endocrinopathies or other known predisposing factors (Dunkel and McKenzie, 2003; Dunkel *et al.*, 2014). In these horses, frequent monitoring of circulating triglyceride concentration is recommended as hypertriglyceridaemia can be an incidental finding in populations at risk. For example, in miniature horses presented for colic, up to 70% had increased triglyceride concentrations indicating that nutritional support should be provided before hyperlipaemia develops (Hughes *et al.*, 2003).

When possible, risk factors should be eliminated. Management of obesity has been covered in Chapter 5 and the same principles apply in the prevention of hyperlipaemia. In addition, feeding fat-supplemented diets to horses and ponies has been shown to increase lipoprotein–lipase activity which would improve triglyceride clearance and help decrease the incidence of hyperlipaemia (Geelen *et al.*, 1999; Schmidt *et al.*, 2001). However, the effect of fat supplementation on insulin sensitivity has been questioned, with one study suggesting that it would reduce insulin sensitivity while others have failed to find a significant effect (Schmidt *et al.*, 2001; Bamford *et al.*, 2016).

Other Lipid Metabolism Disorders

In sick foals, a syndrome resembling hyperlipaemia has been described (Myers *et al.*, 2009; Berryhill *et al.*, 2017). In these cases, the increase in circulating triglycerides is usually milder, up to 4.3 mmol/l, and associated with sepsis and a positive blood culture (Berryhill *et al.*, 2017). In one study, foals with circulating triglyceride concentrations above 2.3 mmol/l were less likely to survive, suggesting that the pathogenesis of this disorder could be different from what is reported in adult horses (Myers *et al.*, 2009). Unlike adults, foals would have some degree of primary liver dysfunction, caused by sepsis or neonatal isoerythrolysis, limiting the hepatic uptake of triglycerides and their metabolism (Tan *et al.*, 2005; Myers *et al.*, 2009). Treatment is similar to hyperlipaemia in adult horses, including management of the primary condition and nutritional support, acknowledging that daily energy requirements in sick foals would drop by 40% compared to healthy foals and would be around 210 kJ/kg/day (50 kcal/kg/day) instead of 335 kJ/kg/day (80 kcal/kg/day) (Ousey *et al.*, 1996; Jose-Cunilleras *et al.*, 2012).

References

Argenzio, R.A. and Hintz, H.F. (1972) Effect of diet on glucose entry and oxidation rates in ponies. *The Journal of Nutrition* 102(7), 879–892. DOI: 10.1093/jn/102.7.879.

Bamford, N.J., Potter, S.J., Harris, P.A. and Bailey, S.R. (2016) Effect of increased adiposity on insulin sensitivity and adipokine concentrations in horses and ponies fed a high fat diet, with or without a once daily high glycaemic meal. *Equine Veterinary Journal* 48(3), 368–373. DOI: 10.1111/evj.12434.

Bergman, E.N. (1990) Energy contributions of volatile fatty acids from the gastrointestinal tract in various species. *Physiological Reviews* 70(2), 567–590. DOI: 10.1152/physrev.1990.70.2.567.

Berryhill, E.H., Magdesian, K.G., Kass, P.H. and Edman, J.E. (2017) Triglyceride concentrations in neonatal foals: serial measurement and effects of age and illness. *The Veterinary Journal* 227, 23–29. DOI: 10.1016/j.tvjl.2017.08.002.

Breidenbach, A., Fuhrmann, H., Deegen, E., Lindholm, A. and Sallmann, H.P. (1999) Studies on equine lipid metabolism. 2. Lipolytic activities of plasma and tissue lipases in large horses and ponies. *Journal of Veterinary Medicine Series A* 46(1), 39–48. DOI: 10.1046/j.1439-0442.1999.00186.x.

Conwell, R. (2010) Hyperlipaemia in a pregnant mare with suspected masseter myodegeneration. *Veterinary Record* 166(4), 116–117. DOI: 10.1136/vr.c359.

Council, N.R. (2007) *Nutrient Requirements of Horses: Sixth Revised Edition*. The National Academies Press, Washington, DC.

Cruz, A.M., Coté, N., McDonell, W.N., Geor, R.J., Wilson, B.A. *et al.* (2006) Postoperative effects of anesthesia and surgery on resting energy expenditure in horses as measured by indirect calorimetry. *Canadian Journal of Veterinary Research-Revue Canadienne De Recherche Veterinaire* 70(4), 257–262.

de Laat, M.A., McGree, J.M. and Sillence, M.N. (2016) Equine hyperinsulinemia: investigation of the entero-insular axis during insulin dysregulation. *American Journal of Physiology-Endocrinology and Metabolism* 310(1), E61–E72. DOI: 10.1152/ajpendo.00362.2015.

Díez, E., López, I., Pérez, C., Pineda, C. and Aguilera-Tejero, E. (2012) Plasma leptin concentration in donkeys. *Veterinary Quarterly* 32(1), 13–16. DOI: 10.1080/01652176.2012.677867.

Dunkel, B. and McKenzie, H.C. (2003) Severe hypertriglyceridaemia in clinically ill horses: diagnosis, treatment and outcome. *Equine Veterinary Journal* 35(6), 590–595. DOI: 10.2746/042516403775467270.

Dunkel, B.M. and Wilkins, P.A. (2004) Nutrition and the critically ill horse. *Veterinary Clinics of North America: Equine Practice* 20(1), 107–126. DOI: 10.1016/j.cveq.2003.12.002.

Dunkel, B., Wilford, S.A., Parkinson, N.J., Ward, C., Smith, P. *et al*. (2014) Severe hypertriglyceridaemia in horses and ponies with endocrine disorders. *Equine Veterinary Journal* 46(1), 118–122. DOI: 10.1111/evj.12089.

Durham, A.E. (2006) Clinical application of parenteral nutrition in the treatment of five ponies and one donkey with hyperlipaemia. *Veterinary Record* 158(5), 159–164. DOI: 10.1136/vr.158.5.159.

Durham, A.E., Phillips, T.J., Walmsley, J.P. and Newton, J.R. (2004) Nutritional and clinicopathological effects of post operative parenteral nutrition following small intestinal resection and anastomosis in the mature horse. *Equine Veterinary Journal* 36(5), 390–396. DOI: 10.2746/0425164044868369.

Forhead, A.J. and Dobson, H. (1997) Plasma glucose and cortisol responses to exogenous insulin in fasted donkeys. *Research in Veterinary Science* 62(3), 265–269. DOI: 10.1016/S0034-5288(97)90202-2.

Forhead, A.J., French, J., Ikin, P., Fowler, J.N. and Dobson, H. (1994) Relationship between plasma insulin and triglyceride concentrations in hypertriglyceridaemic donkeys. *Research in Veterinary Science* 56(3), 389–392. DOI: 10.1016/0034-5288(94)90158-9.

Frank, N., Sojka, J.E. and Latour, M.A. (2002) Effect of withholding feed on concentration and composition of plasma very low density lipoprotein and serum non-esterified fatty acids in horses. *American Journal of Veterinary Research* 63(7), 1018–1021. DOI: 10.2460/ajvr.2002.63.1018.

Freestone, J.F., Wolfsheimer, K.J., Ford, R.B., Church, G. and Bessin, R. (1991) Triglyceride, insulin, and cortisol responses of ponies to fasting and dexamethasone administration. *Journal of Veterinary Internal Medicine* 5(1), 15–22. DOI: 10.1111/j.1939-1676.1991.tb00925.x.

Gay, C.C., Sullivan, N.D., Wilkinson, J.S., McLean, J.D. and Blood, D.C. (1978) Hyperlipaemia in ponies. *Australian Veterinary Journal* 54(10), 459–462. DOI: 10.1111/j.1751-0813.1978.tb00284.x.

Geelen, S.N., Sloet van Oldruitenborgh-Oosterbaan, M.M. and Beynen, A.C. (1999) Dietary fat supplementation and equine plasma lipid metabolism. *Equine Veterinary Journal* (30), 475–478. DOI: 10.1111/j.2042-3306.1999.tb05268.x.

Gilbert, R.O. (1986) Congenital hyperlipaemia in a Shetland pony foal. *Equine Veterinary Journal* 18(6), 498–500. DOI: 10.1111/j.2042-3306.1986.tb03704.x.

Golenz, M.R., Knight, D.A. and Yvorchuk-St Jean, K.E. (1992) Use of a human enteral feeding preparation for treatment of hyperlipemia and nutritional support during healing of an esophageal laceration in a miniature horse. *Journal of the American Veterinary Medical Association* 200(7), 951–953.

Hughes, K.J., Hodgson, D.R. and Dart, A.J. (2002) Hyperlipaemia in a 7-week-old miniature pony foal. *Australian Veterinary Journal* 80(6), 350–351. DOI: 10.1111/j.1751-0813.2002.tb14786.x.

Hughes, K.J., Dowling, B.A., Matthews, S.A. and Dart, A.J. (2003) Results of surgical treatment of colic in miniature breed horses: 11 cases. *Australian Veterinary Journal* 81(5), 260–264. DOI: 10.1111/j.1751-0813.2003.tb12566.x.

Hughes, K.J., Hodgson, D.R. and Dart, A.J. (2004) Equine hyperlipaemia: a review. *Australian Veterinary Journal* 82(3), 136–142. DOI: 10.1111/j.1751-0813.2004.tb12636.x.

Jeffcott, L.B. and Field, J.R. (1985a) Current concepts of hyperlipaemia in horses and ponies. *Veterinary Record* 116(17), 461–466. DOI: 10.1136/vr.116.17.461.

Jeffcott, L.B. and Field, J.R. (1985b) Epidemiological aspects of hyperlipaemia in ponies in South Eastern Australia. *Australian Veterinary Journal* 62(4), 140–141. DOI: 10.1111/j.1751-0813.1985.tb07270.x.

Jose-Cunilleras, E., Viu, J., Corradini, I., Armengou, L., Cesarini, C. *et al*. (2012) Energy expenditure of critically ill neonatal foals. *Equine Veterinary Journal* (41), 48–51. DOI: 10.1111/j.2042-3306.2011.00500.x.

Langin, D. (2006) Adipose tissue lipolysis as a metabolic pathway to define pharmacological strategies against obesity and the metabolic syndrome. *Pharmacological Research* 53(6), 482–491. DOI: 10.1016/j.phrs.2006.03.009.

Lavery, G.G. and Glover, P. (2000) The metabolic and nutritional response to critical illness. *Current Opinion in Critical Care* 6(4), 233–238. DOI: 10.1097/00075198-200008000-00001.

Magdesian, K.G. (2010) Parenteral nutrition in the mature horse. *Equine Veterinary Education* 22(7), 364–371. DOI: 10.1111/j.2042-3292.2010.00092.x.

McKenzie, H.C. (2011) Equine hyperlipidemias. *The Veterinary Clinics of North America. Equine Practice* 27(1), 59–72. DOI: 10.1016/j.cveq.2010.12.008.

Meier, A.D., de Laat, M.A., Reiche, D.B., Pollitt, C.C., Walsh, D.M. *et al*. (2018) The oral glucose test predicts laminitis risk in ponies fed a diet high in nonstructural carbohydrates. *Domestic Animal Endocrinology* 63, 1–9. DOI: 10.1016/j.domaniend.2017.10.008.

Mogg, T.D. and Palmer, J.E. (1995) Hyperlipidemia, hyperlipemia, and hepatic lipidosis in American miniature horses: 23 cases (1990-1994). *Journal of the American Veterinary Medical Association* 207(5), 604–607.

Moore, B.R., Abood, S.K. and Hinchcliff, K.W. (1994) Hyperlipemia in 9 miniature horses and miniature donkeys. *Journal of Veterinary Internal Medicine* 8(5), 376–381. DOI: 10.1111/j.1939-1676.1994.tb03253.x.

Murray, M. (1985) Hepatic-lipidosis in a post parturient mare. *Equine Veterinary Journal* 17(1), 68–69. DOI: 10.1111/j.2042-3306.1985.tb02047.x.

Myers, C.J., Magdesian, K.G., Kass, P.H., Madigan, J.E., Rhodes, D.M. *et al.* (2009) Parenteral nutrition in neonatal foals: clinical description, complications and outcome in 53 foals (1995-2005). *The Veterinary Journal* 181(2), 137–144. DOI: 10.1016/j.tvjl.2008.02.024.

Naylor, R.J. and Durward-Akhurst, S.A. (2012) Use of the accutrend plus point-of-care monitor for blood triglyceride measurement in horses. *Veterinary Record* 170(9), 228.2–22228. DOI: 10.1136/vr.100530.

Naylor, J.M., Kronfeld, D.S. and Acland, H. (1980) Hyperlipemia in horses: effects of undernutrition and disease. *American Journal of Veterinary Research* 41(6), 899–905.

Oikawa, S., McGuirk, S., Nishibe, K., Higuchi, T., Kurosawa, T. *et al.* (2006) Changes of blood biochemical values in ponies recovering from hyperlipemia in Japan. *Journal of Veterinary Medical Science* 68(4), 353–359. DOI: 10.1292/jvms.68.353.

Ousey, J.C., Holdstock, N., Rossdale, P.D. and McArthur, A.C. (1996) How much energy do sick neonatal foals require compared with healthy foals? *Pferdeheilkunde Equine Medicine* 12(3), 231–237. DOI: 10.21836/PEM19960313.

Pagan, J.D. and Hintz, H.F. (1986) Equine energetics. I. Relationship between body weight and energy requirements in horses. *Journal of Animal Science* 63(3), 815–821. DOI: 10.2527/jas1986.633815x.

Pongratz, M.C., Junge, H.K., Riond, B. and Schwarzwald, C.C. (2016) Validation of the Accutrend Plus point-of-care triglyceride analyzer in horses, ponies, and donkeys. *Journal of Veterinary Emergency and Critical Care* 26(5), 682–690. DOI: 10.1111/vec.12512.

Rose, R.J. and Sampson, D. (1982) Changes in certain metabolic parameters in horses associated with food deprivation and endurance exercise. *Research in Veterinary Science* 32(2), 198–202. DOI: 10.1016/S0034-5288(18)32414-7.

Schmidt, O., Deegen, E., Fuhrmann, H., Dühlmeier, R. and Sallmann, H.P. (2001) Effects of fat feeding and energy level on plasma metabolites and hormones in Shetland ponies. *Journal of Veterinary Medicine Series A* 48(1), 39–49. DOI: 10.1046/j.1439-0442.2001.00331.x.

Stokes, S.M., Belknap, J.K., Engiles, J.B., Stefanovski, D., Bertin, F.R. *et al.* (2019) Continuous digital hypothermia prevents lamellar failure in the euglycaemic hyperinsulinaemic clamp model of equine laminitis. *Equine Veterinary Journal* 51(5), 658–664. DOI: 10.1111/evj.13072.

Suagee, J.K., Corl, B.A., Crisman, M.V., Wearn, J.G., McCutcheon, L.J. *et al.* (2010) De novo fatty acid synthesis and NADPH generation in equine adipose and liver tissue. *Comparative Biochemistry and Physiology Part B: Biochemistry and Molecular Biology* 155(3), 322–326. DOI: 10.1016/j.cbpb.2009.11.019.

Tan, R.H.H., Hughes, K.J. and Hodgson, D.R. (2005) Hyperlipaemia, neonatal isoerythrolysis and hepatocellular necrosis in a 3-day-old thoroughbred foal. *Australian Veterinary Journal* 83(12), 740–741. DOI: 10.1111/j.1751-0813.2005.tb11581.x.

Toth, B., Bertin, F.R., Miller, M.A., Charney, V.A. and Kritchevsky, J.E. (2014) Evaluation of a technique for percutaneous endoscopic gastrostomy tube placement in horses. *American Journal of Veterinary Research* 75(4), 354–360. DOI: 10.2460/ajvr.75.4.354.

Tóth, B., Auth, A., Rompos, L. and Bakos, Z. (2018) Effect of feed deprivation on selected parameters of lipid mobilisation and hepatic function in healthy Akhal Teke horses. *Equine Veterinary Journal* 50(1), 98–103. DOI: 10.1111/evj.12730.

van der Kolk, J.H., Wensing, T., Kalsbeek, H.C. and Breukink, H.J. (1995) Lipid metabolism in horses with hyperadrenocorticism. *Journal of the American Veterinary Medical Association* 206(7), 1010–1012.

Waitt, L.H. and Cebra, C.K. (2009) Characterization of hypertriglyceridemia and response to treatment with insulin in horses, ponies, and donkeys: 44 cases (1995–2005). *Journal of the American Veterinary Medical Association* 234(7), 915–919. DOI: 10.2460/javma.234.7.915.

Watson, T.D., Packard, C.J., Shepherd, J. and Fowler, J.N. (1990) An investigation of the relationships between body condition and plasma lipid and lipoprotein concentrations in 24 donkeys. *The Veterinary record* 127(20), 498–500.

Watson, T.D., Burns, L., Love, S., Packard, C.J. and Shepherd, J. (1992a) Plasma lipids, lipoproteins and post-heparin lipases in ponies with hyperlipaemia. *Equine Veterinary Journal* 24(5), 341–346. DOI: 10.1111/j.2042-3306.1992.tb02852.x.

Watson, T.D., Murphy, D. and Love, S. (1992b) Equine hyperlipaemia in the United Kingdom: clinical features and blood biochemistry of 18 cases. *Veterinary Record* 131(3), 48–51. DOI: 10.1136/vr.131.3.48.

Watson, T.D., Burns, L., Packard, C.J. and Shepherd, J. (1993) Effects of pregnancy and lactation on plasma lipid and lipoprotein concentrations, lipoprotein composition and post-heparin lipase activities in Shetland pony mares. *Reproduction* 97(2), 563–568. DOI: 10.1530/jrf.0.0970563.

Wensing, T., van Gent, D.M., Schotman, A.J. and Kroneman, J. (1975) Hyperlipoproteinaemia in ponies: mechanisms and response to therapy. *Clinica Chimica Acta* 58(1), 1–15. DOI: 10.1016/0009-8981(75)90479-9.

7 Additional Endocrinopathies

Diabetes Insipidus

The definition of diabetes insipidus has been quite variable in the veterinary literature. Some authors have included diverse causes of polyuria/polydipsia such as primary renal disease, medullary washout, psychogenic polydipsia, iatrogenic polyuria, pituitary pars intermedia dysfunction (PPID) or diabetes mellitus as diabetes insipidus, while other authors have restricted the definition of the disorder to polyuria/polydipsia caused by the inadequate production or the inadequate action of arginine vasopressin (AVP) (Baylis and Cheetham, 1998; Majzoub and Srivatsa, 2006; Schott, 2011). This chapter will focus only on the latter definition.

AVP, or anti-diuretic hormone, is a major regulator of plasma osmolality. This hormone is a 9-amino-acid peptide produced by magnocellular neurons located in the posterior pituitary gland (neurohypophysis). Once produced, the hormone is stored in large amounts in these neurons and is released in the bloodstream when plasma osmolality increases and arterial pressure decreases (Schott, 2011). Osmoreceptors located in the anterior hypothalamus are triggered by osmotic water shift leading to cell shrinkage which initiates osmoreceptor depolarization and subsequent neurotransmitter release. The neurotransmitters trigger the posterior pituitary gland to release AVP. The degree of stimulation of the osmoreceptors varies with the solute responsible for changes in osmolality: sodium and mannitol are potent osmoreceptor triggers whereas glucose and urea are weak osmoreceptor triggers. The osmotic threshold for AVP release is variable between individuals and species, and ranges from 275 to 290 mOsm/kg (Houpt *et al.*, 1989). Once this threshold is reached, osmoreceptors become highly responsive and AVP concentration increases proportionally (Schott, 2011). Changes in arterial pressure are another trigger for AVP secretion (Hollis *et al.*, 2008; Hurcombe *et al.*, 2008). However, only prolonged and larger haemodynamic changes can relieve the inhibitory effect of baroreceptors on AVP secretion.

Three types of AVP receptors have been described (Holmes *et al.*, 2003):

- *V1A (or V1)*, located on the vascular smooth muscles, the myometrium, hepatocytes and platelets leading to vasoconstriction, uterine contraction, glycogenolysis and platelet aggregation;
- *V1B (or V3)*, located in the anterior pituitary gland and leading to adrenocorticotropic hormone (ACTH) and prolactin (PRL) release; and
- *V2*, located at the basolateral membrane of the principal cells of the renal collecting duct leading to urine concentration.

Arginine vasopressin receptor V2 (AVP2R) is coupled to a transmembrane G protein that activates an adenyl cyclase leading to the increase in cyclic adenosine monophosphate concentration and subsequent translocation of aquaporin-2 into the apical membrane (Holmes *et al.*, 2003). Exposure of aquaporin-2 increases renal water absorption resulting in an increase in urinary osmolality that is proportional to AVP concentration (Schott, 2011).

In cases of diabetes insipidus, either the secretion of AVP is impaired (central or neurogenic diabetes insipidus) or the AVP2R is mutated (nephrogenic diabetes insipidus). In both cases, polyuria/polydipsia develops. Polyuria/polydipsia in horses is characterized by the production of more than 50 ml/kg/day of urine (22.5 l for a 450 kg horse) and the consumption of more than 100 ml/kg/day of water (45 l for a 450 kg horse) (Schott, 2011). The disease is rarely recognized when horses are kept in a herd outside with access to automatic waterers; however, in stable horses or in horses that drink from buckets of water, the problem is readily recognized.

Central or neurogenic diabetes insipidus

This disease is well described in humans, with both hereditary and acquired forms of diabetes insipidus (Baylis and Cheetham, 1998; Majzoub and Srivatsa, 2006). The hereditary form is often an autosomal dominant disease that results in the formation of an inappropriately folded AVP that accumulates in the magnocellular neurons in the posterior pituitary gland and leads to the loss of these neurons. The acquired forms result from trauma, infections, vascular anomalies or tumours leading to disruption, compression or degeneration of the magnocellular neurons (Maccubbin and Vanburen, 1963; Baylis and Cheetham, 1998; Maghnie *et al.*, 2000; Schott, 2011; Di Iorgi *et al.*, 2014). In all these cases, the clinical signs are only obvious when 90% of the magnocellular neurons are lost.

In horses, true cases of neurogenic diabetes insipidus are rare and historical cases are likely occurrences of psychogenic polydipsia (Schott, 2011). Nevertheless, spontaneous cases have been described (Breukink *et al.*, 1983; Vente and Wijsmuller, 1983; Kranenburg *et al.*, 2010). In these cases, a diagnosis of neurogenic diabetes insipidus is suggested by the presence of severe polyuria/polydipsia and persistent iso- or hyposthenuria (1.001 to 1.005). After elimination of primary renal dysfunction and other endocrine disorders such as PPID or diabetes mellitus, the diagnosis is confirmed by failure to concentrate urine after a water deprivation test or a modified water deprivation test (see Chapter 1), low or undetectable AVP (Table 7.1) and response to exogenous AVP administration.

The definitive cause of diabetes insipidus has not been determined in any of the reported cases; however, based on the case history, some authors have suggested a possible congenital defect (Breukink *et al.*, 1983; Kranenburg *et al.*, 2010). Another report suggested an acquired diabetes insipidus subsequent to encephalomyelitis. In that case, the signs resembled those of pony mares in which the pituitary stalk had been transected (Sharp *et al.*, 1982). In the pony mares, extensive fluid and AVP replacement therapy was initially required; however, normal water homeostasis developed after 48 h.

Considering the paucity of cases, therapeutic options are poorly described. Intramuscular injection of 40 units of pitressin tannate in oil has been shown to increase urine specific gravity and to decrease water consumption for 24 h; intraocular administration of 20 µg of desmopressin (10 µg in each eye) has been shown to increase urine specific gravity for 4 h (Breukink *et al.*, 1983; Kranenburg *et al.*, 2010). However, none of the horses treated with AVP analogues received long-term treatment. Carbamazepine has been reported to both stimulate AVP secretion and activate AVP2R in renal collecting ducts and could be of therapeutic benefit (de Bragança *et al.*, 2010). However, although the drug has been evaluated in horses for treatment of head shaking, its indication in the treatment of diabetes insipidus remains unknown (Newton *et al.*, 2000). In other species, spontaneous resolution of idiopathic forms of central diabetes insipidus have been reported, as well as long-term oral treatment with desmopressin acetate (Harb *et al.*, 1996; Maghnie *et al.*, 2000; Aroch *et al.*, 2005; Ooi *et al.*, 2013).

Nephrogenic diabetes insipidus

Primary nephrogenic diabetes insipidus is caused by a mutation leading to an impaired AVP2R or an impaired aquaporin-2. Four groups of mutation have been reported for the AVP2R depending on the localization of the mutant receptor (inserted in the membrane or not) and its ability to bind to AVP or to activate the transmembrane G protein (Schott, 2011). In horses, specific mutations have not been identified but congenital and hereditary nephrogenic diabetes insipidus have been suspected in several cases. (Schott *et al.*, 1993; Brashier, 2006;

Table 7.1. Results of arginine vasopressin (AVP) determinations (pg/ml) in the blood of a pony with diabetes insipidus during two water deprivation tests. Adapted from Breukink *et al.*, 1983.

	Patient		
Time (hours)	1st test	2nd test	Controls (median)
0	<0.9	1.7	12.6
12	1.3	–	5.4
16	1.0	<0.9	–
28	–	–	8.5

Morgan *et al.*, 2012). In these cases, a diagnosis of nephrogenic diabetes insipidus is confirmed by the presence of severe polyuria/polydipsia, failure to concentrate urine after a water deprivation test, adequate AVP response to haemoconcentration and failure to respond to exogenous AVP administration. Similarly to central diabetes insipidus, primary renal disease and other endocrinopathic causes must be ruled out before undertaking a water deprivation test. Polyuria/polydipsia can be dramatic in nephrogenic diabetes insipidus and water deprivation tests must be performed carefully, as such cases can lose up to 15% of their body weight over 12 h (Schott *et al.*, 1993; Brashier, 2006). In only one case, treatment consisting in water and salt restriction was attempted but no long-term follow-up was available (Brashier, 2006). In other species, thiazide diuretics are commonly used to treat nephrogenic diabetes insipidus (Takemura, 1998; Al Nofal and Lteif, 2015). This paradoxical use of a diuretic to treat polyuria/polydipsia is based on the thiazide-induced decreased reabsorption of sodium in the distal tubule. The loss of sodium would decrease the extracellular fluid volume, decrease glomerular filtration rate and increase sodium and water reabsorption in the proximal tubule (Durham, 2017). This effect of thiazide diuretics has, however, not been demonstrated in horses.

Nephrogenic diabetes insipidus can also be secondary to an infectious, mechanical or metabolic processes. These disorders can lead to an alteration of the AVP2R or a down regulation of aquaporin-2 expression (Nielsen *et al.*, 1999; Kwon *et al.*, 2001). These changes are observed in cases of acute kidney injury, chronic kidney disease or medullary washout (Schott, 2011).

Pheochromocytoma

Pheochromocytoma, although infrequent, is the most commonly reported tumour of the equine adrenal gland with a reported prevalence estimated at around 1% (Luethy *et al.*, 2016). Other tumours of the adrenal glands such as adrenocortical adenoma and adrenocortical carcinoma are extremely rare; only incidental necropsy findings are reported in older horses with no or vague clinical signs (mild colic, progressive weight loss) (Fix and Miller, 1987; van Andel *et al.*, 1988; van der Kolk *et al.*, 1994).

Pheochromocytomas develop from the chromaffin cells of the medulla of the adrenal gland, which are postganglionic neurons of the autonomic nervous system and have been diagnosed in a wide variety of domestic animals. In horses, the disease has been described mainly in older horses ranging from 13 to 38 years of age, with the exception of a case report of pheochromocytoma in a 6-month-old filly (Froscher and Power, 1982; Luethy *et al.*, 2016). No breed or sex predisposition has been described.

In about 80% of cases, pheochromocytomas are not associated with clinical signs and are incidental findings at necropsy (Luethy *et al.*, 2016). The other 20% of cases are usually younger with a median age of around 17 years, where patients presented for signs of acute colic associated with persistent tachycardia, marked perspiration, pale mucous membranes, slow capillary refill time and variable tachypnoea (Yovich *et al.*, 1984; Germann *et al.*, 2006; Fouché *et al.*, 2016; Luethy *et al.*, 2016; Monahan and Craig, 2016; Katzman *et al.*, 2018). Tachycardia can be severe and associated with cardiac arrhythmias (Yovich *et al.*, 1984; Fouché *et al.*, 2016). Other, less commonly described clinical signs include lameness, weight loss, ataxia, recumbency and diarrhoea (Gelberg *et al.*, 1979; Froscher and Power, 1982; Luethy *et al.*, 2016; Katzman *et al.*, 2018). Similar to the clinical signs, clinico–pathological findings in cases of pheochromocytoma are unspecific and often confused with severe acute colic: hyperlactataemia, hyperglycaemia (sometimes severe), hypovolaemia, neutrophilia and lymphopoenia (Anderson and Aitken, 1977; Yovich *et al.*, 1984; Luethy *et al.*, 2016; Katzman *et al.*, 2018).

A suspicion of pheochromocytoma can be made in an acutely colicky horse when a mass is transrectally palpated medially to the left kidney or identified transcutaneously with a macro-convex ultrasound probe (Gelberg *et al.*, 1979; Germann *et al.*, 2006; Fouché *et al.*, 2016). Additional ultrasound findings that can be inconsistent include a haemoabdomen or an ileus (Germann *et al.*, 2006; Monahan and Craig, 2016). The diagnosis is often only confirmed at necropsy with immuno–histochemical staining of paraffin-embedded tissue sections with anti-chromogranin A antibody and anti-synaptophysin antibody (Fig. 7.1) (Katzman *et al.*, 2018). Chromogranin A is a glycoprotein expressed in cellular secretory granules, used to identify endocrine tumours, while synaptophysin

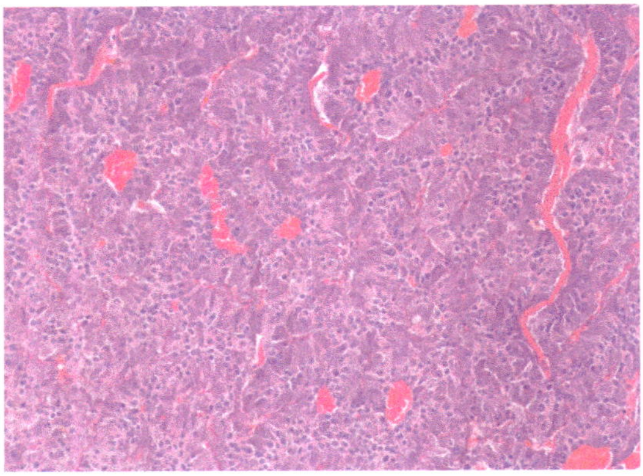

Fig. 7.1. Histopathological diagnosis of pheochromocytoma in a 15-year-old Thoroughbred gelding. Note the neoplastic cells arranged in cords and trabeculae, often palisading along a fine fibrovascular stroma. Neoplastic cells have distinct cell borders, abundant cytoplasm and an irregularly round to oval nucleus with finely stippled chromatin and one distinct nucleolus (courtesy of Dr Chiara Palmieri).

is a membrane glycoprotein expressed in normal and neoplastic neuroendocrine cells including pheochromocytomas and paragangliomas (Wiedenmann *et al.*, 1986; Campana *et al.*, 2007). A positive staining for both is considered diagnostic for pheochromocytoma (Gelberg *et al.*, 1979).

In many cases, multiple endocrine neoplasias are identified at necropsy. The most commonly described endocrine tumours associated with pheochromocytoma are pituitary pars intermedia adenoma (or hyperplasia), thyroid adenoma, parathyroid C-cell carcinoma and corticoadrenal hyperplasia (De Cock and MacLachlan, 1999; Luethy *et al.*, 2016; Monahan and Craig, 2016). In humans, multiple endocrine neoplasia syndromes have been described and, although the numbers of equine cases are low, they appear to share many similarities. Wermer's syndrome or type-1 multiple endocrine neoplasia syndrome is characterized by hyperparathyroidism, pancreatic islet hyperplasia and pituitary gland adenomas (De Cock and MacLachlan, 1999). Sipple's syndrome or type-2a multiple endocrine neoplasia syndrome is characterized by parathyroid C-cell carcinoma, hyperparathyroidism and pheochromocytoma, while type-2b multiple endocrine neoplasia syndrome is characterized by parathyroid C-cell carcinoma, pheochromocytoma and extra-endocrine changes including mucosal neuromas or ganglioneuromas. In one case of aggressive pheochromocytoma in both adrenal glands, metastases to the liver, lungs, vertebral canal, azygous vein and left scapula were reported (Froscher and Power, 1982).

In a few cases, an ante-mortem diagnosis was achieved by measuring plasma and urinary catecholamines. As catecholamines are very unstable, analysis of collected samples within minutes of collection is paramount (Germann *et al.*, 2006). Plasma and urinary epinephrine, norepinephrine, normetanephrine (free and total fractions) and metanephrine (free and total fractions) can be determined by high-performance liquid chromatography tandem mass spectrometry (Fouché *et al.*, 2016). Ideally, samples should be collected into an ethylenediaminetetraacetic acid (EDTA) tube, containing an antioxidant such as sodium bisulfite, centrifuged and analysed, or frozen at −70°C immediately after collection (Parry, 1984; Yovich *et al.*, 1984). Only a few laboratories are equipped for this type of analysis and confirmation of the sampling protocol with the laboratory is recommended before collection and shipping. Excitement is a potent trigger for catecholamine secretion and can lead to false positive diagnoses and a threefold increase in norepinephrine (Yovich *et al.*, 1984). Proper reference ranges for equine catecholamines have not been published and data from a suspected animal are often compared controls (Table 7.2) (Fouché *et al.*, 2016).

Therapeutic options are limited in cases of pheochromocytoma and many horses die from hypovolaemic shock as the tumour ruptures, or are euthanized during surgery as the tumours cannot be resected (Yovich *et al.*, 1984; Katzman *et al.*, 2018). In one case of a pony with pheochromocytoma, aggressive treatment was undertaken with fluid therapy, non-steroidal anti-inflammatory drugs, propranolol (an adrenergic beta-blocker) and phenoxybenzamine (an adrenergic alpha-blocker) (Fouché *et al.*, 2016). Episodes of ventricular tachycardia were managed with magnesium sulfate and a continuous infusion rate of lidocaine. In this case, the size of the tumour decreased by 60% and the pony improved clinically within a week.

Table 7.2. Results of plasma (P-) catecholamines and plasma total and free metanephrines; urinary (U-) catecholamines; metanephrine to creatinine ratios vanillyl mandelic acid; and homovanillic acid to creatinine ratios, in a pony with suspected pheochromocytoma (PC) and three controls (C1, C2, C3) (Fouché *et al.*, 2016).

Parameter	PC	C1	C2	C3
P-dopamine (nM/l)	0.18	0.10	0.04	0.10
P-epinephrine (nM/l)	0.15	1.03	1.13	0.46
P-norepinephrine (nM/l)	11.62	0.61	1.12	1.15
P-total metanephrine (nM/l) [sulfatase-treated]	0.16	0.97	0.42	0.31
P-total metanephrine (nM/l) [glucuronidase-treated]	1.17	5.94	2.41	2.12
P-free metanephrine (nM/l)	0.16	0.94	0.26	0.25
P-total normetanephrine (nM/l) [sulfatase-treated]	3.82	0.93	1.02	0.84
P-total normetanephrine (nM/l) [glucuronidase-treated]	19.24	3.94	3.84	5.58
P-free normetanephrine (nM/l)	3.29	0.73	0.72	0.66
P-total methoxytyramine (nM/l) [sulfatase-treated]	0.01	0.05	0.08	0.02
P-total methoxytyramine (nM/l) [glucuronidase-treated]	7.32	7.77	7.15	6.08
P-free methoxytyramine (nM/l)	0.02	0.10	0.10	0.06
U-dopamine: creatinine (nM/mM)	20.9	11.6		
U-epinephrine: creatinine (nM/mM)	1.6	2.1		
U-norepinephrine: creatinine (nM/mM)	69.2	3.1		
U-metanephrine: creatinine (nM/mM) [sulfatase-treated]	4	12.2		
U-metanephrine: creatinine (nM/mM) [glucuronidase-treated]	23.1	63.3		
U-normetanephrine: creatinine (nM/mM) [sulfatase-treated]	76.2	13.4		
U-normetanephrine: creatinine (nM/mM) [glucuronidase-treated]	384.9	48.9		
U-vanillyl mandelic acid: creatinine (μM/mM)	1.82	0		
U-homovanillic acid: creatinine (μM/mM)	10.4	1.82		

References

Al Nofal, A. and Lteif, A. (2015) Thiazide diuretics in the management of young children with central diabetes insipidus. *The Journal of Pediatrics* 167(3), 658–661. DOI: 10.1016/j.jpeds.2015.06.002.

Anderson, M.G. and Aitken, M.M. (1977) Biochemical and physiological effects of catecholamine administration in the horse. *Research in Veterinary Science* 22(3), 357–360. DOI: 10.1016/S0034-5288(18)33263-6.

Aroch, I., Mazaki-Tovi, M., Shemesh, O., Sarfaty, H. and Segev, G. (2005) Central diabetes insipidus in five cats: clinical presentation, diagnosis and oral desmopressin therapy. *Journal of Feline Medicine and Surgery* 7(6), 333–339. DOI: 10.1016/j.jfms.2005.03.008.

Baylis, P.H. and Cheetham, T. (1998) Diabetes insipidus. *Archives of Disease in Childhood* 79(1), 84–89. DOI: 10.1136/adc.79.1.84.

Brashier, M. (2006) Polydipsia and polyuria in a weanling colt caused by nephrogenic diabetes insipidus. *The Veterinary Clinics of North America. Equine Practice* 22(1), 219–227. DOI: 10.1016/j.cveq.2005.12.010.

Breukink, H.J., Van Wegen, P. and Schotman, A.J. (1983) Idiopathic diabetes insipidus in a Welsh pony. *Equine Veterinary Journal* 15(3), 284–287. DOI: 10.1111/j.2042-3306.1983.tb01796.x.

Campana, D., Nori, F., Piscitelli, L., Morselli-Labate, A.M., Pezzilli, R. *et al.* (2007) Chromogranin A: is it a useful marker of neuroendocrine tumors? *Journal of Clinical Oncology* 25(15), 1967–1973. DOI: 10.1200/JCO.2006.10.1535.

de Bragança, A.C., Moyses, Z.P. and Magaldi, A.J. (2010) Carbamazepine can induce kidney water absorption by increasing aquaporin 2 expression. *Nephrology Dialysis Transplantation* 25(12), 3840–3845. DOI: 10.1093/ndt/gfq317.

De Cock, H.E. and MacLachlan, N.J. (1999) Simultaneous occurrence of multiple neoplasms and hyperplasias in the adrenal and thyroid gland of the horse resembling multiple endocrine neoplasia syndrome: case report and retrospective identification of additional cases. *Veterinary Pathology* 36(6), 633–636. DOI: 10.1354/vp.36-6-633.

Di Iorgi, N., Allegri, A.E.M., Napoli, F., Calcagno, A., Calandra, E. *et al.* (2014) Central diabetes insipidus in children and young adults: etiological diagnosis and long-term outcome of idiopathic cases. *The Journal* of *Clinical Endocrinology & Metabolism* 99(4), 1264–1272. DOI: 10.1210/jc.2013-3724.

Durham, A.E. (2017) Therapeutics for equine endocrine disorders. *The Veterinary Clinics of North America. Equine Practice* 33(1), 127–139. DOI: 10.1016/j.cveq.2016.11.003.

Fix, A.S. and Miller, L.D. (1987) Equine adrenocortical carcinoma with hypercalcemia. *Veterinary Pathology* 24(2), 190–192. DOI: 10.1177/030098588702400216.

Fouché, N., Gerber, V., Gorgas, D., Marolf, V., Grouzmann, E. *et al.* (2016) Catecholamine metabolism in a Shetland pony with suspected pheochromocytoma and pituitary pars intermedia dysfunction. *Journal of Veterinary Internal Medicine* 30(6), 1872–1878. DOI: 10.1111/jvim.14606.

Froscher, B.G. and Power, H.T. (1982) Malignant pheochromocytoma in a foal. *Journal of the American Veterinary Medical Association* 181(5), 494–496.

Gelberg, H., Cockerell, G.L. and Minor, R.R. (1979) A light and electron microscopic study of a normal adrenal medulla and a pheochromocytoma from a horse. *Veterinary Pathology* 16(4), 395–404. DOI: 10.1177/030098587901600401.

Germann, S.E., Rütten, M., Derungs, S.B. and Feige, K. (2006) Multiple endocrine neoplasia-like syndrome in a horse. *Veterinary Record* 159(16), 530–532. DOI: 10.1136/vr.159.16.530.

Harb, M.F., Nelson, R.W., Feldman, E.C., Scott-Moncrieff, J.C. and Griffey, S.M. (1996) Central diabetes insipidus in dogs: 20 cases (1986-1995). *Journal of the American Veterinary Medical Association* 209(11), 1884–1888.

Hollis, A.R., Boston, R.C. and Corley, K.T.T. (2008) Plasma aldosterone, vasopressin and atrial natriuretic peptide in hypovolaemia: a preliminary comparative study of neonatal and mature horses. *Equine Veterinary Journal* 40(1), 64–69. DOI: 10.2746/042516407X235795.

Holmes, C.L., Landry, D.W. and Granton, J.T. (2003) Science review: Vasopressin and the cardiovascular system part 1--receptor physiology. *Critical Care* 7(6), 427–434. DOI: 10.1186/cc2337.

Houpt, K.A., Thornton, S.N. and Allen, W.R. (1989) Vasopressin in dehydrated and rehydrated ponies. *Physiology & Behavior* 45(3), 659–661. DOI: 10.1016/0031-9384(89)90087-5.

Hurcombe, S.D.A., Toribio, R.E., Slovis, N., Kohn, C.W., Refsal, K. *et al.* (2008) Blood arginine vasopressin, adrenocorticotropin hormone, and cortisol concentrations at admission in septic and critically ill foals and their association with survival. *Journal of Veterinary Internal Medicine* 22(3), 639–647. DOI: 10.1111/j.1939-1676.2008.0090.x.

Katzman, S.A., Perez-Noguez, M., Pypendop, B.H., Alex, C.E. and Affolter, V.K. (2018) Anesthesia case of the month. *Journal of the American Veterinary Medical Association* 252(3), 286–288. DOI: 10.2460/javma.252.3.286.

Kranenburg, L.C., Thelen, M.H.M., Westermann, C.M., de Graaf-Roelfsema, E. and van der Kolk, J.H. (2010) Use of desmopressin eye drops in the treatment of equine congenital central diabetes insipidus. *Veterinary Record* 167(20), 790–791. DOI: 10.1136/vr.c5125.

Kwon, T.H., Hager, H., Nejsum, L.N., Andersen, M.L., Frøkiaer, J. *et al.* (2001) Physiology and pathophysiology of renal aquaporins. *Seminars in Nephrology* 21(3), 231–238. DOI: 10.1053/snep.2001.21647.

Luethy, D., Habecker, P., Murphy, B. and Nolen-Walston, R. (2016) Clinical and pathological features of pheochromocytoma in the horse: a multi-center retrospective study of 37 cases (2007-2014). *Journal of Veterinary Internal Medicine* 30(1), 309–313. DOI: 10.1111/jvim.13799.

Maccubbin, D.A. and Vanburen, J.M. (1963) A quantitative evaluation of hypothalamic degeneration and its relation to diabetes insipidus following interruption of the human hypophyseal stalk. *Brain* 86, 443–464. DOI: 10.1093/brain/86.3.443.

Maghnie, M., Cosi, G., Genovese, E., Manca-Bitti, M.L., Cohen, A. *et al.* (2000) Central diabetes insipidus in children and young adults. *New England Journal of Medicine* 343(14), 998–1007. DOI: 10.1056/NEJM200010053431403.

Majzoub, J.A. and Srivatsa, A. (2006) Diabetes insipidus: clinical and basic aspects. *Pediatric Endocrinology Reviews : PER* 4(Suppl 1), 60–65.

Monahan, C.F. and Craig, L.E. (2016) Pathology in practice. *Journal of the American Veterinary Medical Association* 248(3), 271–273. DOI: 10.2460/javma.248.3.271.

Morgan, R.A., Malalana, F. and McGowan, C.M. (2012) Nephrogenic diabetes insipidus in a 14-year-old gelding. *New Zealand Veterinary Journal* 60(4), 254–257. DOI: 10.1080/00480169.2012.669723.

Newton, S.A., Knottenbelt, D.C. and Eldridge, P.R. (2000) Headshaking in horses: possible aetiopathogenesis suggested by the results of diagnostic tests and several treatment regimes used in 20 cases. *Equine Veterinary Journal* 32(3), 208–216. DOI: 10.2746/042516400776563617.

Nielsen, S., Kwon, T.H., Christensen, B.M., Promeneur, D., Frøkiaer, J. *et al.* (1999) Physiology and pathophysiology of renal aquaporins. *Journal of the American Society of Nephrology : JASN* 10(3), 647–663.

Ooi, H.L., Maguire, A.M. and Ambler, G.R. (2013) Desmopressin administration in children with central diabetes insipidus: a retrospective review. *Journal of Pediatric Endocrinology and Metabolism* 26(11–12), 1047–1052. DOI: 10.1515/jpem-2013-0078.

Parry, B.W. (1984) Diagnosis of equine pheochromocytoma. *The Canadian Veterinary Journal* 25(8), 333.

Schott, H.C. (2011) Water homeostasis and diabetes insipidus in horses. *Veterinary Clinics of North America: Equine Practice* 27(1), 175–195. DOI: 10.1016/j.cveq.2011.01.002.

Schott, H.C., Bayly, W.M., Reed, S.M. and Brobst, D.F. (1993) Nephrogenic diabetes insipidus in sibling colts. *Journal of Veterinary Internal Medicine* 7(2), 68–72. DOI: 10.1111/j.1939-1676.1993.tb03172.x.

Sharp, D.C., Grubaugh, W., Berglund, L.A., McDowell, K.J., Kilmer, D.M. *et al.* (1982) Effects of pituitary stalk transection on endocrine function in pony mares. *Journal of Reproduction and Fertility. Supplement* 32, 297–302.

Takemura, N. (1998) Successful long-term treatment of congenital nephrogenic diabetes insipidus in a dog. *Journal of Small Animal Practice* 39(12), 592–594. DOI: 10.1111/j.1748-5827.1998.tb03714.x.

van Andel, A.C., Gruys, E., Kroneman, J. and Veerkamp, J. (1988) Amyloid in the horse: a report of nine cases. *Equine Veterinary Journal* 20(4), 277–285. DOI: 10.1111/j.2042-3306.1988.tb01524.x.

van der Kolk, J.H., Mars, M.H. and van der Gaag, I. (1994) Adrenocortical carcinoma in a 12-year-old mare. *Veterinary Record* 134(5), 113–115. DOI: 10.1136/vr.134.5.113.

Vente, J.P. and Wijsmuller, J.M. (1983) [Diabetes insipidus in a filly]. *Tijdschrift Diergeneeskd* 108(5), 210.

Wiedenmann, B., Franke, W.W., Kuhn, C., Moll, R. and Gould, V.E. (1986) Synaptophysin: a marker protein for neuroendocrine cells and neoplasms. *Proceedings of the National Academy of Sciences* 83(10), 3500–3504. DOI: 10.1073/pnas.83.10.3500.

Yovich, J.V., Horney, F.D. and Hardee, G.E. (1984) Pheochromocytoma in the horse and measurement of norepinephrine levels in horses. *The Canadian Veterinary Journal* 25(1), 21–25.

8 Diseases of the Female Reproductive System

Development of the Female Reproductive System

Sexual differentiation can be divided into chromosomal, gonadal and phenotypic sex. Normal female mammals are of chromosome XX makeup, with paired ovaries and normal tubular tract and external genitalia which makes them readily physically differentiable as female mammals.

Genetic sex determination

Chromosomal sex is established at the time of fertilization with the X chromosome bearing spermatozoa and is apparent in the developing zygote. Inactivation of a single X chromosome results in only one of the X chromosomes being transcriptionally active while the other chromosome is mostly silent (Galupa and Heard, 2018); this process has long been studied in humans and mice, but has not been specifically studied in horses to date. Inactivation of a single X chromosome is believed to result in a form of dosage compensation between XX and XY individuals in any species, and failure to induce inactivation results in mortality of affected embryos. This transcriptional silencing is maintained into adulthood (Sierra and Anguera, 2019). In mice and humans, a small percentage (up to 30%) of X-inactivated genes escape the silencing process but this phenomenon and a threshold for biallelic conditions is currently unknown in the mare. X-inactive specific transcript (Xist) was one of the first long non-coding RNAs to be identified in the early 1990s and is primarily responsible for dose regulation of X-linked genes (Loda and Heard, 2019).

Development of gonadal sex

The primordial germ cells develop early in embryogenesis, within the first 15% of gestation (Senger, 2012). The pathway of sex determination begins with the formation of a single pair of morphologically undifferentiated bipotential gonads that can develop into testes or ovaries. The initial development is paired genital ridges, which are a consequence of thickening of the coelomic epithelium on the ventromedial surface of the mesonephros. In mice, primordial germ cells migrate from the hindgut into the mesonephros until day 13 after coitus. These germ cells are supported by somatic cell lineages (steroidogenic precursor cells) that have the potential to differentiate into Leydig or theca cells and support cell precursors that can differentiate into Sertoli or granulosa cells. The forkhead box protein L2 (*FoxL2*) gene is important for development of granulosa cells during gonadal expression (Quinn and Koopman, 2012).

There are two signalling pathways that promote ovarian development and, at the same time, act to repress male development (Quinn and Koopman, 2012). The R-spondin-1 (*Rspo1*) gene is expressed in the coelomic epithelium of the bipotential gonad and is up regulated in XX gonadal somatic cells. Also, *Rspo1* activates *Wnt4*, which suppresses migration of steroidogenic and endothelial cells from the mesonephros. In turn, *Wnt4* up regulates *Dax1*, a gene located on the X chromosome that suppresses expression of *Sf1* and subsequently *Sox9*, which prevents male gonadal differentiation and androgen production. At this stage of development, primitive sex cords and paired Wolffian and Müllerian ducts are formed, which will selectively regress, depending on the fate of the bipotential gonads. If the bipotential gonad is male, the Müllerian ducts regress; conversely, if the bipotential gonad is female, the Wölffian ducts regress.

Historically, development of the ovary was thought to be the default pathway in mammalian development, with development of the testis actively driven by the presence of the Y chromosome sex-determining region (SRY, see Chapter 9). Gonadal differentiation is a balance between the rival influences of XX- and XY-promoting factors.

Up regulation of *Sox9* in supporting precursor cells of an XY gonad down regulates genes involved with ovarian development, including *Rspo1*, *Wnt4* and *FoxL2*. In an XX gonad, *Rspo1*, *Wnt4* and β-*catenin* down regulate genes involved with testicular development and up regulate *Wnt4* (along with *FoxL2*), which acts as an antagonist of the *Sox9* feedback loop. Therefore, female reproductive tract development, including development of the hypothalamic–pituitary–gonadal axis, is actively driven by pro-female genetic control.

Development of the female brain in the embryo

Historically, development of the hypothalamic tonic (male) or surge (female) centres has been thought to arise from the transport of fetal oestrogens and α-fetoprotein across the blood–brain barrier. The default developmental pathway for the hypothalamus is the formation of a surge centre; thus, feminization is the default process relative to male hypothalamic development. However, there is increasing evidence that feminization or masculinization of the brain might at least in part be driven at a genetic level. In the female fetus, oestrogens are bound by α-fetoprotein which prevents oestrogen from crossing the blood–brain barrier. Therefore, oestradiol cannot affect the development of the hypothalamus and the surge centre remains intact. In the male fetus, testosterone readily crosses the blood–brain barrier and is then converted to oestradiol in the brain. This process is described in Chapter 9.

Development of phenotypical sex: tubular tract and external genitalia

In the absence of a Y chromosome and sex-determining region expression, the female pathway is activated, which promotes development of the ovaries. This involves activation of a set of genes specific to female development. Historically, the development of the female reproductive tract was thought to be a default pathway that occurred in the absence of the SRY protein. The development of the female tubular tract and ovary both require active pathways that are under female gene control. Normal tubular tract development involves the activation of two parallel development pathways, both by suppressing male tract development and promoting female tract development.

Expression of *Rspo1* and *Wnt4* is mediated via the β-*catenin* pathway. This pathway is crucial because it antagonizes *Sox9*; overexpression of β-*catenin* promotes female development, and underexpression allows overexpression of *Sox9* and promotes male development. The second pathway, which is activated in parallel, involves the gene forkhead/winged helix transcription factor (*FoxL2*); it remains active throughout adult life and has a role in suppression of *Sox9* (Quinn and Koopman, 2012). Suppression of *Sox9* permits development of the Müllerian ducts or paramesonephric ducts, which form the uterine tubes, uterus, cervix and the cranial portion of the vagina. The urogenital sinus develops into the caudal portion of the vagina and vestibule, the genital tubercle develops into the clitoris and genital swellings develop into the vulva. Thus, the embryonic tissue origin of the uterus, cervix and cranial portion of the vagina is different from the embryonic tissue comprising the caudal vagina and vestibule.

The homeobox family of genes (HOX genes) comprise a group of regulatory molecules that encode highly conserved transcription factors. HOX genes are expressed along anterior–posterior axes and control proper partitioning of the female reproductive tract. Endocrine disruptors, such as diethylstilboestrol, exert their action by changing HOX gene expression. Differential expression of HOX genes in the Müllerian duct results in normal patterning in the developed reproductive tract. The Müllerian ducts will develop into the oviducts, uterus, cervix and the cranial portion of the vagina; thus, these organs are developed from mesoderm. *Hoxa9* is expressed at high levels in areas that will become the oviduct, *Hoxa10* in the areas that will become the uterus, *Hoxa11* in the lower uterus and cervix and *Hoxa13* in the outer cervix and upper vagina; there is no *Hoxa12* gene (Du and Taylor, 2015). This so called HOX gene family code is critically important to the development of proper spatial tissue orientation in the female reproductive tract.

The caudal vagina and vestibule are derived from a portion of the urogenital sinus and thus derived from ectoderm. The junction where these two tissue types fuse becomes the hymen. Given the number of events that must successfully occur in order for genetic, gonadal and phenotypic sex to align, it should not come as a surprise that disorders of sexual differentiation occur in equids. These will be discussed in detail under the section 'Abnormalities of the Oestrous Cycle'.

Oestrous Cycle Physiology

The oestrous cycle of the mare is approximately 21–22 days in length (up to 25 days in ponies), as measured from ovulation to ovulation (Aurich, 2011). The oestrous cycle can be split into physiologic periods: oestrous, the time when the mare is receptive for mating, and dioestrus, when the mare is not receptive. Mares are described as seasonal, long-day breeders; increasing day length has an inhibitory effect on the release of melatonin, which initiates a neurohormonal cascade driving regular cyclicity. Gonadotroph cells present in the pars distalis and pars tuberalis of the pituitary, differentially store luteinizing hormone (LH) and follicle-stimulating hormone (FSH); this becomes the basis for regulation of gonadotroph secretion throughout the oestrous cycle of the mare. The mare will produce one to two follicular waves over the course of the oestrous cycle, with follicles reaching 35–50 mm prior to ovulation occurring. In certain breeds, such as heavy/draft horses, follicles can exceed 50 mm prior to ovulation. Within the structure of the follicle, only the granulosa cells will develop into luteal cells and secrete progesterone (P4) . P4 will increase at the time of ovulation and reach maximal concentrations at 8 days post ovulation.

During the oestrous cycle of the mare, the structure, texture and size of the reproductive tract will undergo substantive changes in response to the hormonal milieu present. Under the influence of oestrogen, the endometrium becomes oedematous, and the presence of uterine oedema can be used as an indirect marker of the presence of oestrogen. Clinical scoring systems vary but are usually assigned a letter or number to a four-part scale, ranging from no oedema, to slight oedema, moderate oedema and heavy oedema. Some scoring systems incorporate an additional category for pathologic oedema, which is generally extremely heavy. The cervix of mares in oestrous is normally wide, soft and relaxed to accommodate the belling of the glans penis of the stallion during natural service. Conversely, in dioestrus and under the influence of P4, the uterus of the mare is toned, with a tight, ropey cervix and no uterine oedema.

The equine ovary is generally very large relative to other species and can vary substantially between the season of the year and the stage of the oestrous cycle. Mares in winter anoestrus have small inactive ovaries which might only be a few centimetres in diameter (grape- to golf-ball-sized). During the vernal transition, mares might have large ovaries with multiple intermediate-sized follicles prior to the initial ovulation of the breeding season proper. Once the breeding season proper commences, defined as the first ovulation of the year, ovarian size is typically determined by the largest follicular structure present.

Kisspeptin

Kisspeptins (Kp) are a family of neuropeptides that act as regulators of gonadotropin-releasing hormone (GnRH), nearly exclusively through stimulation of GnRH (Caraty *et al.*, 2012). Kps are released from neurons in the hypothalamus, but in some species there might be extrahypothalamic (pituitary and ovarian) functions of Kps as well. Kps are encoded by the *KiSS-1* gene; Kps might be vital in signalling seasonal cyclicity during the transition period (Magee *et al.*, 2009). There appear to be species-specific differences in response to Kp administration. For example, Kps used as a constant infusion to treat pony mares failed to induce synchronized ovulation, as opposed to in ewes where a LH surge was induced within 2 h of administration. Additionally, light horse mares administered a single dose of rodent *KiSS* gene (*rKp-10*) showed no difference in time to ovulation compared to those treated with saline administration, and mares treated with human chorionic gonadotropin (hCG) had a shorter interval to ovulation than *rKp-10*-treated mares. Mares receiving multiple, repeated doses of equine Kp did not show differences in time to ovulation, but this appeared to have a strong inhibitory effect on normal sexual behaviour during oestrous (Magee *et al.*, 2012). Therefore, Kps might be a novel tool for regulating GnRH and its downstream hormonal cascade, but further research is required in the mare. There is currently no commercially available formulation for treatment of mares clinically, and optimal doses and treatment schedules are not yet established (Magee *et al.*, 2009). In light of the potential adverse effects on reproductive behaviour, further research is warranted and current understanding of the role of Kps in regulation of GnRH might be oversimplified.

Gonadotropin-releasing hormone

GnRH is a decapeptide that is produced by the hypothalamic surge centre in females, and its target tissue is gonadotroph cells in the anterior lobe of the pituitary. GnRH controls the release of LH and FSH from the pituitary, with subsequent control over production of other sex steroids and gametogenesis in both males and females. Kps appear to be the regulators of GnRH secretion in many mammals. Several GnRH analogues (deslorelin, historelin, buserelin) are available either commercially or from compounding pharmacies. Deslorelin is available as an injectable product or as a slow-release implant in a commercial formula in many countries and is used to reliably programme ovulation in mares in oestrous with a minimum follicle size of 30 mm. Mares respond most reliably to ovulation programming when a minimum follicle size is achieved; there is presence of moderate to heavy uterine oedema; cervical softening has occurred; and the mare is showing signs of behavioural oestrous. Deslorelin implants have become less popular in areas where the injectable formulation is available; although the implants are designed to dissolve, the continued release of a GnRH agonist appears to cause down regulation of the hypothalamic–pituitary–gonadal axis and potentially a prolonged return to oestrous. Historelin and buserelin have been used in an extralabel fashion to induce follicular growth in transitional mares as a means to hasten the first ovulation of the season.

Oestrogen

Oestrogen is a steroid hormone that is produced by the granulosa cells of the follicle. In addition to oestrogen, mares also produce unique ring-B saturated oestrogens during pregnancy (equilin, EQ, and equilenin, EL, below). In female mammals, the target tissues of oestrogen are varied, and most tissue types have oestrogen receptors present. Key target tissues regarding reproduction include the hypothalamus, the entire reproductive tract and the mammary gland. High concentrations of oestrogen are required to stimulate the LH surge to promote ovulation of the dominant follicle. Oestrogen also increases vasodilation and blood flow to the uterus, resulting in the clinical appearance of uterine oedema. Uterine oedema can subsequently be subjectively scored and is an important parameter in monitoring follicular growth and maturity for breeding management of mares. The primary actions of oestrogen in mares include promoting sexual behaviour, elevating secretory activity within the reproductive tract and enhancing uterine motility during both oestrous and parturition.

Equilin and equilenin

EQ, EL and the bioactive metabolites of EQ are ring-B unsaturated oestrogens biosynthesized by the fetoplacental unit of the mare. The metabolic pathway producing these steroids is different from that of oestrone and oestradiol, as it is cholesterol independent (Numazawa and Osawa, 1987). These compounds are derived from 7-dehydroepiandrosterone and 5,7-androstadien-3,17diol, rather than dehydroepiandrosterone (DHEA) as is the case for the classical oestrogens: oestrone, oestradiol-17α and oestradiol-17β.

Progesterone

P4 is a steroid hormone produced by the corpus luteum (CL) of the mare. The mare also produces a wide variety of species-specific progestogens during pregnancy from the fetoplacental unit, discussed later in this chapter. The primary target tissues of P4 include the endometrium, mammary gland, myometrium and hypothalamus. The actions of P4 are generally related to maintenance of pregnancy, endometrial secretion and inhibition of reproductive behaviour. In many species, P4 has a negative feedback on GnRH secretion, but in the mare this does not appear to be true. Mares that are being synchronized for embryo transfer programmes typically require both exogenous oestrogen and P4 to suppress the follicular wave adequately, to permit emergence to occur in multiple mares at a predictable time.

Luteinizing hormone

LH is a glycoprotein that is released from the anterior lobe of the pituitary. Its target tissue in females is the cells of the theca interna and luteal cells on the ovary. LH promotes the final phases of follicular growth/maturation and induces ovulation, as well as driving the formation of CL and supporting P4 secretion. Mares have a very distinct ovulatory gonadotropin profile relative to other species, which is clinically relevant. In most species, the LH surge is rapid and lasts for 12–24 h, but in mares the LH surge can last for 3–5 days and peaks after ovulation has occurred (Whitmore *et al.*, 1973). Thus, no short, distinct periovulatory LH surge occurs in mares (Aurich, 2011). A suggested mechanism for the ability to maintain the prolonged LH surge is resistance to desensitization of the GnRH receptor. Due to this unique physiology, agents used to induce ovulation in the mare for breeding management must also be long acting with a similar prolonged effect.

Repeated administration of glucocorticoids, particularly dexamethasone, has the potential to decrease LH and negatively affect ovulation (Ferris and McCue, 2010). Care should be taken when administering dexamethasone to mares for treatment of post-mating-induced endometritis, to limit the number of doses administered and to use the lower end of the dose range.

Follicle-stimulating hormone

FSH is a glycoprotein that is produced by gonadotroph cells in the anterior lobe of the pituitary. Its target tissue is the granulosa cells of the ovary, where it drives follicular development and synthesis of oestrogen.

Inhibin

Inhibin is a glycoprotein that is produced by the granulosa cells of the dominant follicle and exerts its action on the gonadotrophs in the anterior lobe of the pituitary. It inhibits FSH secretion, thus playing a role in the development of the dominant follicle. In monovulatory species such as mares, inhibin helps ensure that only a single follicle achieves dominance during any one follicular wave.

Prostaglandin F2α

Prostaglandin F2α (PGF2α) is prostaglandin hormone derived from the arachidonic acid pathway and is a C-20 fatty acid. It is produced by the endometrium and is released in response to failure of maternal recognition of pregnancy. It has multiple target tissues including the CL, where it induces luteolysis; the uterine myometrium, where it induces myometrial contractions and acts as an ecbolic agent; and the ovulatory follicle, where it aids in degradation of the follicular wall and plays a role in ovulation. Exogenous prostaglandins can be used very effectively as ecbolic agents during breeding management of mares and have a longer duration of effect relative to oxytocin. Care must be taken if administering prostaglandins after ovulation has occurred. Although the equine CL is considered resistant to the effects of prostaglandins for 5–6 days after ovulation, research has shown that repeated doses of prostaglandins shortly after ovulation result in inhibition of the formation of the CL. Similarly, mares treated with prostaglandins shortly after ovulation had lower serum P4 concentrations and lower pregnancy rates at 14 days. Use of prostaglandins as ecbolic agents after ovulation must be carefully weighed under a risk–benefit ratio to the individual patient, as mares that continue to retain uterine fluid despite standard treatment with uterine lavage and oxytocin are unlikely to become pregnant, regardless.

Oxytocin

Oxytocin is a neuropeptide synthesized in the hypothalamus. It is stored and released from the posterior pituitary and is also synthesized by the CL in most species. In mares, there is no significant amount of oxytocin produced by the CL, yet exogenous administration of oxytocin appears to have some positive effect on extending the lifespan of the CL (Aurich, 2011). Its target tissues are the myometrium, endometrium and myoepithelial cells of the mammary gland. Oxytocin promotes uterine motility and promotes endometrial PGF2α synthesis. Oxytocin is frequently administered as an ecbolic agent as it is very effective at inducing uterine contractions and expulsion of intraluminal fluid. Milk ejection (letdown) is regulated by oxytocin, and the sight, smell and tactile responses of the foal will result in oxytocin release.

Prolactin

Prolactin (PRL) is a protein hormone that is produced in the anterior lobe of the pituitary. Its target tissue is mammary cells and it promotes lactation. PRL likely also plays a role in regulation of seasonality in mares, as administration of dopamine antagonists such as domperidone or sulpiride can result in a shortening of the transition period and hastening the first ovulation of the year.

Equine chorionic gonadotropin

Equids and some primates are the only species known to produce chorionic gonadotropins. Equine chorionic gonadotropin (eCG) is produced by the chorionic girdle cells of the developing placenta, starting at approximately 35 days' gestation. eCG acts similarly to the other endogenous gonadotropins, FSH and LH, in that it recruits additional follicular waves and luteinizes the dominant follicle. This results in the formation of accessory and supplementary CLs, which maintain the equine pregnancy until the fetoplacental unit takes over generation of progestogens in sufficient quantities to maintain pregnancy. hCG is frequently used in broodmare practice to programme ovulation. In mares, hCG acts like LH and results in a predictable time to ovulation, 36–48 h after administration. Interestingly, there is individual species variation in response to both eCG and hCG. For example, in cattle hCG binds to LH receptors on the granulosa and theca cells of ovarian follicles with high affinity and has been used to induce ovulation, but does not produce the same stimulatory effect on follicle growth as eCG (Prata *et al.*, 2018). In dairy cattle, administration of eCG post insemination reduces pregnancy loss, presumably through the formation of accessory CL, but treatment with hCG actually reduces fertility (Bartolome *et al.*, 2012).

Follicular dynamics

Mares can develop both major ovulatory and major or minor anovulatory follicular waves over the course of a typical 21-day oestrous cycle. A major follicular wave is classified as one where a dominant follicle develops (Ginther, 2012). Development of the follicular wave in mammals is controlled by both FSH and LH and involves both growth and regression/apoptosis of follicles. Follicular dynamics occur throughout the oestrous cycle, despite the fact that oestrous comprises only approximately 33% of the equine oestrous cycle. A typical follicular wave can be divided into four main phases: recruitment or emergence, selection, dominance and/or atresia. In mares, regressing follicles from a previous wave overlap with follicles in the common growth phase of the ovulatory wave approximately 25% of the time (Ginther *et al.*, 2004).

During recruitment, a cohort of small antral follicles begin to grow; ultimately, the majority of these follicles will undergo atresia. The group of growing follicles that remains has undergone selection; in the mare, generally a single follicle from the selected group will go on to become dominant while the remainder of the follicle cohort undergo atresia. The major wave that produces the dominant (ovulatory) follicle is the most consistent follicular wave in mares and is initiated in the middle of the interovulatory interval (Ginther, 2012). FSH begins to increase as oestradiol is decreasing; this is likely to be related to the negative effect of oestradiol administration on FSH in mares (Jacob *et al.*, 2009). Just prior to follicular deviation, both oestrogen and LH will increase.

Approximately 25% of oestrous cycles will result in ovulation of multiple (typically two) follicles. Multiple ovulations can occur unilaterally or bilaterally, and there appears to be a strong influence of breed. Mares that have spontaneously ovulated multiple follicles in the past might be at higher risk of doing so in the future, and this can be an important clinical factor to consider regarding the risk of developing twins and the need for increased vigilance at pregnancy diagnosis.

Interestingly, there is increasing evidence that exercise might alter follicular dynamics in mares; this can be clinically relevant as more breed registries are permitting multiple offspring to be registered per mare per year. Therefore, more performance mares are eligible to produce multiple foals per season through assisted reproductive technologies such as embryo transfer and intracytoplasmic sperm injection (ICSI), and alterations in follicular dynamics related to exercise might play a role in the success of these procedures in such mares. Kelley *et al.* demonstrated that mares undergoing a moderate exercise programme had lower LH concentrations, a longer interovulatory interval and altered follicular deviation compared to control (non-exercised) mares (Kelley *et al.*, 2011).

Sexual Behaviour

Normal sexual behaviour in mares is largely driven by the presence or absence of gonadal steroids. Evaluation of sexual behaviour provides excellent adjunct information regarding ovarian status and is critical in determining readiness for breeding, particularly if natural service is desired or required. Oestrous behaviour of mares includes squatting; clitoral eversion (winking); passive urination; lifting of the tail; and general passive responses to the stallion. Oestrous behaviour is enhanced by the presence of oestrogen; thus, the mare will generally show an increase in oestrous behaviour as she approaches ovulation and oestrogen concentrations continue to rise with the growth of the dominant follicle. After ovulation, oestrous behaviour will decrease over 24–48 h.

P4 produced by the CL has a strong negative influence on oestrous behaviour. Mares in dioestrus will display avoidance or aggression toward the stallion. Typically, behaviours would include kicking, striking and squealing. In mares maintained and teased in a group, dioestrus individuals might simply refuse to come up and interact with the stallion and would display avoidance behaviour rather than active aggression.

Evaluation of sexual behaviour can be confounded by several factors. Maiden mares with limited historical exposure to stallions might take additional time and effort to display normal oestrous behaviour. Typically, patience and continued exposure to the stallion, possibly through continued fence-line contact if possible, will result in normal expression of oestrous behaviour. Lactating mares, particularly those that have recently foaled, might be reluctant to show normal oestrous behaviour when the foal is near and might instead act aggressively toward the stallion in order to protect the foal. Most lactating mares show more reliable teasing behaviour with increasing time after foaling. There can be considerable variation between individual mares, with certain individuals showing clear indications of oestrous on transrectal examination (good oedema scoring, large follicle, etc.) yet only displaying oestrous behaviour fairly close to the time of ovulation or not at all.

Abnormalities of the Oestrous Cycle

The most frequent reason for examination of the reproductive tract in mares is for the purpose of breeding management. However, veterinarians might be requested to investigate complaints regarding abnormalities of the oestrous cycle such as persistent oestrous, erratic teasing behaviour, aggression or failure to display oestrous behaviour. The reproductive examination for abnormalities relating to oestrous should include: a general clinical examination to exclude concurrent disease; transrectal palpation of the reproductive tract to assess the size, position and tone of reproductive structures; ultrasonography of the reproductive organs; and endocrine testing, as appropriate. Additional diagnostic testing such as endometrial culture and cytology, endometrial biopsy, vaginal speculum examination and/or hysteroscopy might be indicated, depending on the specific condition.

Failure to ovulate (anovulation)

Failure to ovulate is a normal physiologic process in the mare, in the vernal and autumnal transition periods. Transition to the breeding season proper is preceded by the development of several follicular waves prior to ovulation finally occurring. Extension of photoperiod is the primary means to enable mares to cycle during late winter and early spring to meet the needs of registry body birthdates (1 January in the northern hemisphere and 1 August in the southern hemisphere). There are several pharmacologic protocols that can be used to hasten or perhaps even slightly shorten the transition period, but drug protocols are insufficient to stimulate ovarian activity in mares that are in deep anoestrus. In order to be most effective, phototherapy must be initiated prior to the winter solstice. Little research has been performed on the factors controlling the autumnal transition period as this is not considered economically important, thus the precise mechanisms that govern what will ultimately become the last ovulation of the season remain unknown.

Anovulatory follicles will also occasionally occur during the breeding season proper, and the cause for this remains unknown. This can be a particularly frustrating phenomenon to deal with during the breeding management of mares. Some anovulatory follicles will simply regress; more common is the development of a haemorrhagic anovulatory follicle (HAF). Typically, HAFs are associated with signs of impending ovulation such as LH peak and decrease in oestradiol (Ginther *et al.*, 2007). Endometrial oedema decreases in association with decreasing oestrogen, and the subsequent dioestrus is of normal length. Ultrasonographically, HAFs are very similar in ultrasound appearance to experimentally induced, luteinized unruptured follicles (LUF) (Cuervo-Arango and Newcombe, 2012). Although shortening of dioestrus by administration of prostaglandins is a common strategy in the breeding management of mares, there might be an increased incidence of HAFs in cycles where oestrous is induced via administration of cloprostenol

(Cuervo-Arango and Newcombe, 2009). Anti-Mullerian hormone (AMH) concentrations are lower in mares with HAF, reflecting diminished follicular activity, and might be resultant of diminished granulosa cell function (Gharagozlou *et al.*, 2014).

Persistent corpus luteum

The CL forms at the site of ovulation and secretes P4. A *persistent CL* is any CL that remains functional beyond the 14–15 days of dioestrus. This condition can affect up to 10% of cycles during the breeding season proper and might occur at a higher frequency during the autumnal transition (Santos *et al.*, 2015). Clinical conditions that are associated with persistent CL include pyometra, where the endometrium might be too diseased to secrete PGF2α in the normal fashion, or where pregnancy loss occurs after maternal recognition of pregnancy. Mares with suspected persistent CL should undergo transrectal palpation and ultrasonography to determine pregnancy status, as pregnancy would be a normal clinical condition associated with persistent CL. When the aetiology of persistent CL is unknown, the terms *idiopathic* or *spontaneous persistent CL* might be used. The pathophysiology regarding persistent CL in mares has been attributed to either a defect in PGF2α secretion or a response to PGF2α. The lifespan of the persistent CL is approximately 60 days.

A clinical condition that might result in prolonged persistence of multiple CL occurs when pregnancy loss takes place after the formation of endometrial cups. As the endometrial cups continue to produce eCG, there is a continuation of follicular development and luteinization, forming the accessory and supplementary CL. In some mares, endometrial cups will persist beyond the normal expected time frame, and can be identified on hysteroscopy and removed using surgical laser.

Ovarian haematoma

Ovarian haematomas are a common cause of unilateral ovarian enlargement and might be confused with granulosa cell tumours (GCT). Haemorrhage occurs into the follicular lumen following ovulation, and these structures are essentially very large corpora haemorrhagica. The contralateral ovary is normal in size, shape and function, and the mare continues to cycle normally. Over time, the ovarian haematoma will organize and begin to regress; in addition to endocrinologic testing, serial monitoring can be used to distinguish ovarian haematomas from ovarian neoplasia, as ovarian haematomas will gradually decrease in size and the mare should still continue to cycle.

Chromosomal abnormalities and developmental disorders

The normal karyotype of the mare is 64,XX. Chromosome abnormalities of the sex chromosomes are associated with infertility in the horse. The most common abnormality, 63,XO, results in gonadal agenesis from the absence of a second sex chromosome. This is similar to Turner's syndrome in humans. Mares with this condition develop a female phenotype as there is no Y chromosome to direct development toward a male phenotype. Affected mares have small inactive ovaries and an underdeveloped tubular tract and might show erratic or unpredictable oestrous behaviour. Occasionally, mosaicism occurs where the mare has a 63,XO/64,XX phenotype, and there have been reports of mosaic mares producing foals. 64,XXX genotypes have been reported in mares but are rare, and these mares are uniformly infertile. Karyotyping (chromosomal analysis) can easily be performed on blood or hair samples to confirm the diagnosis.

Female pseudohermaphrodites, with a 64,XX genotype but a male-like phenotype, are very rare but do occur. Male pseudohermaphrodites are much more common and are discussed in the following chapter. Female pseudohermaphrodites have ovaries and might have components of a female tubular tract but have external male genitalia. XX sex reversal syndrome occurs when the chromosomal and gonadal sex do not align and might result from mutation of autosomal genes that allows testicular development to occur.

Pituitary pars intermedia dysfunction

Mares with pituitary pars intermedia dysfunction (PPID) have been reported to have abnormal oestrous cycles and/or infertility (Rohrbach *et al.*, 2012; Horn *et al.*, 2019). Generally, mares with PPID are older and might have other reproductive comorbidities influencing fertility, as well as decreased fertility resulting from age-related reduction in oocyte quality. The causative mechanism for how PPID reduces fertility in mares is currently unknown, but mares might have improved fertility after successful treatment for PPID. Mares that are treated with pergolide and become pregnant might need therapy to be discontinued approaching lactation, due to the effects of this medication on PRL.

Endocrinology of Pregnancy

During the first 150 days of pregnancy, P4 is produced by the primary and secondary CL of the ovary, resulting in high plasma concentrations of P4. In the last third of gestation, P4 concentrations drop to baseline, and uterine quiescence is maintained by progestogens produced by the fetoplacental unit (metabolites of pregnenolone, P5).

Since most of the progestogens present in the plasma of the mare are derived from the fetal placental unit, maternal progestogen concentrations drop rapidly when acute fetal death occurs. Quantitatively, the most important progestogens measurable in the mare's blood in mid- to late gestation are 5α-pregnane-3,20-dione (5αDHP) and its derivatives (Fowden *et al.*, 2008). Pregnane metabolites such as 5αDHP might be more important than P4 in maintaining uterine quiescence in mares during late gestation, as it has a much higher binding affinity for P4 receptor in the uterus. There are two complex biosynthetic pathways for production of 5αDHP, and it can be produced by the fetoplacental unit from mid-gestation onward.

Precursors to oestrogen synthesis in the pregnant mare are derived from the fetal gonads; thus, concentrations of oestrogens present in maternal blood closely parallel the growth and regression of the fetal gonads and peak around day 200 of gestation. Since both fetal ovaries and testes produce the precursors, there is no difference in total oestrogen concentration between mares carrying colt vs filly foals.

Endocrinology of Parturition

In general, the hormonal cascade of fetal and maternal endocrine events approaching parturition is similar among species, with some differences in placental hormone synthesis and in the timing of key prepartum events. Mares are unusual in that there is very little P4 circulating in maternal plasma at the time of parturition and that both progestogens and oestrogens are produced by precursor molecules from the fetus. Many of the steroids produced by the fetoplacental unit during gestation are unique to the horse, and the progestogens produced do not cross-react with traditional assays for P4. Although the fetal hypothalamo–pituitary–adrenocortical axis is required for parturition in sheep, its role in initiation of parturition in horses is less clear. Fetal cortisol secretion in response to adrenocorticotropic hormone (ACTH) is poor until several days prior to term. Basal fetal cortisol concentrations only rise in the final 24–36 h prior to parturition, meaning the fetal cortisol rise is confined to the last 1–2% of gestation. The role of the fetal hypothalamo–pituitary–adrenocortical axis in sheep results in prematurity being very uncommon in this species, yet in horses prematurity and dysmaturity in foals are common clinical problems. Thus, fetal maturation and myometrial activity in mares might not occur as a direct result of the final rise in fetal cortisol as it does in sheep.

In most domestic species, P4 concentrations drop precipitously toward the end of gestation and just prior to parturition, but in mares progestogen concentrations actually rise in the last month of gestation and only fall in the 24–48 h preceding delivery of the foal. At time of delivery, progestogen concentrations will continue to fall for several hours after parturition. Also, in contrast to other mammals, total oestrogen concentrations decrease before parturition rather than increase. Oestrogens are believed to play an important role in the labour process by augmenting myometrial contraction. Mares that have low total oestrogen concentrations experimentally induced due to fetal gonadectomy, have weak myometrial contractions. Concentrations of oestradiol-17B, which has the highest receptor binding affinity for any of the equine oestrogens, double in the last 24–48 h prior to parturition. Therefore, despite relatively low concentrations of oestrogens compared to other species, they still appear to play an important role in enhancement of prostaglandin production and activation of the myometrium. Prostaglandins play a role in cervical ripening (prostaglandin E2) and myometrial contractions (PGF2α) by increasing intracellular calcium in myometrial cells. The fall in progestogens and rise in oestradiol-17B just prior to parturition might alter the ratio of prostaglandin synthesis, resulting in cervical ripening and an increase in myometrial contractions.

Endocrinology of Lactation

Development of the mammary gland and the onset of lactation are under the control of the complex interactions between many hormones, including ovarian and adrenal steroids, PRL, oxytocin, growth hormone, insulin, thyroid hormones and other factors. The development of the mammary ducts is influenced by oestrogens, while P4 stimulates lobuloalveolar growth and inhibits lactogenesis. The rise of progestogens in the last month of gestation is associated with mammary gland development which occurs 4–8 weeks prior to parturition. The subsequent rapid decline in progestogens that occurs just prior to parturition is associated with the change in mammary secretion electrolytes that can be used as an indicator of impending parturition. Just prior to foaling, sodium and potassium invert, calcium concentrations rise dramatically and pH drops. Serum PRL concentrations are highest in mares 24 h after foaling (Krakowski *et al.*, 2020).

Mares with concurrent PPID that are being treated with pergolide mesylate will need to have treatment discontinued prior to foaling, as pergolide inhibits the secretion of PRL. It is the author's preference to discontinue treatment 4–6 weeks prior to foaling, and to restart treatment with pergolide after the mare is lactating well, approximately 30 days after foaling. If the mare is experiencing adverse effects from the withdrawal of pergolide (such as laminitis), pergolide can be reinstituted sooner. Foals from mares treated with pergolide should be regularly monitored for weight gain and adequate nutrition; a surrogate mare might need to be considered in some cases. Mares with untreated PPID might present with inappropriate lactation that responds to therapy with pergolide.

Lactation can be induced in non-pregnant mares that have previously foaled and lactated successfully. Final development of the mammary gland does not occur until the final stages of gestation, thus using maiden mares is less effective for this purpose. There are several major advantages to lactation-induced nurse mares: they can be prepared as needed; they do not need to be rebred as in the case of commercial wet nurse mares; and there are no ethical dilemmas over removal of a healthy foal from a lactating commercial wet mare. There are several reported protocols for lactation induction in mares, and all include a combination of oestrogen, P4 and a dopamine D2 antagonist (sulpiride or domperidone) (Chavatte-Palmer *et al.*, 2002; Porter *et al.*, 2002). A major disadvantage of this technique is the delay in reaching peak lactation; without supplemental feeding, foals raised by lactation-induced mares typically show reduced growth early on but catch up to their naturally-raised cohort by the time of weaning. Continued treatment with dopamine D2 antagonists might reduce this lag period to some extent.

The author's preferred protocol is as follows: altrenogest at 0.088 mg/kg by mouth every 24 h for 7–10 days; oestradiol benzoate 50 mg by intramuscular injection once on the first day of treatment; and domperidone at 1.1 mg/kg by mouth twice daily for 7–14 days until lactation is sufficient to maintain the foal. Mares are hand milked every 3–6 h on the second or third day after starting treatment, and oxytocin can be administered during hand milking to improve milk letdown if needed. Generally, once udder stimulation begins, the mare rapidly starts to increase mammary secretions. Ideally, the mare should be housed in sight and sound of the foal and be able to interact with it over a safety barrier. On day 5–7 of treatment when sufficient udder development is present, behavioural grafting can be performed. The mare is administered 500 mg cloprostenol intramuscularly and allowed to become colicky and sweaty. Sweat from the mare is rubbed on to the foal to increase acceptance of the foal. The perineum of the mare is aseptically prepared, and the cervix is manually dilated for 1–2 min, twice, at 10 min intervals. The foal is then presented to the front of the mare and allowed to nurse. Experience at our hospital suggests that mare selection is critical to success; calm, quiet mares in good body condition that have successfully raised foals are good candidates for lactation induction. Many of the mares in our nurse mare programme show interest and maternal behaviour within several days of being allowed to interact with the foal; we have a purpose built mare–foal box that allows the mare to be housed completely separate from the orphan foal, but interact over a half door so she can lick, nuzzle and otherwise connect with the foal without the risk of injuring it. In our hospital, the above protocol results in rapid acceptance of the foal. Once grafting is complete, altrenogest therapy is discontinued and the mare is maintained on domperidone for several more days. The foal is weighed daily and supplemented with additional milk if clinically indicated. However, it is important to remember that the stimulus of the foal aggressively nursing will cause the mare to produce more milk, so if the foal is otherwise vigorous a small decrease in weight might be an acceptable trade-off to encourage more rapid lactation in the first few days of treatment.

Ovarian Tumours

The equine ovary is a highly dynamic structure, with considerable changes in size relative to season of year, stage of oestrous cycle, nutritional status or disease. Ovarian neoplasia must be differentiated from normal or transient causes of ovarian enlargement and other non-neoplastic conditions. Persistent transitional follicles, paraovarian cysts, ovarian haematomas and supplementary CL are all physiological structures causing ovarian enlargement that might be confused with ovarian tumours. Although ovarian enlargement is often used as a clinical indicator of ovarian neoplasia, not all tumour types cause significant enlargement. Ovarian tumours in the mare include GCTs, teratomas, cystadenomas, adenocarcinomas, dysgerminomas, arrhenoblastomas and other metastatic tumours. Overall, the incidence of ovarian neoplasia is rare in mares. Occasionally, more than one tumour type is found within the affected ovary (Pinna *et al.*, 2019).

Granulosa cell tumours

There are many different types of ovarian tumour in mares, but the most common ovarian tumours are GCTs. GCTs typically only involve one ovary, although bilateral disease has been reported, and they are generally slow growing. Mares might be presented for evaluation due to behavioural changes such as aggression and/or stallion-like behaviour or abnormal oestrous cycles. In the author's experience, clients are poorly aware of what constitutes stallion-like behaviour, and mares might be presented for a variety of symptoms related to poor training or manners. Therefore, it is critically important that appropriate diagnostic testing is performed prior to treatment, rather than simply removing the larger of the two ovaries in a mare presented for stallion-like behaviour. Irregularities of the oestrous cycle are normal during the vernal and autumnal transition periods, for example, and occasionally pregnant mares will show aggressive behaviour during mid-gestation, secondary to testosterone production from the fetus.

Presumptive diagnosis of GCT can be attained by combining clinical examination, behavioural assessment and endocrine testing. The classic examination finding is a mare with an enlarged ovary, often without a palpable ovulation fossa, with a contralateral small, inactive ovary. The ultrasonographic appearance of GCTs are variable; classically, a honeycomb structure has been described, but the tumours can have a highly variable appearance grossly and might show as a single mass or have a large cystic cavity. The ultrasonographic appearance of ovarian haematomas can closely resemble that of GCTs. Mares with thecal cell involvement and subsequent testosterone production are more likely to show stallion-like behaviour and might even tease and attempt to serve oestrous mares. The affected ovary can be submitted for histology for definitive diagnosis.

Endocrine profiles in mares with GCTs typically show markedly elevated AMH and inhibin concentrations. Prior to the advent of AMH testing, mares were often concurrently tested for serum concentrations of inhibin, testosterone and P4. In affected mares, P4 is generally low, as they do not have normal ovulatory oestrous cycles or normal follicular development, and thus no CL is present. Inhibin concentration is increased in 90% of mares, and testosterone concentration is increased in 50–60% of mares. For increased testosterone concentrations to occur, the mare must have theca cells present in the tumour. The current preferred endocrine test to confirm GCTs in mares is AMH (Claes and Ball, 2016). The sensitivity of AMH is significantly greater than either inhibin or testosterone, or the combination of inhibin and testosterone, and results are not affected by season of year (Ball *et al.*, 2013). Occasionally, mares will yield AMH test results that are inconclusive (higher than normal but not sufficiently increased to be consistent with GCT). If clinical signs of GCTs are present, inhibin testing might be useful. Alternatively, AMH can be retested several months later.

Treatment involves removal of the affected ovary. If left untreated, GCTs can grow impressively large: the largest seen by the author was roughly the size of a beagle and spanned the entire width of the abdomen. Some mares with large tumours will present with abdominal colic due to the size of the mass. The ovary can be removed by ventral midline surgery under general anaesthesia, or as a standing procedure via the flank, or by colpotomy if the tumour is small. The author's preferred method of surgical removal is via laparoscopy of the flank; even large tumours can be removed through a relatively small incision by macerating the tumour inside a sterile plastic sleeve within the abdomen, allowing the large tissue mass to be removed in smaller pieces. Laparoscopic ovariectomy in standing sedated mares is associated with low morbidity and few complications (Röcken *et al.*, 2011). After removal of the affected ovary, most mares will resume normal reproductive function, become pregnant and carry a foal to term, assuming the absence of other reproductive disease. It often takes 6 months or more for the mare to return to reproductive cyclicity, so the opportunity for breeding is generally lost in the season when the tumour is removed.

Other ovarian tumours

Ovarian neoplasms that cause enlargement of the ovary are divided into four classes by the World Health Organization:

- *gonadostromal tumours* (GCTs, interstitial cell tumours);
- *epithelial cell tumours* (papillary adenocarcinoma);
- *mesenchymal tumours* (haemangioma, leiomyoma); and
- *germ cell tumours* (teratoma, dysgerminoma).

Some tumour types, such as mesenchymal tumours, might occur on the ovary as a primary tumour, or metastasize from different sites. Primary tumours such as adenocarcinoma, lymphoma or melanoma can metastasize to the ovary from distant sites.

Teratomas are the second most common ovarian tumour in mares, but they are still considered rare. Mares with teratomas continue to have normal oestrous cycles, and the tumours are benign and not hormonally active. Teratomas are comprised of pluripotential germ cells that undergo neoplastic differentiation into multiple germinal cell types. These different tissue types are arranged variably within the tumour such that adipose, epidermal, dental, musculoskeletal and/or nervous tissue could be found within a single mass. Teratomas can be incidental findings, but larger tumours might be associated with colic signs. Ultrasonographic appearance is variably echogenic and dependent on the tissue types comprising the mass (Catone *et al.*, 2004).

Cystadenomas are benign, rare tumours of the equine ovary. They arise from the epithelium of the follicle, medullary or cortical embryonic cords, rete ovarii, influndibulum or ovarian serosa. Cystadenomas have the ultrasonographic appearance of persistent follicles on serial examination. Generally, cystadenomas are not hormonally active, but some might secrete testosterone.

Adenocarcinoma is an extremely rare but malignant tumour of the equine ovary that arises from surface epithelial cells. These tumours metastasize by rupture and leakage of cyst contents into the peritoneal cavity. In addition to metastasis, lymphatic obstruction can occur resulting in ascites secondary to tumour seeding. Hypertrophic osteopathy secondary to metastatic ovarian adenocarcinoma has been reported in a mare (Browne *et al.*, 2016). Dysgerminomas are also malignant and exceedingly rare tumours that are not hormonally active. Mares often present with weight loss, and metastasis is rapid. Mares presenting with weight loss and unilateral ovarian enlargement should undergo thoracic radiography, and thoracic and abdominal ultrasonography to look for metastatic lesions. Metastasis to the thorax has been associated with hypertrophic osteopathy. Prognosis for both these tumour types is generally poor. In one reported case of dysgerminoma, the mare lived at least 7 months after surgical removal of the mass and became pregnant during that time. No further follow-up from the owner was provided (Harland *et al.*, 2009).

References

Aurich, C. (2011) Reproductive cycles of horses. *Animal Reproduction Science* 124(3–4), 220–228. DOI: 10.1016/j.anireprosci.2011.02.005.

Ball, B.A., Almeida, J. and Conley, A.J. (2013) Determination of serum anti-Müllerian hormone concentrations for the diagnosis of granulosa-cell tumours in mares. *Equine Veterinary Journal* 45(2), 199–203. DOI: 10.1111/j.2042-3306.2012.00594.x.

Bartolome, J.A., Wallace, S.P., de la Sota, R.L. and Thatcher, W.W. (2012) The effect of administering equine chorionic gonadotropin (eCG) and human chorionic gonadotropin (hCG) post artificial insemination on fertility of lactating dairy cows. *Theriogenology* 78(5), 1110–1116. DOI: 10.1016/j.theriogenology.2012.05.006.

Browne, N.S., Scarratt, W.K. and Robertson, J. (2016) Hypertrophic osteopathy secondary to metastatic ovarian adenocarcinoma in a mare. *The Canadian Veterinary Journal* 57(12), 1237–1241.

Caraty, A., Decourt, C., Briant, C. and Beltramo, M. (2012) Kisspeptins and the reproductive axis: potential applications to manage reproduction in farm animals.

Domestic Animal Endocrinology 43(2), 95–102. DOI: 10.1016/j.domaniend.2012.03.002.

Catone, G., Marino, G., Mancuso, R. and Zanghì, A. (2004) Clinicopathological features of an equine ovarian teratoma. *Reproduction in Domestic Animals = Zuchthygiene* 39(2), 65–69. DOI: 10.1111/j.1439-0531.2003.00476.x.

Chavatte-Palmer, P., Arnaud, G., Duvaux-Ponter, C., Brosse, L., Bougel, S. *et al.* (2002) Quantitative and qualitative assessment of milk production after pharmaceutical induction of lactation in the mare. *Journal of Veterinary Internal Medicine* 16(4), 472–477. DOI: 10.1892/0891-6640(2002)016<0472:qaqaom>2.3.co;2.

Claes, A.N.J. and Ball, B.A. (2016) Biological functions and clinical applications of anti-Müllerian hormone in stallions and mares. *The Veterinary Clinics of North America. Equine Practice* 32(3), 451–464. DOI: 10.1016/j.cveq.2016.07.004.

Cuervo-Arango, J. and Newcombe, J.R. (2009) The effect of hormone treatments (hCG and cloprostenol) and season on the incidence of hemorrhagic anovulatory follicles in the mare: a field study. *Theriogenology* 72(9), 1262–1267. DOI: 10.1016/j.theriogenology.2009.07.022.

Cuervo-Arango, J. and Newcombe, J.R. (2012) Ultrasound characteristics of experimentally induced luteinized unruptured follicles (LUF) and naturally occurring hemorrhagic anovulatory follicles (HAF) in the mare. *Theriogenology* 77(3), 514–524. DOI: 10.1016/j.theriogenology.2011.08.026.

Du, H. and Taylor, H.S. (2015) The role of Hox genes in female reproductive tract development, adult function, and fertility. *Cold Spring Harbor Perspectives in Medicine* 6(1), a023002–a023002. DOI: 10.1101/cshperspect.a023002.

Ferris, R.A. and McCue, P.M. (2010) The effects of dexamethasone and prednisolone on pituitary and ovarian function in the mare. *Equine Veterinary Journal* 42(5), 438–443. DOI: 10.1111/j.2042-3306.2010.00034.x.

Fowden, A.L., Forhead, A.J. and Ousey, J.C. (2008) The endocrinology of equine parturition. *Experimental and Clinical Endocrinology* 116, 393–403.

Galupa, R. and Heard, E. (2018) X-chromosome inactivation: a crossroads between chromosome architecture and gene regulation. *Annual Review of Genetics* 52, 535–566. DOI: 10.1146/annurev-genet-120116-024611.

Gharagozlou, F., Akbarinejad, V., Youssefi, R., Masoudifard, M. and Hasani, N. (2014) Reduced anti-Müllerian hormone (AMH) in mares with hemorrhagic anovulatory follicles. *Iranian Journal of Veterinary Research* 15(4), 336–340.

Ginther, O.J., Gastal, E.L., Gastal, M.O., Bergfelt, D.R., Baerwald, A.R. *et al.* (2004) Comparative study of the dynamics of follicular waves in mares and women. *Biology of Reproduction* 71(4), 1195–1201. DOI: 10.1095/biolreprod.104.031054.

Ginther, O.J., Gastal, E.L., Gastal, M.O. Beg, M.A, Beg, M.J.J.O.E.V.S. (2007) Incidence, endocrinology, vascularity, and morphology of hemorrhagic anovulatory follicles in mares. *Journal of Equine Veterinary Science* 27(3), 130–139. DOI: 10.1016/j.jevs.2007.01.009.

Ginther, O.J. (2012) The mare: a 1000-pound guinea pig for study of the ovulatory follicular wave in women. *Theriogenology* 77, 818–828.

Harland, S., Smith, C., Mogg, T., Horadagoda, N. and Dart, A. (2009) Surgical resection of a dysgerminoma in a mare. *Australian Veterinary Journal* 87(3), 110–112. DOI: 10.1111/j.1751-0813.2009.00392.x.

Horn, R., Bamford, N.J., Afonso, T., Sutherland, M., Buckerfield, J. *et al.* (2019) Factors associated with survival, laminitis and insulin dysregulation in horses diagnosed with equine pituitary pars intermedia dysfunction. *Equine Veterinary Journal* 51(4), 440–445. DOI: 10.1111/evj.13041.

Jacob, J.C., Gastal, E.L., Gastal, M.O., Carvalho, G.R., Beg, M.A. *et al.* (2009) Temporal relationships and repeatability of follicle diameters and hormone concentrations within individuals in mares. *Reproduction in Domestic Animals* 44(1), 92–99. DOI: 10.1111/j.1439-0531.2007.01003.x.

Kelley, D.E., Gibbons, J.R., Smith, R., Vernon, K.L., Pratt-Phillip, S.E. *et al.* (2011) Exercise affects both ovarian follicular dynamics and hormone concentrations in mares. *Theriogenology* 76, 615–622.

Krakowski, L., Brodzki, P., Krakowska, I., Opielak, G., Marczuk, J. *et al.* (2020) The level of prolactin, serum amyloid A, and selected biochemical markers in mares before and after parturition and foal heat. *Journal of Equine Veterinary Science* 84, 102854. DOI: 10.1016/j.jevs.2019.102854.

Loda, A. and Heard, E. (2019) Xist RNA in action: past, present, and future. *PLOS Genetics* 15, e1008333.

Magee, C., Foradori, C.D., Bruemmer, J.E., Arreguin-Arevalo, J.A., McCue, P.M. *et al.* (2009) Biological and anatomical evidence for kisspeptin regulation of the hypothalamic-pituitary-gonadal axis of estrous horse mares. *Endocrinology* 150, 2813–2821.

Magee, C., Bruemmer, J.E., Nett, T.M., Squires, E.L. and Clay, C.M. (2012) Kisspeptide in the estrous mare: is it an appropriate ovulation-inducing agent? *Theriogenology* 78, 1987–1996.

Numazawa, M. and Osawa, Y. (1987) Equilin and equilenin biosynthesis. Stereochemistry of aromatization of 3-hydroxy-3,5,7-androstatrien-17-one by horse placenta. *Journal of Steroid Biochemistry* 26(1), 137–143. DOI: 10.1016/0022-4731(87)90042-2.

Pinna, A.E., Okada, C.T.C., Ferreira, C.S.C., Campos, D.G., Possidente, K.S. *et al.* (2019) Double ovarian tumour in the mare: case report. *Reproduction in Domestic Animals* 54(6), 912–916. DOI: 10.1111/rda.13433.

Porter, R.H., Duchamp, G., Nowak, R. and Daels, P.F. (2002) Induction of maternal behavior in non-parturient adoptive mares. *Physiology & Behavior* 77(1), 151–154. DOI: 10.1016/S0031-9384(02)00819-3.

Prata, A.B., Drum, J.N., Melo, L.F., Araujo, E.R. and Sartori, R. (2018) Effect of different chorionic gonadotropins on final growth of the dominant follicle in Bos indicus cows. *Theriogenology* 111, 52–55.

Quinn, A. and Koopman, P. (2012) The molecular genetics of sex determination and sex reversal in mammals. *Seminars in Reproductive Medicine* 30(5), 351–363. DOI: 10.1055/s-0032-1324718.

Röcken, M., Mosel, G., Seyrek-Intas, K., Seyrek-Intas, D., Litzke, F. *et al*. (2011) Unilateral and bilateral laparoscopic ovariectomy in 157 mares: a retrospective multicenter study. *Veterinary Surgery* 40(8), n/a–1014. DOI: 10.1111/j.1532-950X.2011.00884.x.

Rohrbach, B.W., Stafford, J.R., Clermont, R.S.W., Reed, S.M., Schott, H.C. *et al*. (2012) Diagnostic frequency, response to therapy, and long-term prognosis among horses and ponies with pituitary par intermedia dysfunction, 1993-2004. *Journal of Veterinary Internal Medicine* 26(4), 1027–1034. DOI: 10.1111/j.1939-1676.2012.00932.x.

Santos, V.G., Bettencourt, E.M. and Ginther, O.J. (2015) Long-term characteristics of idiopathic persistent corpus luteum in the mare. *Theriogenology* 84, 242–251.

Senger, P.L. (2012) *Pathways to Pregnancy & Parturition*. Current Conceptions, Redmond, OR.

Sierra, I. and Anguera, M.C. (2019) Enjoy the silence: X-chromosome inactivation diversity in somatic cells. *Current Opinion in Genetics & Development* 55, 26–31. DOI: 10.1016/j.gde.2019.04.012.

Whitmore, H.L., Wentworth, B.C. and Ginther, O.J. (1973) Circulating concentrations of luteinizing hormone during estrous cycle of mares as determined by radioimmunoassay. *American Journal of Veterinary Research* 34(5), 631–636.

9 Diseases of the Male Reproductive System

Development of the Male Reproductive System

Normal sexual differentiation is dependent on establishment of normal genetic, gonadal and phenotypic sex. Genetic sex determination is established at the time of fertilization, and normal male genetic sex is an XY genotype. The initial developmental pathway is shared between both male and female mammals; primordial germ cells develop, originating from the base of the hindgut, and migrate to the gonadal ridge. These primordial germ cells will ultimately reside in the bipotential gonad, which can develop into either an ovary or testis dependent on which developmental pathway is ultimately activated.

Brain development and responsiveness to gonadotropin-releasing hormone (GnRH) is very different between male and female mammals. Whereas females develop a 'surge centre' during fetal development, testosterone produced by the fetal testis 'defeminizes' the brain and inhibits the formation of the surge centre in the male hypothalamus. In the male fetus, testosterone readily crosses the blood–brain barrier where it is converted to oestradiol (E2). Oestradiol likely acts through multiple oestrogen receptors with different specific impacts on defeminization and male behaviour (Kudwa *et al.*, 2005). Completion of the defeminization process seems to require exposure to androgens in the post-natal period, and continued exposure to these androgens ensures the surge centre remains non-functional.

The reproductive system in both sexes develops spatially and proximally close to the renal system. The developing embryo utilizes three distinct renal systems: the pronephros, mesonephros and metanephros. The pronephros is the first renal structure to develop and regresses early in embryogenesis. The mesonephros, a bilaterally-paired intermediate kidney, replaces the pronephros and begins to produce urine. Urine is diverted from the mesonephros by the bilateral mesonephric ducts, or Wölffian ducts, which extend to the urogenital sinus. The metanephros, the final form of the kidney, will develop and be functional approximately 30% of the way through gestation; the paramesonephric ducts, or Müllerian ducts, develop at approximately the same time. The development of the mesonephric and paramesonephric ducts is important as these structures will either develop into the tubular portion of the reproductive tract or regress, depending on the sex of the embryo.

In males, sexual differentiation is regulated by the sex-determining region on the Y chromosome (SRY). Production of sex-determining region protein by the primitive gonad stimulates the development of the male reproductive tract. Portions of the male reproductive tract are derived from the mesonephros; the mesonephric tubules will penetrate into the primitive gonad and form the efferent ducts, and the mesonephric ducts will develop into the epididymis and ductus deferens. Anti-Müllerian hormone (AMH) is secreted by the Sertoli cells of the developing testis and plays a critical role in the development of the male reproductive tract, resulting in the regression of the paramesonephric (Müllerian) ducts, which in females form part of the tubular reproductive tract. Serum AMH concentrations are significantly higher in neonatal colts than neonatal fillies (Claes *et al.*, 2013).

The developing testis continues to secrete AMH and dihydrotestosterone (DHT). Undifferentiated mesenchymal-like stem cells, or stem Leydig cells, are present in the interstitial compartment of the developing testis. The differentiation of these stem Leydig cells into functional adult Leydig cells is positively regulated by Desert hedgehog (DHH), lithium-induced signalling, and activating, and is negatively regulated by tumour growth factor beta (TGF-β), platelet-derived growth factor BB (PDGF-BB), fibroblast growth factor 2 (FGF-2) and the *Notch* and *Wnt* pathways (Chen *et al.*, 2017). Production of testosterone and DHT by the fetal testis is required for continued development of the male tubular tract and external genitalia. Testosterone drives the development of the male ductal (tubular) system, and DHT drives the development of the penis, scrotum and accessory sex glands. Circulating levels of testosterone also play a role in the degeneration of the paramesonephric ducts, thus inhibiting the formation of a female tubular tract.

The genital tubercle is the precursor to the penis in males or the clitoris in females. Development of the genital tubercle can be roughly divided into a 3-phase process; this developmental process has been most closely studied in mice (Haller and Ma, 2019). The first phase is the pre-androgen phase. The bilateral genital swellings emerge on either side of the cloacal membrane and continue to grow until sexually dimorphic divergence. The second phase is regulated by masculinizing genes and androgen signalling; at this phase, the developing embryo cannot readily be distinguished as male or female. In humans, defects in these phases result in abnormalities such as ambiguous genitalia or micropenis and may be related to abnormal androgen secretion. The third phase of development is more important in males than in females, due to increased distal outgrowth of the tubercle and development of the urethra throughout the length of the penis. In the equine fetus after day 40 of gestation, the tubercle begins its migration to its final anatomical position: toward the umbilicus in males or toward the tail in females (Crişan *et al.*, 2016). The position of this structure is commonly utilized to determine fetal sex after day 55 of gestation via transrectal or transabdominal ultrasonography.

Post-natally, the critical developmental periods of the stallion reproductive tract can be divided into several distinct phases: the commencement of steroidogenesis (birth to 10 months); initiation of spermatogenesis (puberty, 10–24 months); and finally, maturation (2–5 years of age) (Hess and Roser, 2005). Follicle-stimulating hormone (FSH) and luteinizing hormone (LH) play important roles in normal testicular development. FSH secretion during the fetal and post-natal periods stimulates Sertoli cell proliferation and allows for differentiation of Sertoli cells during puberty. FSH also regulates the production of paracrine factors by the Sertoli cells, which activate Leydig cell function and allow for normal testosterone production by the Leydig cells. The presence of FSH receptors in the seminiferous tubules of prepubertal colts suggests that the pregerminal cells are stimulated by the increasing FSH levels found before puberty and indicates that FSH plays a critical role in initiating and developing spermatogenesis around the time of puberty (Herrera-Luna *et al.*, 2016). LH stimulates the production of both testosterone and oestrogens by the Leydig cells. LH receptor is present in prepubertal equine seminiferous tubules, which is essential for the initiation and maintenance of testicular development post-natally, allowing testicular receptivity to LH stimulation at the time of puberty (Herrera-Luna *et al.*, 2016). In cell culture models, the Leydig cells of prepubertal colts secreted higher amounts of testosterone but lower amounts of oestrogens compared with the Leydig cells from pubertal and post-pubertal animals (Hess and Roser, 2005). The irreversible bioconversion of androgens to oestrogens is performed by aromatase P450; unusual among male mammals, the stallion testis synthesizes high amounts of oestrogens and this is required for normal regulation of reproductive function including germ cell survival and development (Hess and Roser, 2005; Carreau and Hess, 2010). As age increases, there is an increase in the expression of aromatase, indicating the importance of oestrogens for maintenance of normal testicular function in the stallion (Herrera-Luna *et al.*, 2016). Evaluation of histology sections has revealed that both Sertoli cells and Leydig cells participate in oestrogen synthesis (Sipahutar *et al.*, 2003).

Puberty and the attainment of sexual maturity have been less well studied in horses than in production species, as they are less economically relevant to the horse industry. The onset of puberty has been defined in colts as the ability to produce an ejaculate containing ≥50 million total spermatozoa, with ≥10% motile sperm in one study (Naden *et al.*, 1990); however, this is not a practical benchmark as using semen parameters to define puberty in colts would require that the colt is mature enough to display good libido and breeding behaviour for semen collection. Puberty in colts is associated with increases in serum testosterone and rapid growth, and has been shown to correspond with exponential testicular growth, an increase in body weight and increased plasma inhibin B, but unlike in ruminants, does not correspond with increases in body fat, insulin-like growth factor 1 (IGF-1), or leptin (Ellerbrock *et al.*, 2018). This suggests that body fat may not regulate the onset of puberty in the same manner as in ruminants.

Endocrine–Autocrine–Paracrine Regulation of Reproductive Function

Normal testicular function in stallions requires a functional feedback loop between the hypothalamus, pituitary and testes. The hypothalamic–pituitary–gonadal axis is regulated by the actions of several key hormones including GnRH, LH, FSH, testosterone, oestradiol and inhibin. These hormones play key roles in both male and female reproduction and are discussed in greater detail in Chapter 8. Discussion here will be limited to the specific functions of these hormones in the male reproductive tract. Prolactin (PRL) concentration fluctuates seasonally in stallions and is suspected to play an important role in seasonality in mares, but its function in stallions has not yet been fully elucidated (Thompson *et al.*, 1987; Roser, 2008). Inhibin B is the major bioactive form of inhibin in the equine testes and is secreted by both the Leydig and Sertoli cells (Taya *et al.*, 2000).

Seasonality shows less of an effect on reproduction in stallions compared to other seasonally-reproducing species, such as sheep. For example, although there are histological changes in the stallion testis during periods of short day length, he continues to produce sufficient numbers of spermatozoa to retain fertility year round. The most notable change is the increase in daily sperm production directly associated with an increase in type-A spermatogonia (Johnson and Thompson, 1983; Johnson, 1985). The primary regulator of seasonal changes is day length, and subsequently melatonin; melatonin is produced in periods of relative darkness, and therefore is produced in higher levels during autumn and winter months. Melatonin suppresses GnRH output. As day length increases after the winter solstice, this GnRH suppression is reduced and GnRH can then be produced at high levels to optimize testicular function. LH stimulates the production of testosterone from the Leydig cells in the testis, and FSH stimulates production of oestradiol, inhibin and activin from the Sertoli cells. Since the male mammalian brain does not develop a GnRH surge centre, LH is produced in a pulsatile fashion approximately every 2 h. The production of testosterone results in a classic feedback loop, inhibiting further LH secretion. Secretion of key reproductive hormones, such as inhibin, steroid hormones and gonadotropins, are higher during the breeding season than during the non-breeding season (Taya *et al.*, 2000). The steroid content of ejaculated semen also varies with season, with an oestrogenic profile during the breeding season and a higher oestrogen/androgen ratio than in the non-breeding season (Lemazurier *et al.*, 2002).

The effect of the potent GnRH agonist, deslorelin, was investigated in Shetland pony stallions (Gautier *et al.*, 2018). In dogs, a commercially available product is available for non-surgical control of reproduction via its down regulation of the hypothalamic–pituitary–gonadal axis. In stallions, deslorelin implants have been shown to modulate pituitary function but do not down regulate spermatogenesis.

Spermatogenesis

Spermatogenesis is the process of division and differentiation of germ cells within the seminiferous tubules, resulting in the production of spermatozoa. The seminiferous tubules contain two large cell populations: the somatic cells and the germ cells. The somatic cells include myoid cells and Sertoli cells, which are the 'caretakers' of the developing spermatozoa. In stallions, Sertoli cell number is not fixed but fluctuates with season (Johnson *et al.*, 2008). The germ cells include the spermatogonia, spermatocytes and spermatids. Unlike the mare, which is born without the capacity to develop more oocytes with age, stallions will continue to produce spermatozoa throughout their lifetime. In stallions and other male mammals, spermatogenesis and steroidogenesis are controlled largely by the actions of LH and FSH, acting through their receptors. Sertoli cell function is regulated by FSH; thus, FSH plays a major role in regulating spermatogenesis.

Spermatogenesis can be further divided into spermatocytogenesis, meiosis and spermiogenesis. During spermatocytogenesis, the mitosis occurs, allowing continued division and replication of spermatogenic stem cells and primary spermatocytes. These cell types are diploid, containing 64 chromosomes. The spermatogonia are located at the base of the seminiferous tubules and continue to undergo mitosis to continue the stem cell lineage. Five subtypes of spermatogonia have been described in stallions: A1, A2, A3, B1 and B2. Each subtype is described by differences in nuclear structure. The type-B2 spermatogonia divide into the preleptotene primary spermatocytes. Degeneration of excess germ cells is required at this stage to ensure that the

Sertoli cell population can sustain continued development of the spermatozoa.

Meiosis is required in order to reduce the diploid spermatocytes into haploid spermatids. During meiosis, genetic material is also exchanged between homologous chromosomes. Chromosomal duplication occurs in the preleptotene phase; genetic material is exchanged during the zygotene phase. As the chromosomes duplicate once and undergo two meiotic divisions, the resulting product is the haploid spermatid.

During spermiogenesis, the spermatids undergo morphologic differentiation into spermatozoa. The spermatids produced in the second meiotic division differentiate from spherical cells with spherical nuclei into a highly specialized cell with a streamlined head containing condensed nuclei and a specialized flagellum. The acrosome of the spermatozoon is a vesicle of hydrolytic enzymes which envelops its nucleus; it is derived from the Golgi apparatus. The tail of the spermatozoon is comprised of: a capitulum, which fits into the implantation socket in the head, the middle piece, principle piece and terminal piece. The proximal portions of the tail consist of laminated columns, allowing flexibility and the generation of the flagellar beat. The axoneme is comprised of nine pairs of microtubules that are arranged radially around the two central filaments. The mitochondrial helix is located on the middle piece and provides an energy source for generation of the flagellar beat.

The stallion produces gametes continually and relatively uniformly with minor variations in spermatogonia populations related to season. The cycle of the seminiferous epithelium is the progression through a complete series of stages at one location along the seminiferous tubule. The time required for this progression is 12.2 days in stallions (Senger, 2012). The complete process of spermatogenesis from type-A spermatogonia to fully differentiated spermatozoa is approximately 55 days in stallions, or 4.5 cycles of the seminiferous epithelium.

The blood–testis barrier is an important structure in the mammalian testis that separates the diploid spermatocytes from haploid spermatozoa during development. This structure also protects the haploid sperm cells from recognition and destruction by the immune system, as their haploid structure would otherwise be recognized as foreign tissue. The blood–testis barrier is formed between adjacent Sertoli cells during puberty by a complex of different junction types and divides the seminiferous epithelium into the basal compartment with spermatogonia and primary spermatocytes, and an adluminal compartment containing more developing germ cells. The equine junctional complex contains claudin-11, ZO-1, N-cadherin and Cx43; these junctional proteins shift from a diffuse distribution to a basal distribution as tubular development progresses during puberty (Rode *et al.*, 2015).

There are several factors that can affect spermatogenesis in stallions, including dietary deficiency, infectious disease, toxins, stress-related hormones and thermal stress. Some toxins that have been found to alter the normal process of spermatogenesis include anabolic steroids, heavy metals such as cadmium and lead, radiation and dioxin (Johnson *et al.*, 1997). Toxic ergot alkaloids, such as those found in tall fescue grass, do not appear to have an effect on spermatogenesis in adult stallions but have altered sex chromosomes in pachytene spermatocytes in yearling colts (Fayrer-Hosken *et al.*, 2012). In stallions, as in most mammals, the testes are located extra-abdominally. This allows the testes to be maintained at a slightly cooler temperature compared to core body temperature, and this temperature gradient is required for normal spermatogenesis to occur. In an experimental model where the scrota of pony stallions were insulated to increase scrotal temperature, thermal injury resulted in decreases in plasma testosterone, LH, oestradiol and FSH for variable periods of time after the insulation was removed (Blanchard *et al.*, 2000). The potential daily sperm output was also decreased for early primary spermatocytes and late primary spermatocytes; testosterone supplementation did not mitigate the effects of insulation, implying that impaired spermatogenesis was not solely due to altered steroid concentrations. The effect of treatment with therapeutic doses of dexamethasone in stallions was recently investigated; stallions receiving dexamethasone treatment had decreased serum testosterone levels up to 94% from 4–20 h after treatment and alterations in heat shock protein *DNAJC4* and sperm-specific calcium channel *CATSPER1* mRNA (Ing *et al.*, 2015). Both of these genes have been related to male fertility in other species.

Examination of the different cell populations within the testis can be a useful diagnostic test to determine if spermatogenesis is occurring normally, to investigate azoospermia or oligozoospermia, or to assess palpable or ultrasound abnormalities such as a testicular mass or degeneration. Several methods of testicular biopsy have been described in stallions, including fine needle aspirate of testicular tissue, open surgical biopsy, punch biopsy and needle biopsy. Fine needle aspirates are inexpensive and easy to obtain but provide the least amount of diagnostic information and no information on testicular architecture. Open biopsy, such as a wedge resection or surgical biopsy, is performed under general anaesthesia and carries the highest risk of complications, although these complications do resolve with time (Delvento *et al.*, 1992). The open technique is not recommended as there are simpler techniques with lower complication rates that provide excellent quality diagnostic samples. Testicular biopsy can be performed in stallions using standing sedation and local anaesthesia. Spring-loaded needle biopsy using a commercially available instrument (14 g needle instrument) yields a small core of testicular tissue that can be used to evaluate spermatogenesis or other pathology within the testis. The safety of this procedure in stallions has been long established, with no apparent detrimental effects on stallion fertility (Faber and Roser, 2000; Pearson *et al.*, 2011). Needle biopsy can be performed under ultrasound guidance to select a tissue sample from a specific lesion or site. Care must be taken in placing the needle tip to avoid the head of the epididymis, major blood vessels or central vein. Although needle biopsy is well tolerated, reported complications include haemorrhage, scrotal adhesion and infection. Non-steroidal anti-inflammatory drugs administered post procedure may help reduce scrotal swelling and patient discomfort.

Cryopreservation of spermatozoa is routinely performed in clinical practice, with variable success largely dependent on the individual stallion factors. Recently, researchers investigated the feasibility of cryopreserving spermatogonial stem cells, which would allow unlimited production of spermatogenic cell lineages (Costa *et al.*, 2017). This technique would provide major advantages in fertility preservation as the genetic potential of an individual stallion could be continually replenished. Experimentally, an efficient protocol for preservation of equine spermatogonial stem cells has been established, with a slow-freezing method using dimethyl sulfoxide as a cryoprotectant having the best results. This biotechnology is still in its infancy and is not yet readily clinically available but holds great promise for assisted reproductive technologies in the stallion.

Cryptorchidism

Cryptorchidism is the failure of one or both testes to descend into the scrotum and is the most common reproductive disorder seen in stallions. Approximately 2–8% of male horses are affected by this disorder. In other species, cryptorchidism is strongly suspected to be a heritable disorder, and thus affected males are not used for breeding purposes. Definitive evidence is lacking in stallions as to the heritability of this condition, but the majority of breed registries require that stallions be examined to have two normally descended testes in order to be registered for breeding purposes. Bilaterally cryptorchid animals are extremely subfertile or sterile as the testes are maintained at too high a temperature for normal spermatogenesis to occur.

Normal testicular descent occurs in two phases: the transabdominal phase and the inguinal-scrotal phase. During embryogenesis, the testes lie in a retroperitoneal position within the abdomen, and development during the transabdominal phase is regulated by insulin-like growth factor 3 (IGF-3). The gubernaculum, a ligamentous structure, is attached caudally to the testis. The gubernaculum is infiltrated by cells from the peritoneum, which attach the gubernaculum to the body wall. The distal gubernaculum grows toward and into the scrotal region; once it penetrates the inguinal ring, there is rapid growth of the distal portion of the gubernaculum.

The rapid growth of the gubernaculum drives the testis into the inguinal canal; this initiates the beginning of the inguinal-scrotal phase and is androgen dependent. Once the testes are in the inguinal ring, they will continue to descend through the inguinal canal as the gubernaculum retracts and shrinks. Growth of the abdominal viscera may also help 'push' the testes through the inguinal canal due to a reduction of space in the abdomen. As the gubernaculum continues to shrink, the testes are pulled further into the scrotum, and each testis is encapsulated by a layer of peritoneum which will become the visceral vaginal tunic. Once the testis is fully descended, the gubernaculum will regress and anchor the testis.

Cryptorchidism is diagnosed by a combination of careful history, clinical examination, endocrine testing and ultrasonography. A colt or stallion with no history of castration or attempted castration, with a single, or no, palpable testes within the scrotum should be suspected to be cryptorchid. A greater diagnostic challenge is presented by the apparent gelding with stallion-like behaviour and an unknown castration history. A common historical finding in these cases is recent acquisition of the animal, who may have appeared behaviourally normal at the time of purchase. Many owners are not aware of what comprises normal stallion behaviour, and general poor manners are often described as 'stallion-like behaviour'. To further complicate matters, geldings will occasionally serve mares in oestrus and display fairly normal libido and breeding behaviour. This phenomenon is thought to occur more frequently in stallions castrated later in life, as a component of breeding behaviour is learned.

Endocrine testing for diagnosis of cryptorchidism includes evaluation of AMH, human chorionic gonadotropin (hCG) challenge testing or oestrone sulfate measurement. Measurement of random, baseline testosterone is unlikely to yield definitive results due to the pulsatile nature of its release, but a single elevated testosterone level is supportive of the presence of testicular tissue. Histologically, cryptorchid tests show characteristics of failure of maturation of the Sertoli cells and/or lack of testosterone suppression, demonstrated by an increase in AMH and AMH receptor 2 immunolabelling (Almeida *et al.*, 2013). AMH testing is the preferred endocrine diagnostic test for cryptorchidism in post-pubertal stallions as it is readily available and only requires a single blood sample. Serum AMH concentrations are higher in cryptorchid stallions than in either normal stallions or geldings, making this a very useful biomarker for cryptorchidism (Claes *et al.*, 2013). Due to its role in normal reproductive development, AMH is elevated in young colts and is an inconclusive biomarker for cryptorchidism in prepubertal colts (Scarlet *et al.*, 2018). There is a single case report of a cryptorchid Thoroughbred stallion that had negative AMH and hCG challenge test results, despite having a small testis present in the abdomen (Murase *et al.*, 2020). The authors of the study suggested that the failure of detection of either AMH or testosterone from hCG challenge may have been due to low numbers of Sertoli and/or Leydig cells present in the tissue. Oestrone sulfate can be measured in a single plasma sample as an indicator for testicular tissue in suspected cryptorchids; it is not accurate in donkeys or in horses less than 3 years of age (Cox *et al.*, 1986). Challenge testing with hCG can be utilized to identify testicular tissue in horses, as its LH-like effect results in increased testosterone production. An initial baseline testosterone sample is collected, then 10,000 IU hCG is administered intravenously. A second blood sample is collected 2 h after administration of hCG; testosterone levels will continue to rise for 24–48 h after injection, so the second blood sample can be collected the following day if necessary.

In addition to endocrine testing, abdominal or transrectal ultrasonography can be used to visualize the presence of the testis. Ultrasound examination should include the inguinal rings, as the cryptorchid testis can be located in either the abdomen or inguinal areas. The left and right testes are retained with equal frequency; the left testis is more likely to be found abdominally than in the inguinal space. A technique for reliably locating an abdominal testis using ultrasound has been described (Jann and Rains, 1990; Schambourg *et al.*, 2006); however, in the author's experience, locating the testis using this technique is more variable than the reported results. Transrectal palpation of the inguinal rings and ampullae can be used as landmarks to aid in finding an abdominal testis using either palpation or transrectal ultrasonography. The major disadvantage to transrectal ultrasonography is the risk of injury to the operator or rectal tears in the patient, but this can be reduced or mitigated with sedation and adequate restraint in many cases.

Treatment of cryptorchidism is straightforward in cases with no prior surgical history, as the laterality of the hidden testis is known. The author prefers to perform cryptordectomy via laparoscopy, although other techniques including blind, inguinal approaches have been described. Detailed surgical instruction is beyond the scope of this text, and many equine surgical centres routinely perform laparoscopic cryptordectomy. In all cases, it is advised that the cryptorchid rather than descended testis is removed first; if for some reason the cryptorchid testis cannot be located, the horse is still obviously cryptorchid on clinical examination. If the descended testis was removed first and complications were encountered in locating or removing the cryptorchid testis, the horse could then be mistaken for a gelding in the future.

Testicular Neoplasia

Testicular neoplasia occurs relatively infrequently in horses, but the true incidence is difficult to determine as the majority of young colts are castrated early in life (Schumacher, 1999). Clinical signs of testicular neoplasia include non-painful scrotal swelling. Testicular tumours must be differentiated from other causes of non-painful scrotal swelling such as hydrocele. At least one case has reported a stallion presenting with acute colic due to testicular neoplasia in a descended testis (May *et al.*, 1999). Ultrasonography can be very useful at both identifying testicular tumours and identifying other causes of scrotal enlargement; normal testicular parenchyma is uniformly echogenic. Infectious or inflammatory diseases of the testes typically cause palpable heat and discomfort. Equine testicular neoplasms can be broadly classified as germinal or non-germinal tumours. Germinal tumours include seminomas, teratomas, teratocarcinomas and embryonic carcinomas. Non-germinal testicular neoplasms reported in equines include Leydig cell tumours, Sertoli cell tumours, lipomas and mast cell tumours.

Seminomas

Seminomas are the most frequently reported tumours of adult stallions (Brinsko, 1998). Seminomas do not appear to be hormonally active and arise from the neoplastic transformation of germ cells. Sonographically, seminomas appear less echogenic than the surrounding testicular parenchyma, are uniform and homogenous in appearance, have sharply demarcated borders and are frequently multifocal (Beck *et al.*, 2001). This tumour type typically grows rapidly and often occupies the majority of the testicular parenchyma by the time of diagnosis. Seminomas can form in descended or cryptorchid testes and can occur unilaterally or bilaterally. The development of seminomas in cryptorchid testes is common in humans and dogs, and there may be a similar association in stallions (Brinsko, 1998). However, a direct causal relationship between cryptorchidism and seminomas has not been established (Schumacher, 1999). Seminomas typically occur in middle-aged to older stallions and seem to have a greater malignant tendency than in other species. Thus, although the majority of seminomas are benign they should be regarded as potentially malignant (Brinsko, 1998). Metastasis, when it occurs, is typically in the abdominal or thoracic viscera and carries a poor prognosis.

Teratomas

Teratomas are benign tumours that are more commonly found in the cryptorchid testes of young horses. These tumours occur most commonly in horses and are rare in other species. Teratomas arise from pluripotential stem cells and comprise multiple non-testicular tissue types. Teratomas can contain tissues that arise from any embryonic germ cell layer including bone, cartilage, epithelium, hair or teeth. Due to their cystic nature and unique ultrasonographic and morphological features, transabdominal ultrasonography may be helpful in surgical planning (Pasolini *et al.*, 2016). Other tumours that arise from pluripotential stem cells include teratocarcinomas and embryonal carcinomas, but both are considered extremely rare (Brinsko, 1998). Teratocarcinomas will contain both primitive and mature germ cell tissue. Embryonal carcinomas develop from poorly differentiated germ cells. Both are considered highly malignant as the undifferentiated tissue components will continue to proliferate.

Leydig cell tumours

Leydig cell tumours are also referred to as *interstitial tumours* or *interstitial cell adenomas*. They arise from the Leydig (interstitial) cells of the testis, and can be unilateral, bilateral, single or multiple masses. These are slow-growing tumours with a low potential to metastasize. As the Leydig cell tumour grows, it results in pressure atrophy and degeneration of the surrounding seminiferous tubules, resulting in negative impacts to semen quality. Despite their origin in androgen-producing Leydig cells, these tumours rarely result in abnormal levels of androgen production (Brinsko, 1998).

Sertoli cell tumours

Sertoli cell tumours are also known as *sustenacular tumours* and arise from the Sertoli cells of the seminiferous tubules. They are considered rare in stallions and appear grossly similar to seminomas. The testicular feminization syndrome reported in dogs with Sertoli cell tumours does not appear to occur in stallions.

Treatment of testicular tumours

Treatment of testicular tumours is the same regardless of tumour type; gonadectomy of the affected testis is recommended. The entire testis should be submitted for histopathology. A combination of testicular neoplasms is uncommonly reported in horses but occurs commonly in other species such as dogs and humans (Brinsko, 1998). A bilateral mixed germ cell–sex cord stromal tumour has been reported in a stallion (Brito *et al.*, 2009). In the case of abdominal or cryptorchid testes, laparoscopy has been described as a minimally invasive technique for removing even large testicular tumours (Cribb and Bouré, 2010). Hemicastration, performed when the remaining testis is otherwise normal, can preserve fertility in breeding stallions with unilateral testicular neoplasia.

Hypogonadism

Hypogonadism is a pathological disorder of the hypothalamic–pituitary–gonadal axis whereby the testes do not produce sufficient testosterone or adequate spermatozoa (Yeap *et al.*, 2016); this condition is well recognized in the human literature, but not as well characterized in domestic animals. Hypogonadism can be due to congenital or acquired defects of the testes, or a failure of hypothalamic–pituitary stimulation. Hypotrophic hypogonadism has not been reported in the stallion, but therapy with GnRH has improved fertility in a limited number of horses (Brinsko, 1996). GnRH therapy is unlikely to be helpful in most cases but is also unlikely to be harmful; stallions should be thoroughly investigated for other causes of subfertility before considering this therapy.

Idiopathic Testicular Degeneration

Although stallions continue to produce spermatozoa throughout their lifetime, age-related decline in spermatozoa quality and testicular function is not uncommon. This is commonly referred to as age-related or idiopathic testicular degeneration, differentiating this condition from the testicular degeneration that can occur after a specific event, such as heat stress or trauma. Typically, stallions with idiopathic testicular degeneration are presented for evaluation of reduced fertility or reduced pregnancy rates as opposed to noticeable changes due to reduced levels of circulating androgens. Early in the disease process, improved management of the stallion and/or the addition of assisted reproductive techniques may allow continuation of the stallion's breeding career for a period of time.

The onset of testicular degeneration is variable; although some stallions maintain high fertility into their twenties, others will begin to show evidence of decline in fertility from the mid-teen years. Accurate clinical diagnosis requires a history of declining fertility, as the histopathological lesions associated with testicular degeneration cannot be distinguished from testicular hypoplasia. Careful assessment of the stallion's history is necessary to determine if testicular degeneration is indeed idiopathic or age related, or if there is an identifiable inciting cause. Evaluation of historical breeding records, including the per cycle pregnancy rate for mares bred to the stallion, can help identify early trends in fertility.

Serial evaluation of several parameters can be helpful in diagnosis. Over time, stallions with testicular degeneration will demonstrate a decrease in testicular volume. Repeated testicular volume measurements performed at regular intervals will help determine if a decreasing trend is present. Care must be taken to account for season of year, as stallions will have changes in testicular volume between the breeding and non-breeding seasons. Serial semen analysis can monitor for total sperm number in the ejaculate as well as for trends in motility and morphologically normal spermatozoa. The presence of immature spermatogenic cells (round cells) in the spermiogram is characteristic of testicular degeneration (Turner, 2019).

Endocrinology evaluation is typically unrewarding. Seasonal and daily variations in circulating hormones have been well established in stallions, making interpretation of endocrine testing difficult. In severe cases, elevated FSH and LH and low oestradiol may be seen (Turner, 2019). Typically, endocrine changes are preceded by changes in testicular size and character as well as spermiogram characteristics, making hormonal assay unnecessary. Recently, AMH was evaluated as a marker of testicular damage in stallions due to toxic insults that lead to testicular degeneration (Pozor *et al.*, 2018); further research is required to determine if AMH can also be used as a biomarker of idiopathic testicular degeneration.

Treatment of stallions with idiopathic testicular degeneration is largely focused on better management to improve breeding efficiency, as there is no treatment available to reverse the process of testicular degeneration. Lack of gonadotropins does not appear to be the underlying cause of this disease process (Turner and Zeng, 2012; Turner, 2019). Docosahexaenoic acid (DHA), a fat-soluble antioxidant, is frequently recommended in cases of idiopathic testicular degeneration, but there is no literature supporting its benefit in improving function in diseased testes. If the disease process is unilateral, hemicastration can be attempted. Proponents of this treatment advocate that hemicastration reduces the risk of anti-sperm antibody formation from the diseased testis and allows the contralateral testis to undergo hypertrophy for improved semen output. Hypertrophy is only likely to occur in a normal testis; unilateral castration is not recommended if the contralateral testis is showing signs of disease. Semen cryopreservation can be performed in stallions whose breed registries allow the use of artificial insemination as a means of prolonging the breeding career of that stallion.

Intersex Conditions

A true hermaphrodite, where both testicular and ovarian tissue are present, is extremely rare in horses. Male pseudohermaphrodites, still uncommon, have an XY genotype and ambiguous external genitalia. Most commonly, the external genitalia appear as a vulva with an enlarged clitoris or glans penis. There is one reported case of an agonadal colt with a male karyotype and pseudohermaphrodite phenotype (Kuiper *et al.*, 2010).

Klinefelter's syndrome has also been reported in horses (Kubień *et al.*, 1993; Mäkinen *et al.*, 2000). Klinefelter's syndrome is a clinical disorder characterized by gonadal dysgenesis and infertility and is associated with extra X chromosomes in males. Males with Klinefelter's syndrome generally have a normal phenotype. The most frequent chromosomal configuration is XXY. One animal had an XXXY genotype, hypoplastic abdominal testes, an infantile female tubular tract and vulvar lips with glans penis protruding at the ventral aspect (Gluhovschi *et al.*, 1970). Klinefelter's syndrome can be difficult to diagnose in stallions prior to puberty.

Intersex conditions in horses can be diagnosed via clinical examination, karyotyping, endocrine testing and histopathology of the gonads. Typical complaints in intersex animals with a Y chromosome are related to stallion-like behaviour, secondary to testosterone production by the gonads in an 'apparently female' animal. Castration will likely resolve the offending behaviours, and although affected animals are unsuitable for breeding they can generally be used for other sport or leisure activities.

References

Almeida, J., Conley, A.J. and Ball, B.A. (2013) Expression of anti-Müllerian hormone, CDKN1B, connexin 43, androgen receptor and steroidogenic enzymes in the equine cryptorchid testis. *Equine Veterinary Journal* 45(5), 538–545. DOI: 10.1111/evj.12013.

Beck, C., Charles, J.A. and Maclean, A.A. (2001) Ultrasound appearance of an equine testicular seminoma. *Veterinary Radiology Ultrasound* 42(4), 355–357. DOI: 10.1111/j.1740-8261.2001.tb00954.x.

Blanchard, T., Varner, D., Johnson, L., Roser, J., Hill, J. *et al.* (2000) Testicular and hormonal changes in stallions with thermally induced testicular degeneration. *Journal of Reproduction and Fertility. Supplement* (56), 51–59.

Brinsko, S.P. (1996) Gnrh therapy for subfertile stallions. *The Veterinary Clinics of North America. Equine Practice* 12(1), 149–160. DOI: 10.1016/s0749-0739(17)30301-2.

Brinsko, S.P. (1998) Neoplasia of the male reproductive tract. *The Veterinary Clinics of North America. Equine Practice* 14(3), 517–533. DOI: 10.1016/S0749-0739(17)30184-0.

Brito, L.F.C., Engiles, J.B., Turner, R.M., Getman, L.M. and Ebling, A. (2009) Bilateral testicular mixed germ cell-sex cord-stromal tumours in a stallion. *Reproduction in Domestic Animals* 44(5), 846–851. DOI: 10.1111/j.1439-0531.2008.01090.x.

Carreau, S. and Hess, R.A. (2010) Oestrogens and spermatogenesis. *Philosophical Transactions of the Royal Society B: Biological Sciences* 365(1546), 1517–1535. DOI: 10.1098/rstb.2009.0235.

Chen, H., Wang, Y., Ge, R. and Zirkin, B.R. (2017) Leydig cell stem cells: identification, proliferation and differentiation. *Molecular and Cellular Endocrinology* 445, 65–73. DOI: 10.1016/j.mce.2016.10.010.

Claes, A., Ball, B.A., Almeida, J., Corbin, C.J. and Conley, A.J. (2013) Serum anti-Müllerian hormone concentrations in stallions: developmental changes, seasonal variation, and differences between intact stallions, cryptorchid stallions, and geldings. *Theriogenology* 79(9), 1229–1235. DOI: 10.1016/j.theriogenology.2013.03.019.

Costa, G.M.J., Avelar, G.F., Lacerda, S.M.S.N., Figueiredo, A.F.A., Tavares, A.O. *et al.* (2017) Horse spermatogonial stem cell cryopreservation: feasible protocols and potential biotechnological applications. *Cell and Tissue Research* 370(3), 489–500. DOI: 10.1007/s00441-017-2673-1.

Cox, J.E., Redhead, P.H. and Dawson, F.E. (1986) Comparison of the measurement of plasma testosterone and plasma oestrogens for the diagnosis of cryptorchidism in the horse. *Equine Veterinary Journal* 18(3), 179–182. DOI: 10.1111/j.2042-3306.1986.tb03589.x.

Cribb, N.C. and Bouré, L.P. (2010) Laparoscopic removal of a large abdominal testicular teratoma in a standing horse. *Veterinary Surgery* 39(1), 131–135. DOI: 10.1111/j.1532-950X.2009.00618.x.

Crișan, M.I., Damian, A., Morar, I., Páll, E., Peștean, C. *et al.* (2016) Equine Embryo Sexing and Ultrasonographic Foetal Sexing - Interests and Applicability. *Anatomia, Histologia, Embryologia* 45(5), 329–337. DOI: 10.1111/ahe.12205.

Delvento, V.R., Amann, R.P., Trotter, G.W., Veeramachaneni, D.N. and Squires, E.L. (1992) Ultrasonographic and quantitative histologic assessment of sequelae to testicular biopsy in stallions. *American Journal of Veterinary Research* 53(11), 2094–2101.

Ellerbrock, R.E., Canisso, I.F., Lima, F.S., Shipley, C.F., Thompson, D.L. *et al.* (2018) Endocrine and metabolic profile of peripubertal standardbred colts. *Theriogenology* 117, 78–84. DOI: 10.1016/j.theriogenology.2018.05.006.

Faber, N.F. and Roser, J.F. (2000) Testicular biopsy in stallions: diagnostic potential and effects on prospective fertility. *Journal of reproduction and fertility. Supplement* (56), 31–42.

Fayrer-Hosken, R., Stanley, A., Hill, N., Heusner, G., Christian, M. *et al.* (2012) Effect of feeding fescue seed containing ergot alkaloid toxins on stallion spermatogenesis and sperm cells. *Reproduction in Domestic Animals* 47(6), 1017–1026. DOI: 10.1111/j.1439-0531.2012.02008.x.

Gautier, C., Schmidt, K., Aurich, J. and Aurich, C. (2018) Effects of implants containing the GnRH agonist deslorelin on testosterone release and semen characteristics in Shetland stallions. *Animal Reproduction Science* 195, 230–241. DOI: 10.1016/j.anireprosci.2018.05.027.

Gluhovschi, N., Bistriceanu, M., Suciu, A. and Bratu, M. (1970) A case of intersexuality in the horse with type 2A+XXXY chromosome formula. *British Veterinary Journal* 126(10), 522–525. DOI: 10.1016/S0007-1935(17)48137-1.

Haller, M. and Ma, L. (2019) Temporal, spatial, and genetic regulation of external genitalia development. *Differentiation* 110, 1–7. DOI: 10.1016/j.diff.2019.08.003.

Herrera-Luna, C.V., Scarlet, D., Walter, I. and Aurich, C. (2016) Effect of stallion age on the expression of LH and FSH receptors and aromatase P450 in equine male reproductive tissues. *Reproduction, Fertility and Development* 28(12), 2016–2026. DOI: 10.1071/RD15027.

Hess, M.F. and Roser, J.F. (2005) A comparison of the effects of equine luteinizing hormone (eLH), equine growth hormone (eGH) and human recombinant insulin-like growth factor (hrIGF-I) on steroid production in cultured equine Leydig cells during sexual maturation. *Animal Reproduction Science* 89(1–4), 7–19. DOI: 10.1016/j.anireprosci.2005.06.014.

Ing, N.H., Brinsko, S.P., Curley, K.O., Forrest, D.W., Love, C.C. *et al.* (2015) Dexamethasone acutely regulates endocrine parameters in stallions and subsequently affects gene expression in testicular germ cells. *Animal Reproduction Science* 152, 47–54. DOI: 10.1016/j.anireprosci.2014.11.007.

Jann, H.W. and Rains, J.R. (1990) Diagnostic ultrasonography for evaluation of cryptorchidism in horses. *Journal of the American Veterinary Medical Association* 196(2), 297–300.

Johnson, L. (1985) Increased daily sperm production in the breeding season of stallions is explained by an elevated population of spermatogonia. *Biology of Reproduction* 32(5), 1181–1190. DOI: 10.1095/biolreprod32.5.1181.

Johnson, L. and Thompson, D.L. (1983) Age-related and seasonal variation in the Sertoli cell population, daily sperm production and serum concentrations of follicle-stimulating hormone, luteinizing hormone and testosterone in stallions. *Biology of Reproduction* 29(3), 777–789. DOI: 10.1095/biolreprod29.3.777.

Johnson, L., Blanchard, T.L., Varner, D.D. and Scrutchfield, W.L. (1997) Factors affecting spermatogenesis in the stallion. *Theriogenology* 48(7), 1199–1216. DOI: 10.1016/S0093-691X(97)00353-1.

Johnson, L., Thompson, D.L. and Varner, D.D. (2008) Role of Sertoli cell number and function on regulation of spermatogenesis. *Animal Reproduction Science* 105(1–2), 23–51. DOI: 10.1016/j.anireprosci.2007.11.029.

Kubień, E.M., Pozor, M.A. and Tischner, M. (1993) Clinical, cytogenetic and endocrine evaluation of a horse with a 65,XXY karyotype. *Equine Veterinary Journal* 25(4), 333–335. DOI: 10.1111/j.2042-3306.1993.tb02976.x.

Kudwa, A.E., Bodo, C., Gustafsson, J.-A. and Rissman, E.F. (2005) A previously uncharacterized role for estrogen receptor beta: defeminization of male brain and behavior. *Proceedings of the National Academy of Sciences* 102(12), 4608–4612. DOI: 10.1073/pnas.0500752102.

Kuiper, H., Blum, N. and Distl, C. (2010) An XY agonadal Oldenburg warmblood horse exhibiting a male phenotype. *Sexual Development* 4(6), 348–351. DOI: 10.1159/000321075.

Lemazurier, E., Moslemi, S., Sourdaine, P., Desjardins, I., Plainfosse, B. *et al.* (2002) Free and conjugated estrogens and androgens in stallion semen. *General and Comparative Endocrinology* 125(2), 272–282. DOI: 10.1006/gcen.2001.7747.

May, K.A., Moll, H.D., Duncan, R.B., Pleasant, R.S. and Purswell, B.J. (1999) Unilateral Leydig cell tumour resulting in acute colic and scrotal swelling in a stallion with descended testes. *Equine Veterinary Journal* 31(4), 343–345. DOI: 10.1111/j.2042-3306.1999.tb03828.x.

Murase, H., Ochi, A., Tozaki, T., Kakoi, H., Munkhtuul, T. *et al*. (2020) A case of equine cryptorchidism with undetectable serum anti-Müllerian hormone. *Journal of Veterinary Medical Science* 82(2), 209–211. DOI: 10.1292/jvms.18-0057.

Mäkinen, A., Katila, T., Andersson, M. and Gustavsson, I. (2000) Two sterile stallions with XXY-syndrome. *Equine Veterinary Journal* 32(4), 358–360. DOI: 10.2746/042516400777032138.

Naden, J., Amann, R.P. and Squires, E.L. (1990) Testicular growth, hormone concentrations, seminal characteristics and sexual behaviour in stallions. *Reproduction* 88(1), 167–176. DOI: 10.1530/jrf.0.0880167.

Pasolini, M.P., Della Valle, G., Pagano, T.B., Miele, F., Paciello, O. *et al*. (2016) Mature teratoma arising from an undescended testis in a horse: comparison between ultrasonographic and morphological features. *Folia Morphologica* 75(2), 211–215. DOI: 10.5603/FM.a2015.0088.

Pearson, L., Rodriguez, J. and Tibary, A. (2011) How to obtain a stallion testicular biopsy using a spring-loaded split-needle biopsy instrument. *Proceedings of the 57th Annual Convention of the American Association of Equine Practitioners*, San Antonio, Texas, USA, 18–22 November 2011. American Association of Equine Practitioners (AAEP), pp. 219–225.

Pozor, M., Conley, A.J., Roser, J.F., Nolin, M., Zambrano, G.L. *et al*. (2018) Anti-Müllerian hormone as a biomarker for acute testicular degeneration caused by toxic insults to stallion testes. *Theriogenology* 116, 95–102. DOI: 10.1016/j.theriogenology.2018.05.009.

Rode, K., Sieme, H., Richterich, P. and Brehm, R. (2015) Characterization of the equine blood-testis barrier during tubular development in normal and cryptorchid stallions. *Theriogenology* 84(5), 763–772. DOI: 10.1016/j.theriogenology.2015.05.009.

Roser, J.F. (2008) Regulation of testicular function in the stallion: an intricate network of endocrine, paracrine and autocrine systems. *Animal Reproduction Science* 107(3–4), 179–196. DOI: 10.1016/j.anireprosci.2008.05.004.

Scarlet, D., Wulf, M., Kuhl, J., Köhne, M., Ille, N. *et al*. (2018) Anti-Müllerian hormone profiling in prepubertal horses and its relationship with gonadal function. *Theriogenology* 117, 72–77. DOI: 10.1016/j.theriogenology.2018.05.012.

Schambourg, M.A., Farley, J.A., Marcoux, M. and Laverty, S. (2006) Use of transabdominal ultrasonography to determine the location of cryptorchid testes in the horse. *Equine Veterinary Journal* 38(3), 242–245. DOI: 10.2746/042516406776866354.

Schumacher, J. (1999) Testicular neoplasia of horses: an underreported condition. *Equine Veterinary Journal* 31(4), 270–272. DOI: 10.1111/j.2042-3306.1999.tb03815.x.

Senger, P.L. (2012) *Pathways to Pregnancy & Parturition*, Current Conceptions. Redmond, OR.

Sipahutar, H., Sourdaine, P., Moslemi, S., Plainfossé, B. and Séralini, G.-E. (2003) Immunolocalization of aromatase in stallion Leydig cells and seminiferous tubules. *Journal of Histochemistry & Cytochemistry* 51(3), 311–318. DOI: 10.1177/002215540305100306.

Taya, K., Nagata, S., Tsunoda, N., Nagamine, N., Tanaka, Y. *et al*. (2000) Testicular secretion of inhibin in stallions. *Journal of Reproduction and Fertility* (Suppl), 43–50.

Thompson, D.L., Johnson, L. and Wiest, J.J. (1987) Effects of month and age on prolactin concentrations in stallion serum. *Journal of Reproduction and Fertility. Supplement* 35, 67–70.

Turner, R.M. (2019) Declining testicular function in the aging stallion: management options and future therapies. *Animal Reproduction Science* 207, 171–179. DOI: 10.1016/j.anireprosci.2019.06.009.

Turner, R.M. and Zeng, W. (2012) The emerging pathophysiology of age-related testicular degeneration with a focus on the stallion and an update on potential therapies. *Reproduction in Domestic Animals* 47(Suppl 4), 178–186. DOI: 10.1111/j.1439-0531.2012.02073.x.

Yeap, B.B., Grossmann, M., McLachlan, R.I., Handelsman, D.J., Wittert, G.A. *et al*. (2016) Endocrine Society of Australia position statement on male hypogonadism (Part 1): assessment and indications for testosterone therapy. *Medical Journal of Australia* 205(4), 173–178. DOI: 10.5694/mja16.00393.

Index

Page numbers in *italics* refer to illustrations

www.ingramcontent.com/pod-product-compliance
Lightning Source LLC
LaVergne TN
LVHW070854210926
848482LV00016B/936